Fundamentals of Traditional Chinese Medicine

Written by Yin Huihe and others
Edited & translated by Associate Professor Shuai Xuezhong

FOREIGN LANGUAGES PRESS   BEIJING

First Edition   1992
Second Printing   1995

ISBN 7-119-01398-X

© Foreign Languages Press, Beijing, China, 1992

Published by Foreign Languages Press
24 Baiwanzhuang Road, Beijing 100037, China

Printed by Beijing Foreign Languages Printing House
19 Chegongzhuang Xilu, Beijing 100044, China

Distributed by China International Book Trading Corporation
35 Chegongzhuang Xilu, Beijing 100044, China
P.O. Box 399, Beijing, China

Printed in the People's Republic of China

PREFACE

Last year, the Chinese Ministry of Public Health started a two-year project to teach traditional Chinese doctors English in a specialized course. The aim of the course is to bridge the gap between foreign acupuncture students and their Chinese teachers, and to improve future international courses and scientific exchanges. By teaching in English loss of teaching time because of translation is eliminated, and the content is clearer.

I was invited to give a four-month course on the fundamentals of traditional Chinese medicine (TCM) in English. When I finished my courses, some of my students encouraged me to publish my lecture notes, for the benefit of readers at home and abroad. Immediately after returning from Beijing; I started to compile and supplement my lecture notes with the help of the comments I received from many hours spent discussing acupuncture with doctors from all over China. This enabled me to improve my writing with new facts and to develop a holistic and systematic structure similar to the TCM concept.

Now that I have completed my book, I hope that it will be helpful to readers. My main motivation for writing this book was to spread TCM all over the world. This may help increase efficacy in the struggle against disease.

There are some difficult interpretations of the ancient classics that have led to misunderstandings and even misapplications in clinical work. I hope I have been able to dispel any misunderstandings.

The theories and fundamental knowledge described in this book is the basis for other branches of Chinese medicine and pharmacology, as well as a must for both domestic and foreign readers that intend to further study this traditional health system which is more than 2,000 years old.

In the process of my writing, I have referred to a lot of classics and texts for traditional Chinese medicine and pharmacology, such as the *Fundamentals of Traditional Chinese Medicine* published by the Shanghai Science & Technology Press, the *Basic Theories of Traditional Chinese Medicine* also published by the Shanghai Science & Technology Press, the *Practical Chinese Medicine* published by the Beijing Press, and others.

My book is mainly written for two groups of readers. The first one is the domestic professionals, to help them teach TCM in English, as well as to provide a framework for international scientific exchange that is necessary to further development and optimal use of historical health research.

This book is useful not only for foreign readers who already have some knowledge of TCM, but also for interested laymen who need a comprehensive approach.

During my writing I was aware that confusion in the past was due to misinterpretation or wrong translations of TCM terms, since our sources are written in ancient Chinese characters. Since there are no established TCM terms in English, I have referred to my

Chinese-English Terminology of Traditional Chinese Medicine published by the Hunan Science & Technology Press. TCM has its own set of terms. Although some of them are the same as those of Western medicine, the names of the internal organs of TCM are seen as connected to the emotions, as well as having distinct functions in controlling and balancing the flow of *qi* (vital energy) in the body. Some terms cannot be easily translated into English, for instance, *qi*, yin-yang, *zang-fu*, etc. For this reason, foreign readers will understand them better after they are familiar with their historical background. Otherwise they will be inevitably confused with the terms of modern medicine. Main reference books I used in compiling this book include *Basics of Traditional Chinese Medicine*, a textbook edited by noted TCM physician Professor Yin Huihe of Beijing's Sino-Japanese Friendship Hospital for medical colleges and universities throughout the country.

I would like to thank Dr. Adren Berthoud, my dear friend from Switzerland, for his careful reading and his many suggestions, and also Mr. C. F. Martin of Canada for going over the English Text.

Associate Professor Shuai Xuezhong, Acupuncture
Department of Hunan College of Traditional
Chinese Medicine, Changsha, China
November, 1989

CONTENTS

1. GENERAL INTRODUCTION

Traditional Chinese medicine (TCM) has been developing for over two thousand years. It is the accumulation of the experience of the Chinese in the attempt to maintain health and treat disease. It is an important component of Chinese culture. Guided by observation and experience through the ages Chinese medical experts have developed a system of health care for the prevention and treatment of disease.

1-1 Formation and development of the theoretical system of TCM

The science of TCM is the study of human physiopathology, diagnosis, prevention and treatment of disease. It is a theoretical system based on clinical experience and is mainly guided by a holistic concept, based upon the physiopathology of *zang-fu* (viscera)[1] and meridians[2] and treatment is planned according to diagnosis (*bianzheng* and *lunzhi*)[3].

During the Spring and Autumn and Warring States Periods (770-221 B.C.), Chinese society advanced rapidly and during this rapid development *Huangdi's* (Yellow Emperor) *Internal Classic of Medicine*, referred to as *Neijing*, *Internal Classic*, appeared as the earliest book of Chinese medicine that has been preserved up to now. It sums up medical achievements before the Spring and Autumn and Warring States Periods and laid the foundation for Chinese medicine and pharmacology.

Internal Classic and the *Classic on Difficult Medical Problems* (*Nanjing*) are other medical classics which were written before the Han Dynasty (206 B.C. to A.D. 220). They outline physiology, pathology, diagnosis and treatment, and supplement *Neijing* as a theoretical foundation.

In the Western Han Dynasty (206 B.C. to A.D. 24), Chinese medicine made great progress. During the last period of the Eastern Han Dynasty (25 to 220), on the basis of the theoretical foundation of *Neijing* and *Nanjing*, Zhang Zhongjing, a famous medical expert, further summarized medical achievements and wrote the *Treatise on Febrile and Miscellaneous Diseases* (i.e., *Treatise on Febrile Diseases*) and *Synopsis of the Golden Bookcase*. Since it is the first specialized book to successfully apply *bianzheng* and *lunzhi* (planning treatment according to diagnosis) in TCM, *Treatise on Febrile Diseases* establishes a guiding principle of "identifying the syndromes with the names of the six meridians" and identifies the syndromes according to each meridian on the basis of "Treatise on Heat," a chapter in *Plain Questions*. In *Synopsis of the Golden Bookcase*, the syndromes are identified according to the pathogenic theory of *zang-fu* (viscera) and more than 40 diseases and 262 prescriptions are recorded. It elaborates on the etiology theory in *Neijing* and has influenced the theory of the three causes of diseases in later generations.

Using *Internal Classic* and *Treatise on Febrile and Miscellaneous Diseases*, medical experts further developed Chinese medical theories. For instance, *Treatise on the Causes and Symptoms of Various Diseases* written by Cao Yuanfang of the Sui Dynasty

1

(581-618) is the first specialized book about etiology, pathogenesis and symptoms in TCM. In *Treatise on the Three Categories of Pathogenic Factors* by Chen Wuze of the Song Dynasty (960-1279), the "theory of the three causes of diseases" was introduced. *Key to Therapeutics of Children's Diseases* is the first book dealing with the diagnosis and treatment of *zang-fu* (viscera). During the Jin and Yuan dynasties (1271-1368), different schools of medicine appeared, among which the representatives were Liu Wansu, Zhang Chongzheng, Li Gao and Zhu Danxi, called the "Four Major Schools" by later generations. The *mingmen* (vital portal) theory put forth by Zhao Xianke, Zhang Jingyue, etc., in the Ming Dynasty (1368-1644) further elaborated upon the visceral symptoms theory. It originated from *Internal Classic* and *Classic on Difficult Medical Problems*, *Treatise on Febrile and Miscellaneous Diseases*, etc., and gradually formed an independent subject after the Han Dynasty. Wu Youke of the Ming Dynasty promoted the development of the etiology of acute febrile diseases (particularly pestilential diseases) in his *Treatise on Pestilence*. The science of acute febrile disease formed an integral theoretical system in etiology, syndromes, pulse and treatment.

Wang Qingren, a medical expert of the Qing Dynasty (1644-1911), paid special attention to anatomy and in his *Errors in Medicine Corrected* he corrected the anatomical errors that had been made in the ancient medical books and promoted the development of the theory that stagnant blood can cause disease, thus the development of fundamental theories of TCM.

After the founding of the People's Republic of China, members of both traditional Chinese and Western medicine have made great advances in research on the meridians and *zang-fu* (viscera) by a study on fundamental theories of TCM with modern scientific methods and techniques, while systematizing and studying the medical literature of the dynasties.

1-2 The materialistic and dialectical outlook in the theoretical system of TCM

This outlook was formed and developed on the basis of medical practice and greatly influenced by ancient materialism and dialectics, which permeates its theoretical system.

1-2-1 The materialistic outlook

1-2-1-1 The human body is formed by *qi* between heaven and earth

The world consists of matter and is a result of the interaction of yin and yang. *Qi* is energy that moves. Everything in the universe is a result of *qi* movement.

TCM holds that *jing* (vital principle) is the primordial substance of life, which is congenital as well as hereditary. It refers to the vital principle that is received by the offspring from its parents. It is therefore called the "congenital essence." The parents' vital principles combine and form the substance from which the embryo develops. After birth, the cultivation and supplement of congenital and acquired *jing* is responsible for the continuous activities of the body. *Qi* maintains bodily activity. Its motion and change and accompanying energy transformation are termed *qihua*, which is basic to life. There would be no life if it did not exist. The essence of *qihua* is the movement of yin and yang which decline and transform themselves within the body. *Qi* ascends and descends within the body, and leaves and enters the body.

1-2-1-2 Mutual dependence of *xing* (body) and *shen* (spirit)

The theory of the body's structural form and the spirit is one of the basic theories of TCM. It is formed on the basis of the materialistic Chinese outlook of the natural world. Spirit comprises emotional and mental activities.

The relationship between the body and the spirit is the relationship between material and spirit. The body is primary and materialistic and the spirit animates the body. Their unity is essential to maintain health and prevent disease.

1-2-1-3 The prevention and treatment of disease

Disease can be treated after finding its primary cause. After a pathogenic factor has invaded the body, it breaks the balance between the body's yin and yang resulting in disease. But, whether disease flourishes or not depends upon "whether the anti-pathogenic factor is predominant or not. The reason why the pathogenic factor succeeds in invading the body is that the anti-pathogenic factor is comparatively weak." Before the invasion of disease, special attention is paid to regulating and nourishing the body and spirit. People should adapt to weather changes, keep the emotions normal and live in a comfortable place, regulate yin and yang and strengthen their body resistance. After the occurrence of disease, stress is laid on diagnosing the disease, treating it at its initial stage and preventing it from taking a turn for the worse.

1-2-2 The dialectical outlook

All things are not static and isolated but interconnected. This implies not only the viewpoint of materialism, but that of dialectics. The body is an organic integral that constantly moves. The motion of everything in the natural world is governed by the contradictory forces of yin and yang. Life is also governed by *qi* and there would be no life if there was no *qi*.

Emotions act upon the body: TCM has recognized the connection between mind and body, e.g., "anger injures the liver, joy injures the heart, worry injures the spleen, anxiety injures the lung and fright injures the kidney."

Routine and contrary treatment: After distinguishing the cause of a disease and determining the sequence of its treatment, therapeutic measures should be adopted to regain the equilibrium between yin and yang. A therapeutic method is applied to regulate the imbalance of yin and yang, for instance, "healing the cold, tonifying the deficiency and purging the excess" in order to resume the balance of the body. The therapeutic principle of treatment by application of drugs contrary to the symptoms and signs, is to use the principle of dialectics, that contradictions are not only opposing, but supporting. Different therapies are adopted according to different conditions.

In TCM, the disease and conditions of the patient are complex and various. Therapies should differ in treatment of the same disease because the climate, living conditions, environment, profession and constitution vary with different cases. The case should be treated according to its particular circumstances. The same disease may be treated differently according to different individuals. The same treatment can be adopted for different diseases when the change of the same pathogenesis occur in the process of its development. In TCM attention is paid to different stages of a disease.

1-3 Chief features of TCM

1-3-1 The holistic concept

In TCM the integrity of the body is emphasized, and its relationship with the natural world. The body is an organic integral, and its functions are interconnected. There is a close relationship between the body and the natural environment. The body maintains its normal activities by adapting itself to the environment. Remoulding the natural environment so as to preserve the integrity of the body, is the holistic concept. This viewpoint manifests itself in the thought of ancient materialism and dialectics, and permeates physiology, pathology, diagnosis, identification of syndromes and treatment of disease.

1-3-1-1 The body is an integral whole

The body consists of a number of viscera, tissues and organs with different functions. These functions interconnect to maintain the harmony of physiological activities. The unity of the body is formed with the five yin viscera at its centre. These are also associated with the yang viscera, and the action of the meridians that internally pertain to the viscera, and externally connect with the limbs. The five yin viscera represent the five systems of the body and all the organs of the body are included within them. With the five yin viscera[4] as the centre, the body's tissues and organs are connected, such as the six yang viscera,[5] five tissues,[6] five sense organs,[7] nine apertures,[8] limbs and bones, etc. through the meridian system, which carry on the functions.

Guided by the holistic concept, TCM holds that the normal physiological activity is dependent on the various viscera and tissues to exercise their functions and they also depend upon the coordinating and restraining action of each viscus, so that a physiological balance can be maintained.

Connecting the whole body, the meridian system links the viscera, meridians, body and limbs, sense organs and nine apertures, etc. as an organic whole. The theory of *qi*, blood and body fluids and that of the unity of body and spirit reflect the integrity of the body's function and structure. The holistic concept is also manifest in the theories such as "yin flourishing smoothly and yang vivified steadily," etc., which means that the transformation and interaction of yin and yang maintain a kinetic balance is the basic condition of normal physiological activity. The inhibition of extreme excess and the interaction among the viscera to keep vitality and kinetic equilibrium are important to the physiology of TCM.

While analysing the pathogenesis of a disease or syndrome, TCM starts first from the whole body and symptoms that are caused by local processes, and takes into account not only the local pathological changes and *zang-fu* (viscera), meridians directly concerned with the illness but also the influence of the affected viscus and meridian upon other viscera and meridians.

Pathological changes in a local area are usually related to the flourishing and decline of *zang-fu* (viscera), *qi* (vital energy), blood and yin and yang of the whole body. The interconnection of various viscera, tissues and organs determine which process of the viscera can be understood and judged through external changes of the five sense organs, body form, skin colour and pulse, etc. so that a correct diagnosis and treatment can be made. Since *xu* (deficiency) and *shi* (excess) of the viscera, flourishing and decline of *qi* and blood and the excess and deficiency of a disease may be reflected by the tongue, the state of the viscera can be discovered by inspecting the tongue.

As the body is an organic whole, proper measures can only be adopted when considering the whole body and also by treating local pathological changes. For example, the tongue is the window of the heart, and the heart is closely related to the small intestine, so an inflamed mouth and tongue can be treated by purifying the heart, and purging pernicious fire (heat) in the small intestine.

1-3-1-2 The unity of man and nature

Man lives in the natural world and changes in the environment influence the body.

The influence of weather and seasons upon health. Spring corresponds with wood and is warm; summer with fire and is hot; late summer with earth and is moist; autumn with metal and is dry; winter with water and is cold. Hence, the warm spring, hot summer, moist late summer, dry autumn and cold winter indicate a general rule of weather patterns in the year. Influenced by these changes, an organism adapts to the changes corresponding to germination in spring, growth in summer, change in late summer, reaping in autumn and storing in winter. Pulse indications change corresponding to the four seasons. For instance, a pulse is felt floating and large in spring and summer, and usually sunken and small in autumn and winter. The changes of pulse indications are the reflection of adaptability of *qi* and blood when the body is influenced by seasonal changes.

Influence of morning and evening, daytime and night. The body must also adapt itself to changes of yin and yang in the morning and evening, daytime and night. Yang *qi* usually lies in the superficial part of the body in the morning, and in the deep part at night, which reflects the adaptability of the body's activities to the process of the natural changes of yin and yang. The environment and way of life influence the body. For instance, since it is wet and hot in the region south of the Changjiang River, the junction between the muscle and skin is loose; since it is dry and cold in north China, the junction is taut. Whenever people suddenly change their living environment, they will feel unable to adapt to their new environment, however they can gradually adapt to it after a certain period of time.

TCM holds that man cannot only actively adapt to nature, but remould it, so as to increase the level of health and reduce disease, e.g., "Do more physical exercise so as not to be affected by pathogenic cold, and live in a shady and cool place to avoid pathogenic summer heat," (*Plain Questions*) and so on.

Sometimes weather changes are unfavourable to an organism. Man's ability to adapt to the natural environment is limited. If the weather changes rapidly and exceeds the limitation of the regulating function of the body, or the function becomes abnormal, so that it fails to adapt to the natural change, disease inevitably occurs. Each season has its own characteristic, hence some seasonal epidemic diseases may often occur along with common illnesses. For instance, "In spring, epistaxis easily occurs; in mid-summer, chest and hypochondriac trouble; in late summer, damp diarrhea; in autumn, wind malaria; in winter, *bijue* syndrome.[9]" In addition, certain chronic diseases may appear or are aggravated when the weather changes rapidly, or the season alternates, e.g., *bi* syndrome,[10] asthma, etc.

The time of day influences diseases. Most common diseases are mild in the daytime, but more severe at night, because of the generation, growth, contraction and concealment of yang *qi* in the body in the morning, noon, evening and midnight. Hence disease is relieved in the morning, does not attack the body at noon, begins to attack the body in the evening and is aggravated at midnight.

Man and nature are interconnected. Treating a disease according to different environments and individuals is an important therapeutic principle in TCM. Attention must be paid to analyse the connection between the external environment and the body in order to find an effective treatment in the process of *bianzheng* and *lunzhi* (planning treatment according to diagnosis).

1-3-2 *Bianzheng* and *lunzhi* (planning treatment according to diagnosis)

Bianzheng and *lunzhi* are basic principles of recognizing and treating disease in TCM. "*Zheng*" includes the location, cause and features of a pathological process, and reflects pathological changes at certain stages of the disease. It shows the course of a disease more wholly and accurately than looking at the symptoms only. *Bianzheng* is the data, symptoms and signs collected through the four diagnostic techniques and then identified as "*zheng*" (symptoms-complex or syndrome). *Zheng* is then analysed to differentiate the cause, features and location of the disease, and the relation between pathogenic and anti-pathogenic factors. "*Lunzhi*" (also called *shizhi*) means that a corresponding therapy is determined in accordance with the result of *bianzheng*. Whether the therapy is correct or not will be shown by its effects.

In recognizing and treating a disease, TCM not only identifies the disease, but also the syndrome. For instance, a common cold with fever, creeping chills and pain in the head and body is located in the superficial part of the body. But, it is often manifested as two different patterns of syndromes, namely, wind-cold or wind-heat because pathogenic factors and body reactions are different. Only by distinguishing the wind-cold pattern from the wind-heat pattern can one determine a diaphoretic therapy with pungent-warm drugs or pungent-cool ones, and can the disease be properly treated. From this it can be seen that *bianzheng* and *lunzhi* differ not only from symptomatic treatment, but also differ from the treatment of which the major and minor diseases and their stages are not differentiated and a single prescription or drug is used.

Bianzheng and *lunzhi* are regarded as a basic principle of guiding diagnosis and treatment of disease in clinic. As it can dialectically deal with the relation between the disease and syndrome, i.e., a disease may include several syndromes and the same syndrome may appear in the course of the development of different diseases, the disease is dealt with by adopting "different treatments for the same disease" or "the same treatment for different diseases" under the guidance of this principle in clinical treatment. "Different treatments for the same disease" is when the same disease is manifested by different syndromes and treated with different therapies corresponding to the time and place of its invasion and as the patient's reaction varies at different stages. Take the common cold as an example. Since it invades the body in different seasons, the therapy varies. Since a summer cold is due to pathogenic summer-heat and damp, it should be treated with aromatics to subdue the turbid substance and eliminate pathogenic summer-heat and damp. When the same pathogenesis appears in the process of different diseases, the same therapy may also be adopted. For instance, prolapse of rectum, prolapse of uterus, etc. can all also be treated by elevating *qi* in the middle energizer if it manifests as the syndrome of trapped *qi*[11] in the middle energizer. From this it can be seen that in treatment TCM does not emphasize the similarity or difference of the disease, but comparable pathogenesis. Diseases with the same pathogenesis may be treated with the same therapy; those with different pathogenesis, different therapies. *Bianzheng* and *lunzhi* mean that different therapies are applied to treat different diseases according to their features in the course of their development.

Notes

1. A general term for the five yin viscera, six yang viscera and unusual organs.

2. Referring to *jing-luo*, including their collaterals. They are the passages through which *qi* and blood circulate, correlate the viscera with limbs, connect the upper and lower parts of the body with the interior and exterior of the body, and regulate the mechanisms of various parts of the body. They include the *jing-mai* (meridians) and *luomai* (their collaterals); hence, viewing the body as an organic whole. Up to now, there has been no definite proof as to the actual existence of *jing-luo*.

3. *Bianzheng* and *lunzhi* mean that the patient's symptoms and signs are analysed and summarized in order to identify the etiology, location of the lesion, pathological change and body condition, according to the result of diagnosis.

4. A collective term for the heart, liver, spleen, lung and kidney. According to TCM, this term may either refer to the actual organs, or chiefly to the external reflections of their activities and pathological progress. Hence, each of them has its own intrinsic characteristics.

5. A collective term for the gallbladder, stomach, small intestine, large intestine, bladder and triple energizer. TCM regards the six yang viscera in the same way as Western medicine does because a yin viscus and yang viscus are superficially and internally interrelated. Each has its own characteristics.

6. Referring to the tendons, vessels, muscles, skin, hair and bones.

7. A collective term for eyes, ears, tongue and mouth.

8. Referring to the nine openings of the body; the eyes, the ears, the nostrils and the mouth, the urethral meatus anteriorly and the anus posteriorly.

9. Referring to *bi* (blockage) syndrome (the pathological manifestations due to sudden changes of the clinical course, internal invasion of pathogenic factors, collapse of primordial *qi*, internal stagnation of pathogens, and obstruction of visceral functions, such as coma, lockjaw, clenched fists, accumulation and obstruction of phlegm, wiry and rapid or full and rapid pulse, etc.) and *jue* (fainting) syndrome (sudden fainting with unconsciousness, cold clammy limbs, and gradual regaining of consciousness).

10. The pathological manifestations due to sudden changes of the clinical course, internal stagnation of pathogens, and obstruction of visceral functions, such as coma, lockjaw, clenched fists, accumulation and obstruction of phlegm, wiry and rapid or full and rapid pulse, etc.

11. Referring to the function of the spleen and stomach that are located in the middle portion of the body. According to TCM, the body is divided into the upper, middle and lower portions, called the upper energizer, middle energizer and lower energizer respectively and the triple energizer collectively.

2. YIN AND YANG, FIVE ELEMENTS (PHASES)

Yin and yang and the five-element (phases) theory, is an ancient Chinese cosmology to explain nature, as well as materialism and dialectics in ancient China. The yin-yang theory holds that the material world is generating, developing and changing due to the interaction of yin and yang. The five-element theory holds that wood, fire, earth, metal and water are the most basic and necessary substances and their movement and change constitute the material world. This view influenced and laid a foundation for the materialistic world outlook and methodology of natural science in ancient China.

Medical experts in ancient China applied the two theories to explain physiological functions and pathological changes in the body, and guide diagnosis and treatment. Owing to the limited social and historical conditions, this ancient philosophy cannot equal modern scientific materialism and dialectics, but it forms the basis of TCM and some modern concepts.

2-1 The yin-yang theory

Yin and yang comprise opposites such as warm and cold weather, the upper and lower, left and right, external and internal, change and stability, darkness and light, etc. Seeing that everything can be divided into two aspects, this concept was applied to explain duality and delineates that by opposition and support and sometimes synthesis, the ebb and flow of yin and yang are intrinsic in everything.

The yin-yang theory holds that the world is a whole, the result of the unity of the opposites, yin and yang. The motion of the opposites is responsible for change in the universe. Yin and yang represent properties which oppose and interconnect. Rapid, outward, ascending movement, warmth, heat and brightness pertain to yang. Stillness and inward, descending movement, coldness and dullness belong to yin. For example, heavenly *qi* is light and pure, thus it pertains to yang; but earthly *qi*, which is heavy and turbid, pertains to yin; water is yin and fire is yang, because the former is cold, moist and downward, but the latter is hot and flares up. When talking of yin and yang in the medical field, functions possessing promoting, warming and exciting actions, etc. all belong to yang, while those responsible for condensing, moistening and restraining actions, etc. belong to yin.

The properties of yin and yang are by no means absolute, but relative. Relativity is maintained by transformation of yin and yang. It is manifest in the unlimited division of everything. For instance, daytime is yang and night, yin. Relatively speaking, the morning is the yang aspect in yang, while the afternoon, the yin aspect in yang; the first half of night is the yin aspect in yin, and the second, the yang aspect in yin. Everything in the universe can be generally classified into yin and yang and further divided into the yin and yang aspects.

2-1-1 Chief contents of the yin-yang theory

2-1-1-1 Opposition and restraint of yin and yang

The yin-yang theory holds that the opposite aspects of yin and yang exists in everything in the natural world, for instance, the upper and lower, left and right positions, heaven and earth, motion and quiescence, outside and inside, ascent and descent, day and night, brilliance and dimness, heat (and fire) and water, etc. Yin and yang are not only in opposition. The opposition of yin and yang is chiefly manifested in their mutual restraining and kinetic balance. The result is that yin and yang achieves a unity, i.e., a kinetic equilibrium, which is called "yin flourishing smoothly and yang vivified steadily."[1] For example, the four seasons vary with the warm, hot, cool and cold weather. In spring and summer yang *qi* flourishes to restrain the cool and cold *qi* of autumn and winter. In autumn and winter yin *qi* flourishes to restrain the warm and hot *qi* of spring and summer.

The body can function as the result of achieving a dynamic state of the yin and yang. Through the restraint and support of yin and yang things develop and change. If there is no opposition and support of yin and yang within an entity, it cannot exist. In a normal physiological state, the opposite aspects, yin and yang do not coexist in an entity in isolation, but are in a dynamic state in which they interact. "Yin flourishing smoothly and yang vivified steadily" is a kinetic equilibrium between yin and yang. When this equilibrium is lost, disease appears.

2-1-1-2 Interdependence of yin and yang

Yin and yang oppose as well as unify. Neither of them can exist in isolation. For instance, the upward direction is yang and downward is yin; the former does not exist without the latter and vice versa. Heat is yang and cold is yin. There is no heat without cold and vice versa. So, yang depends upon yin and vice versa. The existence of one relies on the simultaneous existence of the other.

The interdependent relation between yin and yang is not only manifest in the interdependence of materials. For instance, the relation of *qi* and blood is the most basic material relationship in the human body for maintaining activity. *Qi* pertains to yang and blood to yin, the former is the governor of the latter, and the latter, the dwelling place for all yang functions of the body. For example, basic functions of the body are excitation and restraint. Excitation is yang and restraint yin. Matter pertains to yin while function, to yang. Yang depends upon yin and vice versa. If the interdependent relation between them is destroyed for any reason, the opposite could no longer sustain itself.[2] If the interdependent relation between the material and function of the body or the function and material become abnormal, an exhaustion of essential *qi* because of the dissociation of yin and yang will result.[3]

2-1-1-3 Kinetic equilibrium between yin and yang

The restraint and support between yin and yang is not static, but always moving and changing. Take seasonal and climatic changes as an example. Cold weather gradually turns into warm weather from winter to spring and to hot weather in summer, which is "yin declines and yang rises." Hot weather gradually turns into cool weather from summer to autumn and to cold weather in winter, which is "yang declines and yin rises." Seasonal and climatic changes reflect the interdependence of yin and yang. Yang flourishes in daytime and is inhibited as yin flourishes at night. At midnight yang *qi* is produced and flourishes at noon. Physiological functions gradually turn from inhibition into excitation, i.e., the cause of "yin declines and yang rises;" from noon to evening "yang *qi* gradually declines while yin *qi* flourishes."

Only if yin and yang maintain a constant kinetic balance can physical activity be normally maintained. If they become imbalanced a pathological state would result.

2-1-1-4 Intertransformation of yin and yang

Under certain circumstances opposing yin and yang may transform themselves into each other, i.e., yin may transform itself into yang and vice versa. The transformation generally occurs at the late stage of change. If the "ebb and flow of yin and yang"[4] is regarded as a quantitative change, the transformation of yin and yang, is then a qualitative one based on the quantitative change.

The transformation of inhibition and excitation is similar. In the course of a disease, it may be often seen that yin transforms itself into yang and vice versa. For instance, in certain acute febrile diseases, fatal signs of collapse of yang *qi*, such as lowered body temperature, pallor, cold clammy extremities, faint pulse, etc. may suddenly occur under the condition of a persisting high fever, as pernicious heat is so severe that a large amount of primordial *qi* in the body is consumed and impaired. This pathological change is the transformation of a yang syndrome into a yin one. At this time, if the patient is dealt with properly, the case will take a turn for the better.

2-1-2 Application of the yin-yang theory

2-1-2-1 Tissues and structures of the body

All tissues and structures of the body are connected, and may be divided into the two opposites, yin and yang. The exterior of the body is yang, the interior is yin; the back is yang and the front is yin. The five storing viscera are yin and the six emptying viscera are yang. The five yin viscera are the liver, heart, spleen, lung and kidney and the six yang viscera are the gallbladder, stomach, large intestine, small intestine, bladder and triple energizer[5] according to "Jingui Zhenyuan Lun," a chapter in *Plain Questions*. The upper portion of the body is yang and the lower yin; the body surface is yang and the internal body yin; the lateral aspects of the limbs are yang and the medial ones yin. The five yin viscera are yin because they pertain to the interior, store but do not excrete *jing* (vital principle); the six yang viscera are yang because they pertain to the exterior, transport, but do not store turbid matter. Each of the five yin viscera pertains to yin or yang, i.e., the heart and lung located in the upper part of the chest cavity belong to yang, while the liver, kidney and spleen located in the lower part belong to yin. Each yin or yang viscus can also be divided into yin and yang, i.e., the heart can be subdivided into heart yin and heart yang; the kidney into kidney yin and kidney yang, etc.

In a word, the unity of opposing yin and yang exists between the upper and lower, internal and external, superficial and deep, anterior and posterior portions of the body and its internal organs.

2-1-2-2 Physiological functions of the body

The yin-yang theory is also used to explain the physiological functions of the body. Normal activity is possible when yin and yang are balanced. As far as function and matter are concerned, the functions pertain to yang while the matter pertains to yin. In the case where yin and yang fail to support each other and dissociate, life will inevitably end.

2-1-2-3 Pathological processes of the body

Yin and yang must always be kept between the interior and the exterior, the superficial and deep, the upper and lower parts of the body and between material and function. Harmony between yin and yang is the manifestation of health, while disease is caused by disharmony between yin and yang. However, the occurrence and development of disease relate to two aspects; anti-pathogenic and pathogenic factors. The former refers to the immune system and resistance against disease; the latter, to causative factors.

Anti-pathogenic factors are classified into yin and yang, including yin fluids and yang *qi* while the pathogenic factors are classified into yin pathogenic factors, such as pathogenic cold and damp and yang factors, such as pathogenic wind, summer-heat (fire) and dryness. There are six climatic exogenous pathogenic factors. Disease is the struggle between pathogenic and anti-pathogenic factors, which results in the relative flourishing or decline of yin and yang in the body.

a. The relative flourishing of yin and yang, i.e., excess yin and excess yang, are pathological conditions where either yin or yang are higher than their normal levels. "In Yin Yang Ying Da Xiang Lun," a chapter in *Plain Questions* points out, "Excess yin would lead to a yang disease and excess yang, a yin disease. Excess yang would lead to a heat affection while excess yin, to a cold affection."

Excess yang would lead to a heat affection or yin disease. Hence, excess yang generally refers to the yang pathogenic factor. The flourishing of yang would lead at the same time to a decline of yin. The flourishing of yang consumes yin.

"Excess yang results in a yin disease" implies that the excess yang impairs yin fluids in the body.

Excess yin leads to a cold affection and yang disease. Excess yin refers to the yin pathogenic factor, which results in an excess of yin. As an excess of yang would lead to a decline of yin, an excess of yin leads to a decline of yang.

"Excess yin leads to a cold affection" refers to a disease caused by a yin pathogenic factor, while "excess yin leads to a yang disease" means that excess yin impairs yang *qi* in the body.

b. The relative decline of yin and yang, i.e., yin deficiency and yang deficiency, where either yin or yang is lower than its normal level. "Tiao Jing Lun," a chapter in *Plain Questions*, points out, "A deficiency of yang would lead to an external effect of cold while that of yin, an internal effect of heat." According to the principle of equilibrium between yin and yang, a deficiency of one would lead to a relative excess of the other.

A deficiency of yang would lead to an affection of external cold: A deficiency of yang is due to an excess of yin caused by the failure of deficient yang (impairment of yang *qi* in the body) to restrain yin.

A deficiency of yin would affect internal heat: A deficiency of yin is due to an excess of yang caused by the failure of deficient yin (insufficient yin fluids) to restrain yang.

c. Transmutation of yin and yang: Under certain circumstances, pathological phenomena due to disharmony between yin and yang in the body may transform into each other, i.e., a yang syndrome may transform itself into a yin one and vice versa.

2-1-2-4 Diagnosis

Since the internal cause and development of disease lie in the disharmony between yin and yang, any disease can generally be explained by yin and yang.

There are eight guiding principles: yin, yang, exterior, interior, cold and heat, deficiency and excess in the identification of syndromes; among them yin and yang is

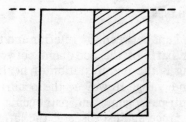

The kinetic equilibrium between yin and yang

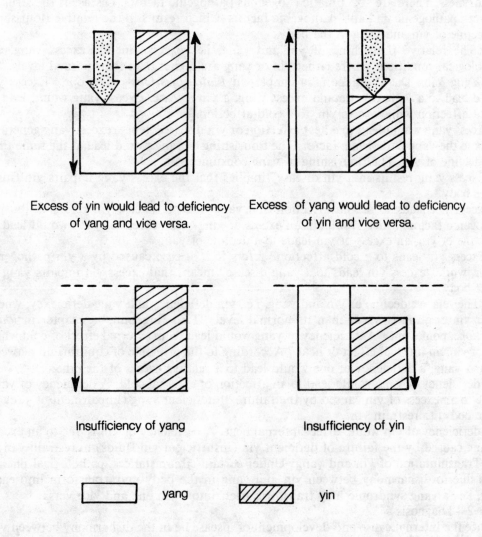

Excess of yin would lead to deficiency of yang and vice versa.

Excess of yang would lead to deficiency of yin and vice versa.

Insufficiency of yang

Insufficiency of yin

yang   yin

Fig. 1. Flourishing and decline of yin and yang.

the general principle. The exterior, excess and heat pertain to yang, while the interior, deficiency and cold to yin. In clinical identification of syndromes, only if yin and yang are first distinguished can the essence of a disease be grasped. Yin and yang can be used not only to determine whether the whole syndrome is yin or yang in nature, but also to analyse pulse indications and symptoms in the four diagnostic techniques. For example, yin and yang complexions; the yin and yang properties of a disease can be differentiated by a bright or dull complexion. The bright one indicates that the disease lies in the yang phase, while a dull complexion indicates that it is in the yin phase. Yin and yang voices: The yin and yang properties of a disease can be differentiated by inspecting the patient's breath and hearing. A high and sonorous voice, talkativeness and restlessness are usually ascribed to an excess or hot yang syndrome, while low feeble speech, speechlessness and calmness, a deficiency or cold indicate a yin disease. A faint breath and coarse voice indicates a yang disease. Yin and yang pulses: according to the location of pulse the *cun* section[6] is yang and the *chi* section[7] yin. According to the course of the pulse, the starting point is yang and the ending one, yin. A rapid pulse is yang and a slow one, yin. A floating, large, full and slippery pulse is yang and a sunken, small, minute, and irregular one, yin.

2-1-2-5 Treatment

As the root cause of disease is the disharmony between yin and yang, the basic therapeutic principle is to regain a balance between yin and yang by regulating them through reinforcing the deficient one and reducing the excess. The yin-yang theory guides the treatment and is used to determine the therapeutical principle and to summarize properties of drugs.

a. To determine therapeutical principles: The therapeutical principles for the relative excesses of yin and yang are "reducing the excess" and "purging the substantial." Excess yang leads to a yin disorder and heat affection; excess yang heat easily consumes yin fluids; excess yin leads to a yang disorder and cold affection, excess yin cold easily consumes yang *qi*. So, attention should be paid to whether a relative decline of corresponding yin or yang exists when regulating excess yin or yang. If yin or yang are excessive and the opposite aspect has not yet been impaired, the therapy of "reducing the excess" may be adopted. If both decline, the therapy of supporting yang or nourishing yin is applied in coordination. "Excess yang leading to a heat affection" belongs to an excess heat syndrome and should be treated with cold or cool drugs to restrain yang. Excess yin leading to a cold affection belongs to a cold excess syndrome and should be treated with warm-hot drugs to restrain yin.

The therapeutical principles for the decline of yin and yang are restraining excess fire (heat) by nourishing yin and reinforcing the kidney and subduing excess yin by reinforcing yang. The case when yang is excessive due to the failure of deficient yin to restrain yang belongs to a deficiency-heat syndrome and cannot be treated by directly relieving pathogenic heat with cold or cool drugs, but by restraining excess fire by nourishing yin and reinforcing the kidney. In the case where yin is excessive due to the failure of deficient yang to restrain it belongs to a deficiency-cold syndrome and should not be treated with pungent warm drugs of dissipating yin cold, but by subduing excess yin by reinforcing yang fire (called a "yin disease treated by treating yang" in "Yin Yang Ying Da Xiang Lun," a chapter in *Plain Questions*).

To sum up, the basic therapeutic principle is to reduce the excess and reinforce the deficiency. Clear up heat in the case of excess yang and eliminate cold in the case of excess yin, reinforce yang when it is deficient and tonify yin when yin is deficient, in order to restore the excess and deficiency of yin and yang to a normal harmonious state.

b. Properties of drugs: The properties of drugs are chiefly cold, hot, warm and cool, also called the four properties, of which the cold and cool pertain to yin and the warm and hot, to yang. The drugs capable of improving or relieving a heat syndrome are generally cold or cool in nature, e.g., *Scutellatis baicalensis*, *capejasmine* (fruit), etc. Those capable of improving or solving a cold syndrome are generally warm or hot in nature, e.g., *radix aconiti*, dried ginger and similar plants.

Five tastes: pungent, sweet, sour, bitter and salty. There are actually more than five tastes of drugs because some of them are moderate or astringent. Pungent, sweet and moderate tastes are yang and the sour, bitter, sweet and salty tastes are yin. Ascending, descending, floating and sinking drugs that generally have the effects of elevation and diaphoresis, dispersing pathogenic wind and cold, emetics and resuscitation that usually go upward and outward are yang drugs. Those that have purgative, anti-pyretic, diuretic, nerve-soothing, yang-restraining, wind-eliminating, depressing and astringent actions that usually run downward and inward and are sinking and descending are yin in nature.

2-2 The five-element theory

The ancient Chinese recognized that wood, fire, earth, metal and water were the most necessary elements, and these were first known as the "five matters."

Based on the "five matters," the five-element theory expounds that everything is formed by the motion and change of these five basic substances. Nothing is isolated and motionless, but everything keeps a kinetic balance in the incessant movement of these elements. Like the yin-yang theory, the five-element theory has become a part of the TCM system of medicine.

2-2-1 Chief contents of the five-element theory

2-2-1-1 Characteristics of the five elements

The characteristics of wood apply to all things which have an action or feature of flourishing growth corresponding to wood. All things characterized by warmth, heat and ascending action correspond to fire. All things which have generating, transmuting, carrying and receiving actions correspond to earth. All things which have clearing, descending and astringent actions correspond to metal. All things which are cold and cool, moist and moving downward correspond to water.

2-2-1-2 Classification according to the five elements

In the five-element theory, an analogy between the features and actions of something and the characteristics of the five elements is made so that the properties of things similar to those of wood are classified into wood; those things similar to fire, into fire, etc. For instance, in classifying according to the five elements, the east is classified as wood because the sun rises from it, which is similar to the ascending and flourishing characteristics of wood; the hot south is classified as fire because it is similar to the flaring-up characteristics of fire; the sun sets in the west, and represents metal because it is similar to the clearing and descending characteristics of metal; the cold north, represents water because it is similar to water in nature.

In the attribution of the five yin viscera to the five elements, the liver corresponds to

Table 1 Five Categories According to the Five Elements

Five Notes	Nature							Human Body					
	Five Tastes	Five Colours	Growth & Development	Five Evils	Five Orientations	Five Seasons	Five Elements	Five Zang Organs	Six Fu Organs	Five Sense Organs	Five Tissues	Five Emotions	Five Voices
Jiao	Sour	Dark blue	Germination	Wind	East	Spring	Wood	Liver	Gallbladder	Eyes	Tendon	Anger	Shouting
Zhi	Bitter	Red	Summer heat	Heat	South	Summer	Fire	Heart	Small Intestine	Tongue	Vessel	Joy	Laughing
Gong	Sweet	Yellow	Transformation	Damp	Middle	Late Summer	Earth	Spleen	Stomach	Mouth	Muscle	Worry	Singing
Shang	Pungent	White	Reaping	Dry	West	Autumn	Metal	Lung	Large Intestine	Nose	Skin & hair	Grief	Wailing
Yu	Salty	Black	Storing	Cold	North	Winter	Water	Kidney	Urinary bladder	Ear	Bone	Fear	Groaning

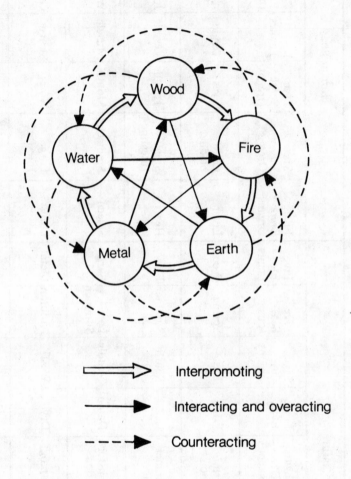

Fig. 2.   The interpromoting, interacting, overacting and
counteracting of the five elements

wood because it is concerned with ascendance; heart yang corresponds to fire because it is warming in action; the spleen corresponds to earth because it is concerned with nourishment; the lung corresponds to metal because it is concerned with descending; the kidney corresponds to water because it governs water.

In addition, the five-element theory also holds that things corresponding to the same element are related. For instance, the east, wind, wood and sour taste are all related to the liver. Therefore it is thought that the five-element theory is the basis for man's relationship to the natural environment, shown in the following table. Tissues and functions can also be categorized into the five physiological and pathological systems which centre upon the five yin viscera.

2-2-1-3 The interrelationship of the five elements

The five-element theory does not attribute things to the five elements mechanically and in isolation but shows the integrity and harmony of things according to the interrelationship of the five elements and shows what happens to the five elements after they have lost their balance.

a. Interpromoting and interacting: "Interpromoting" implies that a thing has an encouraging and generating influence upon another; "interacting" implies that a thing restricts and restrains the growth and function of another. In the five-element theory, both are thought as normal activities. The interrelationships in the environment determine the ecological balance in nature and the physiological balance of the body.

The interpromotion of the five elements is as follows: wood promotes fire, fire promotes earth, earth promotes metal, metal promotes water, and water, in turn, promotes wood.

The sequence of the interaction of the five elements is: wood acts upon earth, earth acts upon water, water acts upon fire, fire acts upon metal and metal, in turn, acts upon wood. The cyclic interaction among the five elements are: "promoted, promoting, acted upon, and acting upon."

In the *Classic on Difficult Medical Problems*, the relation between "promoted" and "promoting" is compared to the maternal and offspring relation. The one that promotes the other is the "mother" while the one that is promoted, the "son." Take fire as an example. As wood promotes fire, the wood is a promoting element; as fire promotes earth, the earth is the promoted element. Thus, wood is the mother of fire and earth is the son of fire. The promoted and promoting elements interact and other elements restrain them. For instance, water is promoted by wood, but water restrains fire. The five-element theory explains that everything is regulated to prevent any excess or deficiency and keep a dynamic ecological balance in the environment and a physiological balance in the body.

b. Counteraction: The concept of counteraction of the five elements was first seen in the *Internal Classic* and refers to the abnormal interaction of the five elements after their balance is upset.

Overaction of the five elements is when one of the five elements acts upon another excessively, resulting in an abnormal reaction. The reasons why the overacting relation occurs are: first of all, one of the five elements is so strong that it acts excessively upon and weakens another, resulting in abnormal interaction of the five elements. For example, wood is so strong that earth is overacted upon by it, causing a deficiency of the latter. Secondly, one of the five elements is so weak that overacting of one by another appears to be stronger, resulting in one getting weaker, e.g., wood is originally not so strong, and when it overacts upon earth it is still within a normal range, but, owing to the deficiency of earth, the wood overacting upon earth becomes relatively strong, causing earth to become deficient.

The counteracting relation of the five elements implies that one of the five elements is so strong that it counteracts another element which then becomes overacted upon. For instance, on the one hand, wood is normally acted upon by metal. When it is particularly strong, it is not acted upon by metal but instead counteracts metal. On the other hand, metal may be too weak to act upon wood, but is counteracted upon by wood. Both overacting and counteracting relations of the five elements are abnormal interactions. For instance, when wood is extremely strong, it can not only overact upon earth, but counteract metal; when metal is extremely weak, it can not only be counteracted by wood but overacted upon by fire. Hence, there is a connection between overaction and counteraction.

2-2-2 Application of the five-element theory in TCM

The applications of the five-element theory in TCM are chiefly analysing and studying the five elements of tissues and organs, such as the *zang-fu* (viscera), meridians of the body etc. and analysing the interconnection of physiological functions among the viscera and meridians, according to the actions of the five elements.

2-2-2-1 The physiological functions of the five yin viscera and their relation

In order to explain the physiological functions of the five yin viscera within the five-element theory, the viscera respectively correspond to the five elements, and the physiological functions of the five yin viscera are explained according to characteristics of the five elements.

Just as trees (wood) may flex and extend and their branches and leaves flourish, so the liver tends to be harmonious and flourishing, dislikes to be depressed and has a dispersing action so the liver corresponds to wood. Since fire is warm, hot and flaring up and heart yang has a warming action, the heart corresponds to fire. Just as earth can produce everything, the spleen transports and digests food, transmits *jing* (vital principle) nourishes the viscera, the four extremities and all tissues and organs and is the resource of generating *qi* and blood, and so the spleen corresponds to earth. Since metal is clearing, descending and contracting and the lung has clearing and descending functions and its *qi* is normal when clearing and descending, the lung corresponds to metal. As water is moist and downward and characterized by cold, moisture and downward movement closing and storing and the kidney has the action of storing *jing* and governing water, the kidney corresponds to water.

In the five-element theory, the body's viscera, tissues and structures correspond to the five elements. At the same time, the five orientations, the five periods of time, the five odours, the five tastes and the five colours are concerned with the five yin viscera, the six yang viscera, the five tissues and the five sense organs. In this way, man and his natural environment are unified. Take the liver as an example. "The east generates wind, the wind generates wood, the wood generates soreness, and the soreness is concerned with the liver, the liver connects with the tendons... the liver is concerned with the eyes." ("Yin Yang Ying Da Xiang Lun," a chapter in *Plain Questions*) Thus, the east, spring, soreness, etc. are connected to the liver, tendons and eyes, illustrating the holistic concept that man is part of nature.

The five yin viscera do not function in isolation but are interconnected. Correspondence of the five yin viscera to the five elements not only outlines the functions of the five yin viscera, but also explains the interconnection of the functions of the viscera.

Interpromotion of the five yin viscera: The liver corresponds to wood and the heart to fire and because wood promotes fire, the liver promotes the heart, e.g., the liver stores blood to support the heart. The heart promotes the spleen because fire promotes earth, e.g., heart yang warms the spleen. The spleen promotes the lung because earth promotes metal, e.g., *jing* (vital principle) dispersed by the spleen ascends to the lung. The lung promotes the kidney because metal promotes water, e.g., the lung (metal) clears and sends air downward to aid the kidney (water). The kidney promotes the liver because water promotes wood, e.g., the kidney stores *jing* to nourish yin blood in the liver, etc.

On the interaction of the five yin viscera "Wu Zang Sheng Cheng Lun," a chapter in *Plain Questions* states, "The heart... is restrained or acted upon by the kidney; the lung is restrained or acted upon by the heart; the spleen...is restrained or acted upon by the liver; the kidney... is restrained by the spleen." The heart corresponds to fire and is restrained by the kidney (water), the kidney is the "governor" of the heart. Since the lung corresponds to metal and is restrained by the heart (fire), the heart is the "governor" of the lung; since the spleen corresponds to earth and is restrained by the liver (wood), the liver is the "governor" of the spleen; since the kidney corresponds to water and is restrained by the spleen (earth), the spleen is the "governor" of the kidney.

To sum up, the five-element theory is used in physiology to explain the interconnection between the viscera and the tissues and the body and its external environment.

2-2-2-2 The influence of pathological changes of the five yin viscera

The five-element theory can be applied to explain not only the interconnection of the viscera, but also the influence of the viscera under various pathological conditions. Disorders of one viscus may transfer to another and vice versa. The interrelated influences in pathology are termed "transformations." The transformation and development of the pathological changes of the five yin viscera explained according to the five-element theory may be divided into that of interpromoting and interacting.

a. Transformation of the interpromoting relation includes the two aspects, "a maternal disease affecting its offspring" and "an offspring stealing its maternal energy." The former refers to a disease that transforms itself and develops with water and the liver corresponds to wood and the water can promote the wood, the kidney is the maternal viscus and the liver the son. It is called a "maternal disease affecting her son" when kidney trouble affects the liver. "Deficient *jing* (vital principle) and blood in the liver and kidney" and "inadequate water (kidney) to nourish wood (liver)" frequently seen in clinic are within the range of a "maternal disease affecting her son." "An offspring stealing its maternal principle" refers to a disease which transforms and develops from the offspring viscus into its maternal one, e.g., as the liver corresponds to wood and the heart with fire, and wood can promote fire, wood is the maternal viscus and the heart the son. Deficient heart and liver blood and excess heart and liver fire are within the range of "a son stealing the maternal principle."

b. Transformation of interaction includes overacting and counteracting. Overacting refers to one element overacting upon another, resulting in a disease. There are two kinds of overacting; one element is overacted upon by its opposite because the latter is too strong; the other is that one element is too weak to be acted upon, resulting in the pathological phenomenon that one is overacted upon. Take the interacting relation of wood and earth as an example. The former is termed "wood overacting upon earth," while the latter, "weak earth is overacted upon by wood." Although the reasons for the two kinds of interaction are different, they may cause an excess of one and a deficiency of another. The invasion of the stomach and spleen by regurgitating liver *qi* is included within the range of overacting.

Interacting refers to one element counteracting upon another and resulting in a disease. In one case one element is too strong to be acted upon by the other, but counteracts upon the other. In another case one element is too weak to act upon the other, causing the pathological phenomenon of counteraction. Although the reasons for the two cases of counteraction are different, they may result in a deficiency of one element and an excess of the other. Take the relation between metal and wood as an example. The lung corresponds to metal and the liver to wood, and the clearing and descending lung *qi* restrains liver *qi* and elevates liver fire under normal physiological circumstances. So it is said that metal interacts with wood. Under the condition of deficient lung (metal) or regurgitating liver fire, pathological counteraction, such as "the invasion of the lung by liver *qi* and fire" may appear.

Harmony among the five yin viscera can be maintained through their interaction in physiological functions. In the condition of disease, the transformation and development of the five yin viscera cannot be carried out entirely according to the sequence of the rule of interpromoting, interacting, overacting and counteracting of the five elements since the pathogenic factor, the patient's constitution and the development of each disease vary.

2-2-2-3 Application of the five-element theory in diagnosis and treatment

a. Diagnosis: If an organ is affected, abnormal changes of the functions of the viscera and their relations may be reflected by their corresponding tissues and on the body surface, etc. because the five yin viscera, five colours, five voices and five tastes, etc. correspond to the five elements. This is the application of the five-element theory in diagnosis. So in clinical diagnosis of disease, a disease can be predicted by synthesizing the data obtained from the four diagnostic techniques, viz., inspection, auscultation, olfaction, inquiry and palpation according to the five elements and their interaction. For instance, the case with dark-bluish complexion, preference for sour food and stringy pulse can be diagnosed as liver trouble; that with flushed face, bitter mouth and full pulse is ascribed to excess heart fire; the patient with a weak spleen and dark-bluish complexion, earth overacted upon .by wood; the patient suffering from heart trouble with dull complexion, fire acted upon by water, etc.

b. Control of the development of disease: An affected yin viscus frequently affects another. Hence, while treating a disease, the interrelation of the viscera should be regulated according to the interaction of the five elements besides dealing with the affected yin viscus. When there is an overactive yin viscus, it should be purged; when there is a deficient yin viscus, it should be tonified in order to normalize it. If the liver is affected, it will affect the heart, spleen, lung and kidney and problems with these viscera affect the liver, too. If liver *qi* is hyperactive, flourishing wood (liver) will overact upon earth (spleen). At this time, the spleen and stomach should first be reinforced. If they are not impaired, the disease will not worsen and the patient will easily recover. Whether the disease develops depends upon the viscera, i.e., the disease will not worsen if all five yin viscera are strong and it will worsen, if they are not.

Therapeutical principles and therapies are determined according to interaction of the viscera: Tonify the maternal viscus and purge its offspring. That is according to "In a deficiency, tonify its maternal viscus and in an excess, purge its offspring." (*Classic on Difficult Medical Problems*)

Tonifying the maternal viscus is mainly used in the deficiency syndrome with a maternal-offspring relation, e.g., it is called "inadequate water to nourish wood" that deficient kidney yin cannot nourish the liver (wood), causing deficient liver yin. It is not treated by directly treating the liver but by tonifying deficient kidney. Since the kidney (water) is the maternal viscus of the liver and promotes the liver (wood), it is tonified to promote the liver. In acupuncture treatment, all the deficiency syndromes can be treated by tonifying the maternal meridian of acupoints they correspond to, e.g., *Yingu* (K 10), the *he*-sea acupoint of the Kidney Meridian, or *Ququan* (Liv 8), the *he*-sea acupoint of Liver Meridian, is punctured.

"Tonify the son" is chiefly used for the treatment of an excess syndrome with a maternal-offspring relation. When liver fire flares up in an excess liver syndrome, the liver (wood) is the mother and the heart (fire) the son. In the treatment of excess liver fire, a heart-purifying therapy can be adopted and purging heart fire aids in purging liver fire. In acupuncture treatment, all the excess syndromes can be treated by clearing the offspring meridian of the acupoints they correspond to, e.g., in an excess liver syndrome, *Shaofu* (H 8), the *ying*-spring (fire) acupoint of the Heart Meridian or *Xingjian* (Liv 2), the *ying*-spring (fire) acupoint of the Liver Meridian are punctured.

Common therapies determined according to the interpromoting action are as follows:

Nourish liver yin by nourishing kidney yin: Suitable for the syndromes, such as deficient liver yin due to consumed kidney yin and relatively excess liver yang.

Tonify spleen yang by nourishing kidney yang: for the case of a weak lung and spleen when the spleen and stomach are too weak to nourish the lung.

Nourish deficient lung and kidney yin: Suitable for the case when the weak lung fails to distribute body fluids to nourish the kidney or essential *qi* cannot upwardly nourish the lung due to insufficient kidney yin, resulting in deficiency yin of lung and kidney.

Liver-restraining and spleen-reinforcing: A therapy for an overactive liver and weak spleen with drugs for soothing the liver and reinforcing the spleen. Suitable for syndromes of an overactive liver overacting upon the spleen.

Restrain the kidney by cultivating the spleen: A therapy for the disorder caused by stagnant aqueous damp with the drugs of warmly invigorating spleen yang or warming edema due to damp caused by the spleen's failure to transport water. If kidney yang is too weak to warm spleen yang, the kidney will not control water and the spleen will not restrain water. It is caused by water (kidney) counteracting upon earth (spleen) and should be treated by chiefly warming the kidney in coordination with the reinforcement of the spleen.

Restrain the overactive liver by purifying lung *qi*: Used for the syndrome of relatively excess liver fire affecting the clearing and descending functions of lung *qi*.

Clear up heart (fire) and nourish kidney (water): Suitable for the disorder of kidney yin deficiency. Heart fire is in relative excess and the heart (fire) and kidney (water) are dissociated.

The five-element theory is widely used in treatment: It suits not only drug therapies, but also acupuncture and moxibustion, psychotherapy, etc.

In moxibustion therapy, the acupoints at the ends of the twelve meridians located in the four extremities were connected with the five elements by ancient acupuncture experts, i.e., well, spring, stream, river, and sea acupoints respectively correspond to wood, fire, earth, metal and water, and they are selected for clinical treatments according to the interpromoting and counteracting of the five elements and different diseases.

The five-element theory is used for treating emotional troubles, since emotions originate from the five yin viscera which are interpromoting and interacting. Emotional changes are interrestraining. For instance, "Overanger injures the liver and overgrief restrains anger ... overjoy injures the heart and overapprehension restrains joy ... overworry injures the spleen and overanger restrains worry ... overanxiety injures the lung and overjoy restrains anxiety ... overapprehension injures the kidney, and overanxiety restrains apprehension." ("Yin Yang Ying Da Xiang Lun," a chapter in *Plain Questions*)

Worry originates from the lung and corresponds to metal; anger, from the liver and corresponds to wood. As metal acts upon the wood, worry restrains anger. Apprehension restrains joy and originates from the heart and corresponds to fire. Water acts upon fire and apprehension restrains joy. Anger originates from the liver and corresponds to wood; worry originates from the spleen and corresponds to earth. As wood acts upon earth, anger restrains worry. Joy originates from the heart and corresponds to fire; anxiety originates from the lung and corresponds to metal. As fire acts upon metal, joy restrains anxiety. Worry originates from the spleen and corresponds to earth; apprehension originates from the kidney and restrains worry.

It should be pointed out that not all diseases can be treated according to the interpromoting and interacting of the five yin viscera. It should be applied according to the actual conditions.

Although the yin-yang and five-element theories have their own characteristics, they are related and applied together. The yin-yang theory explains the kinetic balance and transforming relations between the opposites. As a cosmology, the yin-yang theory holds that the whole universe is a unity of opposites. When applied to explain the body, it holds that the body consists of various kinds of opposite tissues, structures and activities. When applied to explain the relation between man and nature, it holds that man and nature are another unity of opposites.

The five-element theory is a cosmology that considers the universe a unity consisting of the five basic elements (wood, fire, earth, metal, and water) which interact. When applied to the body, it considers the body a unity of five interacting emotions, etc. When applied to explain the relation between man and nature, it considers the natural world and man a unity because the five movements, six *qi*, five orientations, five seasons (summer is divided into midsummer and later summer), etc. in the natural world correspond to the viscera internally and there is an interacting relation between the functions of the viscera and the environment.

It must be pointed out that the yin-yang and five-element theories are concepts of dialectical materialism of ancient China, but both are limited by the social and historical conditions of ancient times. For this reason one cannot only use these concepts. The study of physiological functions and pathological processes must augment TCM so it will further develop and contribute to the health of mankind.

Notes

[1.] The yin principle flourishes smoothly, while the yang principle is vivified steadily. They regulate themselves so as to maintain equilibrium. This is the basic principle for normal activity and health.

[2.] Neither yin nor yang can grow and develop in isolation.

[3.] It denotes a disintegration of the relationship between yin and yang, and is used to express the pathogenesis of death.

[4.] Yin and yang coexist in a dynamic state in which one rises while the other declines. An excess of one will lead to a decline of the other and vice versa.

[5.] One of the six yang viscera. It refers: a) to the body cavity (including the chest cavity, the abdominal cavity, and the pelvic cavity), b) to the lymphatic system, c) to a name with non-existent structure. At present, the consensus leans toward considering it the functional section of the body cavity and not the actual organ. Generally, the segment above the diaphragm, including the heart and lung, belongs to the upper energizer, that between the diaphragm and umbilicus, including the liver, stomach and spleen, belongs to the middle energizer, and that below the umbilicus including the kidney, bladder, and small and large intestines, belongs to the lower energizer.

[6.] The section of the radical artery for pulse diagnosis is divided into three sections. The section distal to the radial styloid process called *guan* is called the *cun* section.

[7.] The section of the radial artery for pulse diagnosis is divided into three sections. The section proximal to the radial styloid process called *guan* is called the *chi* section.

3. VISCERAL SYMPTOMS

The visceral symptoms theory studies the physiological functions and pathological changes of the viscera. This theory is based on *zang-fu* (viscera) a general term for internal organs. They can be classified into the yin viscera, yang viscera and unusual organs according to the characteristics of their physiological functions. The five yin viscera include the heart, lung, spleen, liver and kidney. The six yang viscera include the gallbladder, stomach, small intestine, large intestine, bladder and triple energizer. The unusual organs include the brain, *sui*,[1] bones, vessels, gallbladder and uterus.

The common physiological characteristics of the five yin viscera are: generating and storing essential *qi*. The six yang viscera receive and transport food. The unusual organs do not conform to the six yang viscera and they do not directly process food, but have an action similar to that of the yin viscera which is to store essential *qi*.

The theory is formed chiefly by: a) anatomical knowledge in ancient times, which laid a foundation for morphology; b) observation of physiology, e.g., a common cold results from the cold affection of the skin, with a stuffy or running nose and cough. Thus, the close relation between the skin, nose and lung is recognized. In another example the theory that "the eye is the window of the liver" was derived from that a number of eye troubles were cured by treating the liver for a long period of time.

The theory is chiefly characterized by the holistic concept with the five yin viscera as its centre. This concept is mainly manifest in a) the yin viscera are yin and the yang ones are yang; b) the yin and yang viscera are closely related and are a unity. For instance, the heart and small intestine, lung and large intestine, spleen and stomach, liver and gallbladder, kidney and bladder, pericardium and triple energizer are all closely related.

The five yin viscera connect with various tissues and organs, which is a manifestation of the holistic theory that the five yin viscera are specifically connected with various tissues and organs. According to this theory, the face is the mirror of the heart, the heart is enriched by blood and opens to the tongue; the lung is reflected by the hair and the skin and opens to the nose; the spleen reflects externally on the lips and affects the muscles and opens to the mouth; the liver is reflected by the nails, affects the tendons and opens to the eye; the kidney is reflected by the hair and affects the bones and opens to the ear, external genitalia and anus.

The physiological activities of the five yin viscera are closely related to the spirit and the emotions. Mental and emotional activities are the functions of the brain. However, the theory holds that these activities are closely related to the physiological activities of the five yin viscera which can command the activities of the entire body. Whether physiological activities of the brain are normal or not depends upon the harmony of the five yin viscera. If they are abnormal, the mental and emotional activities of the brain are influenced. An abnormality of the brain will affect the five yin viscera. "Xian Ming Wu Qi Pian," a chapter in *Plain Questions* states, "the heart stores the mind, the lung stores the soul, the liver stores the mood, the spleen stores the emotion and the kidney stores the will." TCM does recognize the function of the brain, but further classifies emotions and explores their relation with various yin viscera.

Harmony between the functions of the five yin viscera is a key link for maintaining stability of the internal system of the body. Equilibrium between the external and internal environments is maintained through the connection between the yin viscera and various tissues and organs and the relation between the five yin viscera and emotions.

3-1 The five yin viscera

The five yin viscera is a collective term for the heart, lung, spleen, liver and kidney. Although they each have their own physiological function, the heart plays a leading role. Harmony among the five yin viscera is mainly based on the yin-yang and five-element theories.

3-1-1 The heart

The heart lies in the chest cavity above the diaphragm, protected by the pericardium. It is the dwelling place of *shen* (Spirit) and regulates the blood and vessels. It corresponds to "fire" in the five-element theory. Its physiological function is governing vessels and mind. The tongue is its window and the face, its mirror. It is closely related to joy and sweat. As the Heart Meridian of Hand-*shaoyin* and the Small Intestine Meridian of Hand-*taiyang* are interconnected, the heart and small intestine are closely related.

3-1-1-1 Main physiological functions of the heart

a. The heart governs blood and vessels. Blood circulates in the vessels and is transported throughout the body. The functions of nutritional *qi* and blood directly influence blood circulation.

In TCM, the normal heartbeat chiefly depends upon heart *qi*. Only if heart *qi* is enriched can a normal heart rate and rhythm be maintained and can blood normally circulate within the vessels continuously and nourish the body, which is shown by a lustrous and bright complexion and a moderate, forceful pulse, etc. Normal blood circulation also depends upon whether the blood is enriched or not. When it is insufficient, the vessels are vacant and normal heartbeat and blood circulation are also influenced. The normal circulation of blood fully depends upon the most basic conditions, such as enriched heart *qi* and blood and unobstructed vessels. If heart *qi* is deficient, blood is consumed and weak, the vessels are obstructed, and an unsmooth flow of blood results, or the vessels are vacant and weak, resulting in dull complexion, minute weak pulse, even stagnant *qi* and blood and blocked vessels, with dark-greyish complexion, dark-bluish lips and tongue, chest distress, stabbing pain and an irregular or regular intermittent pulse appearing.

b. The heart governs the Mind: In its broadest sense, *shen* (Mind) refers to the activities of the body, e.g., appearance, complexion, expression in the eyes, speech, response, manner, etc. In its narrowest sense, "the heart governs the Mind" refers to mental and emotional activities. Since these activities are not only an important component of physiological functions, but can influence the harmony of various physiological functions, "the heart is the prime viscus and governs the Mind" ("Ling Lan Mi Dian Pian," a chapter in *Plain Questions*) and "the heart is the Chief of the five yin and six yang viscera and the residence of Spirit." (*Miraculous Pivot*)

Early in *Internal Classic*, it was described that thoughts and emotions are physiological functions of the brain, i.e., the reaction of the brain to the external environment. Thoughts and emotions are not only ascribed to the brain and the five yin viscera, but also to the physiological function of the heart. Hence, if the heart's regulation of the Mind is normal, one is full of vigour, clear-minded, mentally agile and quick or normal in response to the external environment. If not, symptoms such as insomnia, dreaminess, listlessness, even coma and unconsciousness may appear.

3-1-1-2 Relation of the heart to the emotions, body fluids, tissues and sense organs

a. The heart is related to joy: The physiological function of the heart is closely related to joy. The theory of visceral symptoms holds that joy, anger, anxiety, worry, and fear are the five emotions and correspond to the five yin viscera respectively because emotional changes are produced by the physiological functions of the five yin viscera. In general, joy, a response to external information, belongs to the positive irritations. But, overjoy leads to the injury of the heart (Mind). The hyperfunctional heart would make one laugh persistently; the hypofunctional heart would make one easily sad.

b. The heart is closely related to sweat: Sweat is excreted from the pores after body fluids are activated by the spread of yang *qi*. Excretion of sweat also depends upon the opening and closing action of defensive *qi* or the junction between the muscle and skin. If it opens, sweat would be excreted; if it closes, no sweat would be excreted. As sweat is derived from body fluids and blood that are from the same source, there is a saying that "Sweat and blood have the same source." And because blood is governed by the heart, there is a saying that "Sweat is fluid of the heart."

c. All the vessels belong to the heart and the heart reflects on the face: Since there are many vessels on the head and face, the face is lustrous and moist if heart *qi* flourishes and the vessels are full. Pallor and dull complexion may be seen if blood is insufficient. A dark-bluish complexion may appear if it is congealed.

d. The heart opens to the tongue: "The tongue is the window of the heart." The tongue has tasting and speaking functions, which depend upon the heart to govern blood, vessels and Mind. If the heart functions abnormally, pathological symptoms, such as changes of taste sensation and stiffness of the tongue and dystalia, etc. may result. As the tongue is not covered by the epidermis but is extremely rich in vessels, the circulation of *qi* and blood can be seen and the physiological function of the heart can be judged from the colour of the tongue. "The tongue is the window of the heart" is a theory established by ancient medical experts through their observations. If the cardiac function is normal, the tongue will be red, flexible, brilliant, moist and soft and the sense of taste will be keen and speech will be coherent. If a pathological process of the heart appears, it will reflect on the tongue. For instance, insufficient heart fire, dark-red tongue or even tongue sores; congealed and blocked heart blood, a dark-purplish tongue or the tongue with petechiae; the dysfunction of the heart in governing the Mind, a rolling tongue, stiff tongue, stuttering or aphonia, etc.

In a word, the physiological function of the heart includes not only the regulation of the circulatory system, but also the control of mental and emotional activities.

Appendix: Pericardium

The pericardium, called *xinbao*, or *tanzhong*, is a membrane around the heart to protect it. In the meridian theory, it is also called a viscus because the Heart Meridian of Hand-*jueyin* connects with the pericardium and is closely related to the Triple Energizer Meridian of Hand-*shaoyang*. But, in the theory of viscera symptoms, it is regarded as the surrounding of the heart and protects the heart, so that it is first affected when an exogenous pathogenic factor invades the heart. Mental problems, delirium, etc. appearing in acute febrile diseases are known as "heat invading the pericardium" or "the pericardium misted with heat."

3-1-2 The lung

The lungs are located on each side of the chest cavity. The lungs are called the "roof of the carriage" because they are in a higher position. They are also called delicate organs because the lobars are delicate and cannot tolerate cold and heat and are easily invaded. They are closely related to *hun* (soul). The lungs are the master of *qi* and correspond to metal in the five-element theory. They are concerned with hair, carry on respiration and are concerned with purification and descendance. They control the water duct and all blood passes through them so as to assist the heart to regulate the circulation of *qi* and blood. The lungs are closely related to skin and hair, anxiety, nasal discharge and open to the nose. As the Lung Meridian of Hand-*taiyin* and the Large Intestine Meridian of Hand-*yangming* are connected with each other and pertain to the lung and large intestine respectively, the lung and large intestine are closely related.

3-1-2-1 Main physiological functions of the lung

a. *Qi* is governed by the lung. This is first manifested in the formation of *qi*, particularly chest *qi*,[2] which chiefly depends upon the combination of clear air taken in by the lung with *jing* (vital principle) transported and digested by the spleen and stomach. Hence, whether the respiratory function of the lung is normal or not directly influences the formation of chest *qi* as well as that of *qi* in the whole body. Secondly, the lung also regulates the *qi* of the entire body. Respiration is the ascending, descending, going-out and coming-in movements of *qi*.

The lung is concerned with respiratory *qi* (air), and a place where gases inside and outside of the body exchange. Clear *qi* (air) from the environment is inspired and turbid *qi* from the body, expired. The formation of *qi* is promoted and the movement of *qi* regulated through the incessant expiration of turbid gases and inspiration of air, so that normal metabolism is maintained. The even and moderate respiration of the lung is the primary condition for the formation and normal functioning of *qi*. Abnormal respiration influences the formation of chest *qi* and *qi* movement and weakens the flow of *qi* in the body. Deficient *qi*, abnormal movement of *qi* and abnormal blood circulation and distribution and excretion of body fluids may influence the respiratory movement of the lung, resulting in abnormal respiration.

b. Dispersion, purification and descendance

Dispersion means distribution and spreading of *qi*, that is, the ascending, descending and spreading of lung *qi*. Purification and descendance means the action of lung *qi* to keep the respiratory tract clean.

The actions of dispersion are chiefly: a) to excrete turbid *qi* (gases) from the body; b) to spread body fluids and the refined principle of food transported by the spleen throughout the body, and to the skin and hair; c) to spread defensive *qi*, regulate the opening and shutting of the junction between the skin and muscle and change body fluids that are formed after metabolism into sweat and excrete them out of the body. Thus, if the lung loses its spreading and dispersing action, pathological symptoms, such as dyspnea, chest distress, cough and asthmatic breath, sneezing and anhidrosis, etc. may occur.

The actions of purification and descendance are chiefly: a) to inspire fresh air that has been taken in by the lung and body fluids and the refined food which is transported by the spleen; b) to clear foreign bodies from the lung and respiratory tract. Hence, in case the lung loses its purifying and descending actions, pathological symptoms, such as short or shallow breath, coughing sputum, hemoptysis, etc. may appear.

The dispersing, purifying and descending actions of the lung are opposite, but complementary to each other. The abnormal dispersing, purifying and descending actions of the lung would lead to an obstructed *qi* passage, uneven respiration and abnormal exchange of gases inside and outside the body. If these two functions are in disharmony, pathological changes will occur, with asthmatic breath, cough and regurgitation of lung *qi*.

c. To unblock and regulate water passage: The dispersing, purifying and descending functions of the lung unblock and regulate the distribution, transportation and excretion of body fluids. The lung not only distributes body fluids and the refined principle derived from food to the entire body, but also governs the opening and shutting of the junction between the skin and muscle and regulate excretion of sweat. Lung *qi* not only sends the kidney fresh air, but also continuously transports turbid fluids downward to become urine which is discharged from the body by kidney *qi* and bladder *qi*. This is the action of the lung in regulating water metabolism, as well as its physiological function in unblocking and regulating the water passage. Pathological processes, such as the formation of *tan-yin* (phlegm and excess exudates) due to stagnant aqueous liquid or edema due to overflowing water, etc. may result when the lung fails to regulate the water passage.

d. All blood within the body must pass through the lung: The blood passes through the lung and gases exchange through pulmonary respiration, then are distributed throughout the body. The circulatory system is controlled by the heart and blood circulates in the body by depending upon the impulse of *qi* along with ascending and descending *qi*. The lung governs *qi* in the entire body. As the lung controls respiration and regulates the body's *qi* mechanism, blood circulation is based on the distribution and regulation of lung *qi*.

The governing and regulating functions of the lung are manifest in: a) The lung is concerned with respiration; b) along with respiration the movement of *qi* is regulated by the lung, the heart is assisted in promoting and regulating blood, and fluids are regulated by the dispersing, purifying and descending functions of the lung.

3-1-2-2 Relation of the lung to the emotions, body fluids, tissues and sense organs

a. The lung is related to anxiety: In the respective correspondence of the five emotions to the five yin viscera, the lung is closely related to anxiety. Both anxiety and worry are the reactions of an unfavourable irritation. Anxiety continuously consumes *qi*. As the lung governs *qi*, anxiety and worry can easily injure the lung.

If the lung is weak, tolerance of the body to unfavourable exogenous irritation would become weak, easily causing anxiety and worry.

b. Relation of the lung to nasal discharge: Nasal discharge is mucus secreted by the nasal mucoid membrane which moistens the nostril. The nose is the window of the lung. Under normal conditions, nasal discharge moistens the nostril and does not flow out. If the lung is affected by exogenous pathogenic cold, watery nasal discharge would appear; if affected by pernicious heat, nasal discharge would be yellow and turbid; if affected by dryness, the nose would be dry.

c. The lung corresponds to the skin and reflects on the hair. Here, the skin and hair include the tissues, such as the skin, sweat glands, hair, etc. They are on the surface of the body and depend upon the warming nourishment and moistening of defensive *qi* and body fluids and become a protective screen against the invasion of exogenous pathogenic factors. As the lung governs *qi* and has the action of dispersing defensive *qi*, it transports *jing* (vital principle) to the skin and hair. *Plain Questions* states, "The lung is closely related to the skin and reflects its brilliance on the hair." ("1 *Wu Zang Chen Pian*") If the physiological function of the lung is normal, the skin will be normal and hair shiny, and the skin will better resist exogenous pathogenic factors. If lung *qi* is weak, its distribution of defensive *qi* and transport of *jing* (vital principle) to the skin and hair will be reduced, so the body surface will not be well-protected and its ability to resist an exogenous pathogenic factor weakened, possibly resulting in hyperhidrosis, easily affected by cold and withered skin, etc. Since the lung is concerned with the skin and hair, it is often affected and its *qi* is depressed when the exogenous pathogenic factor invades the skin and hair, the junction between the skin and muscle is blocked and defensive *qi* is stagnant. When the exogenous pathogenic factor invades the lung whose *qi* fails to spread, pathological processes, such as the blocked junction between the skin and muscle and stagnant defensive *qi*, etc. can also be caused.

d. The nose is the window of the lung. Since the nose communicates with the throat and connects with the lung and the nose and throat are the passages for respiration, there is the saying that "the nose is the door of the lung." Both smell and voice are due to the action of lung *qi*. So normal lung *qi* and respiration would lead to a keen smell and beautiful voice. Because the nose is the window of the lung and the lung is directly communicated with the throat, and exogenous pathogenic factor usually invades the lung from the nose and throat. Thus, the pathological processes of the lung are frequently seen in nose and throat troubles, such as a stuffy running nose, sneezing, itching throat, coarse voice, aphonia, etc.

3-1-3 The spleen

The spleen lies in the middle energizer below the diaphragm. The chief function of the spleen is transmission and digestion, sending the purified (nutrient) upward and controlling blood. As the Spleen Meridian of Foot-*taiyin* and Stomach Meridian of Foot-*yangming* pertain to the spleen and stomach respectively, the spleen and stomach are closely related. The spleen and stomach are the main yin viscera in the digestive system. They are called the resource of "acquired foundation," from which *qi* and blood are derived because the activities of the body and generation of *qi*, blood and body fluids all depend upon the refined food that is transported and digested by them. The spleen opens to the mouth, reflects its brilliance on the lips, corresponds to earth, is related to worry and controls the muscle and four extremities according to the five-element theory.

3-1-3-1 Chief physiological functions of the spleen

a. The spleen is concerned with transmission and digestion. The spleen refines food and transmits it to the body. This function can be divided into that of transmission and digestion of food and of liquid.

Transmission and digestion of food refers to the digestion and absorption of food by the spleen. After entering the stomach, food is digested and absorbed in the stomach and small intestine, relying on the transmitting and digesting functions of the spleen. The refined material can be distributed to the whole body by relying on the spleen functions of transmitting and distributing the vital principle. Only if the spleen's transmitting and digesting functions are normal can the spleen supply enough nutrients to generate essential *qi*, blood and body fluids to the viscera, meridians, four extremities and tissues, such as tendons, muscles, skin and hair, etc. and receive nutrients, so they can function normally. Hence, if the spleen is hypofunctional in transmitting and digesting food, the digesting and absorbing functions of the body will be abnormal, arousing pathological processes, such as abdominal distension, loose stools, anorexia, even lassitude, emaciation, deficient *qi* and blood, etc.

Transmission and digestion of liquid refers to the action of the spleen to absorb, transmit and distribute aqueous liquid. The nutrients in food are absorbed when it is in a liquid state. Superfluous moisture in food from which the nutrient is absorbed can be transmitted to the lung and kidney and changed into sweat and urine that are excreted from the body. Superfluous moisture within the body can be prevented from being abnormally stagnant and pathological products such as endogenous damp, *tan-yin* (phlegm and excess exudates), etc. can also be prevented from forming if the spleen's function of transmitting and digesting aqueous liquid is normal. Hypofunction of the spleen in transmitting and digesting liquid would necessarily lead to stagnation of liquid within the body, producing pathological products, such as endogenous damp, *tan-yin*, even edema, etc.

The spleen and stomach are significant in the prevention of disease and the maintenance of health. In daily life, attention must be paid not only to dietary nutrition, but also to protecting the spleen and stomach. For example, certain foods should be avoided when one is sick and the spleen and stomach should be taken into account when taking medications.

b. When the spleen sends the purified (nutrients) upward, they are absorbed and sent upward to the heart, lung, head and eyes, and changed into *qi* and blood by the heart and lung to nourish the entire body.

"Sending the purified (nutrient) upward" and "sending the turbid (matter) downward" are the contrary movements of the *qi* mechanism of the viscera. The spleen function of sending the purified matter upward is the opposite of the gastric function of sending the turbid matter downward. On the other hand, the harmony of ascending and descending functions between the yin and yang viscera is an important factor. Hence, only if the spleen function of sending the purified material upward is normal can the nutritional substance be absorbed and distributed. If spleen *qi* ascends and flourishes visceroptosis will never occur. If spleen *qi* fails to send the purified material upward, food cannot be transmitted and digested and *qi* and blood lose their resource, leading to mental fatigue, lassitude, vertigo, abdominal distension, diarrhea, etc. Prolapse of the rectum and visceroptosis, etc. may be seen if the spleen does not function normally.

c. The spleen controls the blood: The chief mechanism of the spleen's control of the blood is the governing action of *qi*. The reason why the spleen can control blood is that it is the resource of *qi* and blood. If its transmitting and digesting functions are normal, *qi* and blood will be enriched, the governing action of *qi* will be normal, and blood will not extravasate. If it is hypofunctional, *qi* will be hypofunctional, causing hemorrhage.

Bloody stool, hematuria, metrorrhagia, etc. are usually ascribed to the spleen's failure to control blood.

3-1-3-2   Relation of the spleen to the emotions, body fluids, tissues and sense organs

a. The spleen is concerned with worry (or thinking). Under normal conditions, thinking over problems does not influence the body negatively. But, overthinking or extreme worry can affect the body, resulting in stagnation and blockage of *qi*. So far as its influence upon physiological functions of the viscera is concerned, transmitting and digesting functions of the spleen are markedly affected. As blocked *qi* affects the spleen's transmission of the purified material, overthinking can often lead to poor appetite, epigastric distension and fullness, vertigo, etc.

b. Saliva protects the mucus membrane in the mouth and moistens the mouth. During eating plenty of mucus is secreted to aid in swallowing and digesting food. Under normal conditions, it ascends to the mouth, but does not flow outside. In case the spleen and stomach are in disharmony, it will be rapidly secreted, resulting in a spontaneous overflow of saliva.

c. The spleen is concerned with muscles and the four extremities. *Plain Questions* states, "the spleen controls the muscles." This is because the spleen and stomach are the resource of *qi* and blood, and the muscles can be healthy only when nourished by the refined food which is transported and digested by the spleen and stomach. Hence, the strength of the muscles depends upon the transporting and digesting functions of the spleen and stomach and gastrosplenic dysfunction leads to thin, weak or even atrophic muscles.

The transportation of the refined food to the four extremities depends upon the ascending and dispersing functions of pure yang *qi*. Therefore, if splenic *qi* is normal in transporting the nutrients, the muscles of the four extremities will move freely and energetically. If not, the muscles will lack nutrients, and lassitude, weakness and even atrophy may be seen.

d. The spleen opens to the mouth and reflects on the lips. "The spleen opens to the mouth" means that diets and appetite, etc. are closely related to the transporting and digesting functions of the spleen. A normal appetite depends upon whether the normal splenic function of sending the purified material upward and the gastric function of sending the turbid material downward are normal or not. If the spleen and stomach transport food normally, the appetite will be normal. If not, a tasteless, sweet, mucoid, or bitter taste, etc. may appear.

The colour of the mouth and lips indicates whether *qi* and blood are rich or not. As the spleen is the resource of *qi* and blood, whether the mouth and lips are red and moist is not only the reflection of the state of *qi* and blood in the body, but also that of the spleen and stomach's transporting and digesting the refined food.

3-1-4 The liver

The liver lies in the abdomen below the diaphragm in the right hypochondrium. It is the residence of the soul, storehouse of the blood and master of tendons. In the five-element theory it corresponds to wood and is concerned with the movement and predisposed to a flourishing growth. Its chief physiological functions are concerned with dispersing and discharging. The liver opens to the eyes, governs tendons and reflects on nails. It is closely related to anger and tears. As the Liver Meridian of Foot-*jueyin* and the Gallbladder Meridian of Foot-*shaoyang* are respectively connected with the liver and gallbladder, the liver and gallbladder are closely related.

3-1-4-1 Chief physiological functions of the liver

a. The dispersing and discharging functions of the liver refer to the liver's predisposition to a flourishing growth and movement, which is an important link in regulating and unblocking the *qi* mechanism of the entire body and promoting blood circulation and body fluids. They are chiefly: a) Regulating the *qi* mechanism that refers to the movement of *qi*. The movement of the viscera, meridians and organs of the body are based on the movements of *qi*. Since the liver is characterized by flourishing growth and movement, it is an important factor in *qi* movement. Hence, whether its dispersing and discharging functions are normal or not plays a regulating role in balancing and harmonizing the movement of *qi*. If these functions are normal, all *qi* activities will be regulated. *Qi* and blood will be harmonious, the meridian will be unblocked, and the viscera and organs will function normally. If not, a pathological condition may occur. When the liver loses its dispersing and discharging functions, *qi* will fail to flourish and *qi* activities will be blocked, forming pathological obstructions, and stagnant *qi* with local distension, pain and discomfort in the chest and hypochondria, breasts or lower abdomen. When the liver is hyperfunctional, *qi* will become excessive in a flourishing growth and deficient in descending, forming pathological regurgitations of *qi* with distension and pain in the head and eyes, flushed face, congestive eyes, irascibility, etc. If *qi* is excessive in its flourishing growth, blood will flow adversely together with *qi*, causing pathological changes, such as hematemesis, hempotysis, etc., even sudden unconsciousness termed *qi jue* syndrome.

Since circulation of blood and distribution and metabolism of body fluids depend upon movements of *qi*, stagnant *qi* would obstruct blood circulation, forming congealed blood or abdominal masses, lumps or irregular menstrual flow, dysmenorrhea, amenorrhea, etc. in women. It also results in the obstructed distribution and metabolism of body fluids, pathological products, such as *tan-yin* (phlegm and excess exudates), etc. or phlegmatic nodules formed by the blocked meridians[3] or tympanites formed by water retention.

One of the important links for the transporting and digestive functions of the spleen and stomach is the splenic function of sending the turbid matter downward and the dispersing and discharging functions of the liver are closely related to the ascending and descending functions of the spleen and stomach. For splenic *qi* and gastric *qi* to descend normally the dispersing and discharging functions of the liver must be normal. If not, the splenic function of sending the purified matter upward will be influenced (vertigo appearing in the upper part of the body; and diarrhea with undigested food appearing in the lower), and can further influence the gastric function of sending the turbid matter downward (hiccup and belching appearing in the upper part of the body; epigastric distension, fullness and pain in the middle, constipation in the lower). The former is called "liver *qi* invading the spleen" and the latter, "liver *qi* invading the stomach." Both of them are generally termed "overactive wood (liver) overacts upon earth (spleen)." This can also be manifested in secretion and excretion of bile so that the dispersing and discharging functions of the liver aid the transport and digestive functions of the spleen and stomach. The gallbladder is linked with the liver and bile formed by partially accumulated liver *qi*. Bile secretion and excretion are part of the dispersing and discharging functions of the liver. If bile is normally secreted and excreted, the transporting and digesting functions of the spleen and stomach are strengthened. If liver *qi* is stagnant, the bile secretion and excretion may be influenced, with distension and fullness and pain below the hypochondriac region, bitter mouth, dyspepsia, even jaundice, etc. appearing.

Although emotions pertain to the physiological function of the heart to store the Mind, they also closely relate to the dispersing and discharging functions of the liver. That is because a normal emotional state chiefly depends upon the normal circulation of *qi* and blood, but an abnormal state may influence physiological activities, disturbing the normal circulation of *qi* and blood. So, the dispersing and discharging functions of the liver can normalize the emotions, by maintaining normal *qi* activities. If the dispersing and discharging functions of the liver are normal, *qi* activities will be normal. If *qi* and blood are harmonious, one is cheerful; if it is hypofunctional, liver *qi* will be stagnant and depression results; if the liver is hyperfunctional, one will be easily angered and irritated. With repeated and persistent emotional irritation, the dispersing and discharging functions of the liver will also be influenced, leading to problems, such as stagnant or overactive liver *qi*, etc.

In addition, ovulation and menstruation in women and secretion of semen in men are all related to the dispersing and discharging functions of the liver.

b. Some blood must be stored in the liver to restrain overactive liver yang and maintain its dispersing and discharging functions. It also plays an important role in preventing the body from bleeding. If the liver fails to store blood, not only pathological processes, such as insufficient liver blood and overactive yang *qi*, etc. will occur, but hemorrhage may also appear. This function also plays a leading role in distributing blood to various parts of the body, particularly the blood volume in the peripheral parts. With normal physiological activity, emotional and weather changes, etc. the blood volume in various parts of the body changes somewhat. When the body moves rapidly or is highly excited, the liver distributes blood stored in it over the peripheral body in order to meet the body's needs. When one is at rest and calm, the volume of blood needed by the peripheral part of the body decreases so that some blood is stored in the liver. As the liver stores and regulates blood, the activities of various parts of the body are closely related to the liver. In case the liver is in trouble, its function of storing blood will be abnormal and blood deficiency or hemorrhage may result and various parts of the body may not be nourished by blood. If liver blood is too deficient to nourish the eye, dry and uncomfortable eyes and blurred vision or night blindness may result; if it is too deficient to nourish tendons, convulsions of tendons, numbness of limbs and difficulty extending and flexing limbs may result. It is also important in menstruation. When the liver fails to store blood, a decreased amount of menstrual flow, even amenorrhea or an increased amount of menstrual flow, but also metrorrhagia may appear.

There is the saying that "the liver stores *hun* (soul)." According to the visceral symptoms theory *hun* is derived from *shen* (Spirit). Their material basis is blood. As the heart governs blood, it stores the Mind; as the liver stores blood, it stores the soul. If the hepatic function of storing blood is normal, the soul can dwell in the liver. If liver blood and heart blood are impaired, the soul will fail to dwell in the liver, and fright and dreaminess, disturbed sleep, somnambulism and hallucination, etc. will appear.

3-1-4-2 Relation of the liver to the emotions, body fluids, tissues and sense organs

a. The liver is concerned with anger: Anger may make *qi* and blood move adversely and yang *qi* ascend and discharge. Since the liver has the dispersing and discharging functions and yang *qi* is ascending and flourishing, the liver is closely related to anger. If overanger occurs, yang *qi* will ascend and flourish excessively. If liver blood is deficient and liver yang ascends and flourishes excessively, anger may easily appear whenever something is irritating.

b. Relation of the liver to tears: The eye is the window of the liver, so the liver is concerned with tears. Under normal circumstances, tears moisten the eye, but are also secreted when a foreign body invades the eye, to expel it. Under pathological conditions, abnormal secretion of tears can be seen, e.g., dry and uncomfortable eyes due to insufficient liver blood is ascribed to insufficient secretion of tears. Acute conjunctivitis caused by pathogenic wind-fire and Liver Meridian affected by damp-heat may cause lacrimation. Sadness will also cause crying.

c. Tendons and nails. The tendon connects the joints and muscles. The flexion and extension of the body and joints are caused by contraction and relaxation of the tendons and muscles. Tendons are nourished chiefly by liver blood. Only if liver blood is enriched can it be well-nourished and move forcefully and flexibly. The energy of the body originates from the enriched blood stored in the liver. The liver regulates blood volume. If the liver blood is deficient and the fascia lacks nourishment, the fascia will not move so forcefully and smoothly and the hand and foot may tremble and numb trunk and limbs that cannot flex and extend freely, even clonic convulsions,[4] etc. may result.

The flourishing or decline of the liver may influence the nails. If liver blood is enriched, they will be tough, tensible, bright and lustrous. If not, they will be soft, thin and withered, even malformed and fragile.

d. Relation of the liver to the eye. As the Liver Meridian upwardly connects with "ocular connections"[5] and vision depends upon the dispersing and discharging functions of the liver and nourishment of liver blood, it is said, "the eye is the window of the liver." The essential *qi* of the five yin and six yang viscera upwardly reach the eye. Thus, the eye is internally connected with the five yin and six yang viscera.

Because of the intimate relation between the liver and eye, the hepatic function is usually reflected by the eye, e.g., insufficient yin blood of the liver would lead to dry and uncomfortable eyes, blurred vision or night blindness. Wind and heat affection of the Liver Meridian would cause congestive, itching and painful eyes; blazing liver fire would result in congestive eyes with nebula; excess liver yang would lead to vertigo; the internal movement of liver wind would cause deviation and upward fixation of the eye.

3-1-5 The kidney

The kidneys are situated in the lumbar region, each on either side of the spinous column. They are called the "congenital foundation" because they store "congenital *jing* (vital principle)" and are the foundation of yin-yang of the viscera. They correspond to water in the five-element theory. Their physiological function is to store *jing* (vital principle) and they are also concerned with growth, development, generation and water metabolism. They control bones and generate bone marrow, reflect on the hair and open to the ears, external genitalia and anus. As the Kidney Meridian of Foot-*shaoyin* and the Bladder Meridian of Foot-*taiyang* are respectively related to water metabolism, the kidney and bladder are closely related.

3-1-5-1 Chief physiological functions of the kidney

a. Storing *jing* (vital principle), governing growth, development and reproduction. Controlling and storing *jing* is the kidney's chief physiological function. This is mainly to create a favourable condition for the vital principle to be fully effective.

Essential *qi* is the basic substance constituting the body as well as the basis for growth, development and activity. It is stored in the kidney and contains "congenital" *jing* (vital principle) and acquired *jing*. *Qi* is inherited from the parents which is the prime substance for the development of the embryo. *Jing* refers to the nutrients derived from food, transported and digested by the spleen and stomach and the remainder of essential *qi* formed in physiological activities of the viscera and stored in the kidney.

Although they are of different sources, both are stored in the kidney and depend on and complement each other.

The vital principle of the kidney plays an important role in the physiological activities of the body. The vital principle of the kidney is divided into kidney yin and kidney yang. The nourishment and moistening of the viscera, tissues and organs of the body is termed kidney yin; promoting and warming the viscera, tissues and organs is called kidney yang. Both are also known as primordial yin and primordial yang. They are the roots of the yin and yang of all other yin viscera and complement each other to maintain a balance between the yin and yang of the five yin viscera. If balance is regained after it has been lost, deficient kidney yin or yang will form, resulting in symptoms of deficient kidney yin, such as fever, vertigo, tinnitus, sore and weak loin and knee, nocturnal emission, red and dry tongue, etc. or those of deficient kidney yang, such as fatigue, lassitude, cold limbs and trunk, cold, pain and weakness of the loin and knees, watery profuse urine, difficulty in urination or enuresis, incontinence of urine, light-coloured tongue, hypogonadium, edema, etc.

Since kidney yin and kidney yang are the foundations of yin and yang of the viscera, the yin and yang of the viscera may become imbalanced when those of the kidney are disharmonious. For example, if the liver is not nourished by kidney yin, which is called "inadequate water to nourish wood," overactive liver yang or even the internal movement of liver wind may appear. If the heart is not supported by kidney yin, blazing heart fire or yin deficiencies of both the heart and kidney may result. If the lung is not nourished by kidney yin, symptoms of yin deficiencies of the lung and kidney, such as dry throat, dry cough, tidal fever, blazing fire, etc. may appear. If the spleen is not warmed by kidney yang, symptoms of yang deficiencies of the spleen and kidney, such as diarrhea in the morning and aqueous-grainy diarrhea may appear. If the heart is not warmed by kidney yang, there may be symptoms of yang deficiencies of the heart and kidney, such as palpitation, slow pulse, perspiration, cold limbs, short breath, etc. Furthermore, a prolonged disharmony between the yin and yang of the viscera affects the kidney and impairs the vital principle of the kidney, which is the reason for a prolonged disease of the kidney.

When kidney yin becomes deficient, kidney yang may be affected and the disease will develop into deficient yin and yang, called "the deficient yin affecting the yang." When kidney yang becomes weak, kidney yin may also be affected and develop into deficient yin and yang, called "the deficient yang affecting the yin."

The impairment of the vital principle of the kidney is manifest in various ways. Sometimes disharmony between yin and yang is not so obvious even if the vital principle has been impaired, thus called the impairment of the vital principle of the kidney or deficient kidney *jing* and deficient kidney *qi*.

b. Controlling water means that the kidney plays an important role in distributing and excreting body fluids and keeping water metabolism balanced.

Under normal physiological conditions, fluid metabolism is carried on through the ingestion of blood by the stomach, transportation and digestion of nutrients by the spleen, the dispersing functions of the lung and the kidney's functions and transmission of the triple energizer and body fluids that have been metabolized into sweat, urine and gas to be excreted outside the body. The essential *qi* of the kidneys governs the metabolism of body fluids, and the action of the lung and spleen, etc. on body fluids depends on the essential *qi* of the kidney. The formation and discharge of urine plays a vital role in keeping the balance of water metabolism within the body. If the essential *qi* of the kidney becomes abnormal, pathological phenomena, such as the inability of the kidney to control urine, a decreased amount of urine and edema due to the obstructed renal metabolism may appear. If general puffiness occurs, pathological symptoms, such as profuse watery urine, increased amount of urine due to a dysfunctional kidney and bladder, etc. may result.

c. The kidney has the action of receiving clear *qi* (air) that has been taken in by the lung, so as to prevent shallow breath, and keep a normal exchange of gases outside and inside the body. The respiratory function of the body depends on the kidney function of absorbing air although it is controlled by the lung. Theoretically speaking, clear *qi* inhaled by the lung must descend to reach the kidney. The maintenance of deep respiration by the lung depends upon the kidney absorbing air. Hence, if the kidney functions normally, respiration will be even and moderate, but if the kidney is hypofunctional in absorbing *qi*, breath will be shallow, possibly producing pathological symptoms, such as asthmatic breath immediately after exertion, exhaling too much air and little inspiration, etc.

3-1-5-2 Relation of the kidney to the emotions, body fluids, tissues and sense organs

a. The kidney is concerned with fear. Although fear is concerned with the kidney, it also relates to "the heart storing the Mind." As the heart stores the Mind, injury of the Mind would lead to fear. "Fear causing the descent of *qi*" implies that in a stressful situation, the *qi* mechanism of the upper energizer[6] is blocked. *Qi* is pressed to the lower energizer, resulting in distension and fullness of the lower energizer and even enuresis. "Fright causing disorders of *qi*" is when normal physiological activities are disturbed, resulting in mental anxiety, random movements of hands and feet, etc.

b. The kidney is concerned with saliva. Saliva is derived from the vital principle of the kidney and can be swallowed but not spit out. It has the function of replenishing the vital principle of the kidney. If it is frequently or persistently spit out, the vital principle would be easily consumed. So, ancient experts of *daoyin*[7] nourished the vital principle of the kidney by licking their upper palates with their tongues to induce saliva and swallowed it after it filled the mouth.

c. The kidney governs bones, generates marrow and is reflected by the hair. Governing the bones and generating the marrow is an important component of the function of kidney *qi* in promoting growth and development. The growth and development of the bones depends upon the enrichment of bone marrow and the nutrient the marrow supplies. Delayed development of the fontanel, soft and weak bones, fragile bones and easily fractured bones in the aged, etc. all are a result of insufficient essential *qi* in the kidney and bone marrow.

Marrow includes the bone marrow, spinal cord and brain derived from the essential *qi* in the kidney. Hence, the flourishing or decline of the essential *qi* in the kidney not only influences the growth and development of the bones, but also the development and maintenance of the spinal cord and brain. The brain is called the "sea of marrow" because the spinal cord is connected with the brain and forms the brain after it merges into the brain. When essential *qi* in the kidney is full, the sea of marrow will be nourished, the brain will develop and perform normally. If the *qi* is insufficient, the sea of marrow will not be nourished, creating a deficiency. As the teeth and bones are of the same source and the former is nourished by the essential *qi* in the kidney, the "teeth are secondary to the kidney and primary to bones." The growth and loss of the teeth are closely related to the flourishing and decline of the essential *qi*. If the essential *qi* is full, the teeth will be firm and not come out easily; if not, they will become easily loose and drop out before they should. Another influence comes from the meridians of hand-and-foot *yangming* because both enter the teeth. Certain pathological processes of the teeth are thus concerned with these meridians and physiological functions of the intestines and stomach.

The growth of hair depends upon *jing* (vital principle) and blood. Since the kidney stores *jing* (vital principle), it is said that "the kidney reflects its brilliance on hair." As the growing and dropping, moistening and withering of hair depend not only upon the nourishment of essential *qi* in the kidney, but that of blood, it is said that "hair is nourished by blood." In young and middle-aged people, hair is long and brilliant because *jing* (vital principle) and blood are full, while in the elderly hair becomes grey or white and begins to thin. Grey, thinning hair is due to insufficient essential *qi* in the kidney and blood.

d. The kidney is related to the ears, urinary organs, external genitalia and the anus. Whether hearing is normal or not is related to the essential *qi* in the kidney. If the *qi* is full and the sea of the marrow is nourished, the ear will be very sensitive. However, if the *qi* declines and the sea of marrow is not nourished, hearing will be reduced or tinnitus or even deafness will result. In old age, the essential *qi* of the kidney is usually deficient and hearing is reduced.

Yin includes the front yin (urinary organs and external genitalia) and the back yin (the passage through which stools are excreted). Although urine is discharged from the bladder, urination depends upon the functional activities of the kidney. Hence, frequent urination, enuresis, incontinence of urine, oliguria and anuria are all related to the functioning of kidney *qi*. Although the excretion of stools is the function of the large intestine to transmit and transform the waste product, it is also related to the function of the kidney, for instance when kidney yin is deficient, constipation due to a dry intestine may result; when kidney yang is deficient or impaired, constipation or diarrhea caused by deficient yang may appear due to inactive *qi*. When the kidney is hypofunctional, prolonged diarrhea and collapse of the rectum may result. Therefore, it is said that "the kidney opens to the two yin."

Appendix: *Mingmen* (the vital portal)

"*Mingmen*" (the vital portal) was first discussed in "Genjie," a chapter in *Miraculous Pivot. Classic on Difficult Medical Problems* points out that "the two kidneys are not really the kidneys, but the left one is the kidney and the right, *mingmen*, which is the residence of Spirit and the holder of the primordial *qi*. The male's *mingmen* is for storing *jing* (vital principle), and the female's is for maintaining the uterus." Medical experts in later generations took notice of this, and its location and physiological function have become controversial. The chief controversies are as follows:

a. The theory of the right kidney as *mingmen*: It was first seen in *Classic on Difficult Medical Problems* that the kidney has two parts, the left one is the kidney, but the right one is the vital portal. For instance, "The 39th Difficult Medical Problem" of *Classic on Difficult Medical Problems* states, "The left one is the substantial kidney but the right one, the vital portal where various Spirits dwell."

a) The vital portal is so called because "the residence of Spirit" is the foundation of life and the portal to keep life; b) it plays an important role in storing *jing* (vital principle) in the male and maintaining the uterine function in the female and the genital function lies in the vital portal; c) the kidney communicates with the vital portal. Although the two kidneys are divided into the left and the right, they are inseparable in their physiological function. That is to say, the vital portal has the function of the kidney and the kidney, in turn, has the action of the vital portal.

b. The theory that both kidneys are generally called the vital portals. In his *Orthodox Medicine* (*Yixue Zheng Zong*) Lu Bo of the Ming Dynasty (1368-1644) pointed out that "the kidneys are called the vital portals." Although Zhang Jingyue of the Ming Dynasty explained that the vital portal refers to the vestibule of the vagina in a female and the opening of external genitalia in a male, he held that "both the kidneys pertain to the vital portal" and said that "fire in the vital portal is known as primordial *qi*, while water as primordial *jing* (vital principle)."

c. The theory that the area between the two kidneys is regarded as the vital portal. This viewpoint was first put forward by Zao Xianke in his "Ling Lan Mi Dian" ("The Classic Stored Secretly in the Emperor's Library"), a chapter in *Plain Questions*. He also held that the function of the vital portal is to control the body's yang *qi*.

d. The theory of the vital portal as the motive force of *qi* holds that the area between the two kidneys is the vital portal, although there is neither water nor fire, but the motive force of primordial *qi* in it. At the same time, the vital portal is by no means a substantial organ. Su Yikui of the Ming Dynasty held that the motive force of *qi* between the kidney is the vital portal. His viewpoints about the vital portal are as follows: As the vital portal is not a substantial organ, no meridian traverses it and no pulse can be palpated there. The vital portal is located between the two kidneys, and is a residence of the motive force of *qi* between the kidneys as well as a pivot of vitality. Although the motive force of *qi* between the kidneys is the foundation of the viscera, it cannot be thought of as fire.

The above-mentioned controversies of various medical experts about the vital portal include whether it is substantial or not in its morphology, whether it is located between the two kidneys and whether it is concerned with fire in its function. Anyhow, there exists no controversy about its chief physiological functions and the close relation between these functions and the kidney as well. The kidney is the foundation of the five yin viscera, in which the real yin and yang lie, the yin of the five yin and six yang viscera are replenished and supported by kidney yin and warmly nourished by kidney yang. So, kidney yang is fire in the vital portal and kidney yin, "water of the vital portal," so called by Zhang Zhongjing. The kidney yin and kidney yang are the primordial yin and yang. Thus, the reason why ancient medical experts termed the kidney the vital portal was to emphasize the importance of the yin and yang within the kidney.

3-2 The six yang viscera

The six yang viscera is a general term for the gallbladder, stomach, large intestine, small intestine, bladder and triple energizer. Their common physiological functions are to digest food and transmit residues. Food must enter the body and be excreted out of the body through the "seven key passes," so that it may be digested and absorbed. These key passes are called the "seven important portals," the lips, teeth, epiglottis, cardia, pylorus, illeocecal valve and anus. If any of these portals is in disorder, the reception, digestion, absorption and excretion of food will be influenced.

The physiological characteristics of the six yang viscera are normal when their *qi* descends. Deficiency or excess of their "communicating" and "descending" functions are pathological states.

3-2-1 The gallbladder

The gallbladder is the chief of the six yang viscera and also belongs to the unusual organs. It is linked with the liver and appends to the short lobar of the liver. The liver and gallbladder are closely related because they are connected with the meridians.

The formation and excretion of bile is controlled and regulated by the dispersing and discharging functions of the liver. If these functions are normal, bile is excreted normally and the transporting and digesting functions of the spleen and stomach are also normal. If not, the gastrosplenic functions will be influenced, with such signs as distension, hypogastric fullness and pain, poor appetite, abdominal distension, loose stools, etc.; if it ascends adversely, a bitter taste, vomiting yellow dark-bluish bitter fluid may be seen; if it goes wild, jaundice may result.

The chief function of the gallbladder is to store and excrete bile. As bile directly aids digestion the gallbladder is one of the six yang viscera; as the gallbladder does not transmit and digest food, but stores bile, it differs from the yang viscera such as the stomach and intestine, etc. It is also called an unusual organ.

3-2-2 The stomach

The stomach is also termed the "epigastric region" and is divided into the upper, middle and lower portions. The upper portion is called the epigastric region, including the cardia; the middle, the middle epigastrium, the stomach; the lower, the hypogastrium, including the pylorus. Its chief function is to receive and digest food and is normal when its *qi* descends.

3-2-2-1 Digestion

As food enters the mouth, passes through the esophagus and is received by the stomach, it is called the "sea of water, cereals, *qi* and blood" because the physiological activities of the body and derivation of *qi*, blood and body fluids all depend upon food. Food is transmitted downward from the stomach to the small intestine after being digested by the stomach, and its essence nourishes the body after being transported and digested by the spleen. So, only by combining the receiving and digesting functions of the stomach with the transporting and digesting functions of the spleen, can food be changed into nutrients, out of which *qi*, blood and body fluids are generated to supply the body. In clinic, special attention is paid to protecting stomach *qi*.

3-2-2-2 The stomach is concerned with communication and descendance and its *qi* is normal when it descends.

After food is taken in and digested by the stomach, the food descends to enter the small intestine to be further digested and absorbed. It is thus said that the stomach is concerned with communication and descendance and is normal when its *qi* descends. The physiological functions of the digestive system can be generalized as the ascendance of the splenic *qi* and the descendance of the gastric *qi*. In the theory of viscera symptoms, the communicating and descending functions of the stomach also include the function of the small intestine to transport food residues downward to the large intestine, and of the large intestine to transport liquid.

The communicating and descending function of the stomach is to send turbid matter downward, and if it malfunctions this influences appetite and ozostomia, distension and fullness or pain in the epigastric and abdominal region and constipation, etc. may result due to turbid *qi* stagnating in the upper part of the body. If gastric *qi* fails to perform its function, and further causes regurgitation of stomach *qi*, eructation, acid regurgitation, nausea, vomiting, hiccup, etc. may also appear.

3-2-3 The small intestine

The small intestine, a long tract organ, is located in the abdomen. Its upper opening is connected with the lower opening of the stomach at the pylorus, and its lower one is connected with the upper opening of the large intestine at the ileocecal valve. Being connected with the heart by the meridian, it is closely related to the heart. Its chief physiological function is to receive food and differentiate nutrients from waste.

3-2-3-1 The small intestine is concerned with the reception and digestion of food.

It receives food which has been digested by the stomach; to be able to absorb food, food must be retained within the small intestine for a certain time so as to be further digested and absorbed. Its digesting function refers to further digesting food which has already been digested by the stomach, and changes it into purified nutrients.

3-2-3-2 The function of the small intestine is to differentiate the purified (nutrients) from the turbid (waste)

The process is as follows:

a. After being digested by the small intestine, food is divided into the refined material and waste.

b. Absorption of the refined material and transport of waste to the large intestine.

c. When absorbing the refined food, the small intestine also absorbs a large amount of fluids, hence the statement that the small intestine controls fluids. Moreover, this function is concerned with the volume of urine. If this function is normal, defecation and micturation will be normal; if not, stools will become loose and urine scanty. The amount of fluid in the small intestine is related to the volume of urine.

From the above description, it can be seen that the functions of the small intestine to receive and digest food are very important so that nutrients can be derived from food. This is the gastrosplenic function of sending the purified nutrients upward and the turbid waste downward. Hence, a dysfunctional small intestine may cause abnormal distension, abdominal pain, vomiting, constipation, etc. due to turbid matter in the upper portion of the body as well as loose stools, diarrhea, etc. due to purified nutrients in the lower one.

3-2-4 The large intestine

The large intestine is situated in the abdomen, with its upper opening connected with the small intestine at the ileocecal valve and its lower opening with the anus. As it is linked with the lung by the meridian respectively, they are closely connected. Its chief physiological function is to transport and change residues.

After receiving food residues left after the purified nutrients and turbid waste have been differentiated by the small intestine, the large intestine again absorbs the superfluous fluids from them, makes them into stools, and finally excretes them from the body. Its transporting action continues the stomach's function of sending the turbid matter down, and is also related to the clearing and descending functions of the lung. In addition, its transporting actions are also concerned with the functional activities of the kidney.

3-2-5 The bladder

The bladder, located in the middle of the small abdomen, is an internal organ for storing urine. As it is directly linked with the kidney by meridians, they are closely related. Its main function is to store and discharge urine.

Urine is derived from body fluids, formed by kidney *qi* and transported downward to the bladder. Urine is retained within the bladder, until it is discharged from the body.

The function of the bladder depends upon renal *qi*. *Qi* movement in the bladder is also controlled by the kidney. Its pathological condition is chiefly dysuria, or dribbling urine, anuria, enuresis or even incontinence of urine, which are related to the functioning of kidney *qi*.

3-2-6 The triple energizer

The triple energizer is a collective term for the upper, middle and lower energizers. Because of an inaccuracy about this concept controversies have appeared about it in later generations. However, there is agreement on its physiological function. Its main physiological functions are thought to be governing *qi* as well as the passage of water. Its chief physiological functions are the pathway of primordial *qi* and the passage through which body fluids flow.

3-2-6-1 Governing *qi*

As the pathway in which *qi* ascends, descends, goes out and comes in, the triple energizer has the function of governing *qi* activities.

3-2-6-2 The passage through which body fluids pass

The triple energizer has the action of unobstructing the water passage and making body fluids flow, being a pathway in which body fluids ascend, descend, enter and leave. Although water metabolism is governed by the harmonious actions of the viscera, such as the lung, spleen and stomach, intestines, kidney and bladder, etc.; *qi* normally ascends, descends, exits and enters through the pathways of the triple energizer. If the water pathways of the energizer are not kept clear, the water regulating and distributing functions of the lung, spleen, kidney, etc. cannot be realized. Hence, the harmonious action of water metabolism is called the "functional activities of *qi* in the triple energizer."

The functions of the triple energizer are interconnected. This is because the flow of aqueous fluids fully depends upon the movements of *qi* and *qi* depends upon blood and body fluids. Therefore, the pathway for the movement of *qi* must be that of blood or body fluids, and the pathway for the movement of body fluids must be that of *qi*.

3-2-6-3 Location of the upper, middle and lower energizers and their physiological characteristics

a. The upper energizer: In general, the portion above the diaphragm including the heart and lungs, the head and face is called the upper energizer. Its physiological function is to make *qi* flourish and spread and is characterized by the saying "the upper energizer is like an all-pervading vapor."

b. The middle energizer: It is situated in the abdomen below the diaphragm and above the umbilicus. In *Miraculous Pivot*, it refers to the entire stomach. Its physiological characteristics include the transporting and digesting functions of the spleen and stomach. Visually "the middle energizer resembles soaking things in water which causes decomposition and dissolution of substance." The viscera in the middle energizer include not only the spleen and stomach, but also the liver and gallbladder.

c. The lower energizer: According to *Miraculous Pivot*, the internal organs below the stomach, such as the large and small intestines, kidney and bladder, etc. all pertain to the lower energizer. Its physiological characteristics are to excrete the residues and urine and are symbolized as "the lower energizer as an aqueous duct." But the theory of visceral symptoms further developed in later generations and by classifying *jing* (vital principle) and blood of the liver and kidney and primordial *qi* in *mingmen* (the vital portal), etc. into the lower energizer, its physiological characteristics have been widened.

3-3 Unusual organs

The unusual organs include the six organs and tissues, viz., brain, marrow, bones, vessels, gallbladder and uterus. Most of them are not pathways for digestion and excretion of food, but store essential *qi*, which is similar to the physiological functional characteristics of the yin viscera. Another characteristic that differs from the viscera is that they are not closely related except the gallbladder, one of the six yang viscera. As the physiology of the vessels, marrow, bones and gallbladder has been described previously, only those of the brain and uterus are described in this section.

3-3-1 The brain

The brain is located in the skull and formed by "marrow (brains)." Its function was described in *Miraculous Pivot* as the residence of intelligence. Also the relation between the ocular structure and the brain is explained, pathological changes in vision are linked with the brain. Changes of hearing and the mental state are also connected with the brain. Since the brain, ears and eyes are located in the head, insufficient bone marrow may lead to tinnitus, vertigo and listlessness. Li Shizhen of the Ming Dynasty (1368-1644) held that the brain is concerned with mental activities and called the brain "the residence of primordial Spirit." In *Errors on Medicine Corrected* (*Yilin Gai Cuo*) it was recognized that the functions of the sense organs, such as memory, vision, hearing, smelling and speech, etc. are all linked with the brain.

The theory of visceral symptoms holds that the physiopathology of the brain is ascribed to the heart and corresponds respectively to the five yin viscera. The heart is the "Chief of the five yin and six yang viscera and the residence of Spirit." It is said "the heart stores the Mind" because mental and emotional activities are based on the heart (mind), namely, *hun* (mood), *po* (soul), *yi* (will), *zhi* (emotion and spirit), which correspond respectively to the five yin viscera.

3-3-2 The uterus

The fetus grows in the uterus. The uterus has the following features:

a. *Tiankui*: The development of the genital organ fully depends upon *tiankui* which is the product when essential *qi* in the kidney is enriched, and promotes the development and maturity of the sexual gland. Hence, only when promoted by *tiankui* can the female genitals mature and menstruation begin. When the essential *qi* in the kidney of an older woman declines and is deficient, she enters menopause.

b. The Strategic Vessel Meridian and Conception Vessel Meridian: Both the Strategic Vessel Meridian and the Conception Vessel Meridian originate from the uterus. The Strategic Vessel Meridian runs parallel to the Conception Vessel Meridian, is communicated with the *yangming* meridian and can regulate *qi* and blood in the twelve meridians. It is also "the sea of blood." The Conception Vessel Meridian is concerned with the fetus, meets with the three yin meridians at the lower abdomen and can regulate all the body's yin meridians. It is also called the "sea of yin meridians." Only if *qi* and blood in the twelve meridians are full can they irrigate the Strategic Vessel Meridian and the Conception Vessel Meridian, and enter the uterus through the regulation of the two meridians, causing menstruation. The flourishing and decline of the twelve meridians are regulated by *tiankui*. In childhood, as the essential *qi* in the kidney does not flourish, no menstrual flow occurs; in old age, as *tiankui* is gradually exhausted, *qi* and blood in the two meridians decline and in menopause irregular menstruation appears, even amenorrhea. If the two meridians are not in harmony irregular menstruation, even infertility, etc. will appear.

c. The heart, liver and spleen: They regulate the generation and circulation of blood. The heart governs blood, the liver stores blood and the spleen controls blood. As the spleen is the resource of *qi* and blood, menstruation and pregnancy cannot all be separated from normal enrichment of *qi* and blood and regulation of blood. So, menstruation is related to the physiological functions of the heart, liver and spleen. If the liver and spleen are hypofunctional in storing and controlling blood, menorrhagia, early menstruation, prolonged menstruation, even metrorrhagia, etc. may result. If the spleen is hypofunctional in generating *qi* and blood, menses will lack their resource, leading to oligomenorrhea, prolonged menstruation and amenorrhea. If both the heart and Spirit are affected by an emotional factor or if the dispersing and discharging functions of the liver are influenced, pathological symptoms, such as irregular menstruation, etc. can also be caused.

The physiology of menstruation is a complex process. It is closely related to the integral condition of the body and the mental state. The physiological function of the viscera, meridians, etc. is closely related to the heart, liver, kidney and Strategic Vessel Meridian and Conception Vessel Meridian.

3-4 Relation between yin and yang viscera

The relation of the five yin viscera was developed through observation of the interacting relations of the five elements by Chinese medical experts through the ages.

3-4-1 Relation among the five yin viscera

The relation among the five yin viscera was expounded according to the interaction of the five elements by the ancients. At present, this relation is explained according to the physiological functions of the five yin viscera.

3-4-1-1 Relation between the heart and lung

The heart governs blood and the lung governs *qi*. Only if blood circulates normally can the respiratory function of the lung be carried on normally. The key link of heartbeat and respiration is the *qi* that accumulates in the chest. As chest *qi* has the function of clearing the Heart Meridian, controlling respiration and maintaining harmony between blood circulation and respiration, either deficient lung *qi* or the failure of the spreading function of promoting blood circulation, causes abnormal or stagnant blood circulation with pathological symptoms of congealed blood, such as chest diseases, changed heart rate, even dark-bluish lips, dark-purplish tongue, etc. On the other hand, when there is insufficient heart *qi*, heart yang and heart vessels are blocked by congealed blood, the clearing and descending functions may be influenced, resulting in the regurgitation of lung *qi*, such as cough, hasty breath, etc.

3-4-1-2 Relation between the heart and spleen

As the heart controls blood and the spleen governs blood and is the resource of *qi* and blood, the heart is closely related to the spleen. When the spleen's transporting and digesting functions are normal, it can generate blood normally. If blood is enriched, the heart can govern blood. If splenic *qi* and the splenic function of controlling blood are normal, the blood circulates smoothly within vessels. So, the relation between the heart and spleen is chiefly in formation and circulation of blood. Pathologically, the heart and spleen often influence each other, for instance, extreme worry not only consumes blood persistently, but influences the spleen's transporting and digesting functions. If spleen *qi* is too weak to perform its functions, *qi* and blood cannot be generated, leading to deficient blood and lack of control of the blood by the heart. If blood extravasates due to the spleen's failure to control it, insufficient heart blood may also result. All the above-mentioned cases may create deficiencies of both heart and spleen with symptoms such as vertigo, palpitations, insomnia, dreaminess, abdominal distension, poor appetite, lassitude, dull complexion, etc.

3-4-1-3 Relation between the heart and liver

The heart governs blood, while the liver stores blood. Blood is generated by the spleen, stored in the liver and circulates in the body through the heart. If the cardiac function of promoting blood circulation is normal, blood will circulate smoothly and be stored in the liver. If the liver cannot store blood, there will be no blood to be governed by the heart and the blood will circulate abnormally. It is because of the close relationship between the heart and liver in circulation of blood that deficiencies of heart and liver blood often occur simultaneously.

The heart is concerned with the Mind and the liver possesses dispersing and discharging functions. Mental and emotional states are closely related to the liver although they are concerned with the heart. Since emotional injury usually transforms itself into pernicious fire (heat) and consumes yin, deficient heart and liver yin and blazing fire of heart and liver frequently influence each other or appear simultaneously.

3-4-1-4 Relation between the heart and kidney

The heart corresponds to fire according to the five-element theory, lies in the upper portion of the body, and pertains to yang; the kidney corresponds to water, is located in the lower portion of the body, and pertains to yin.

As far as the theory of ascendance and descendance of yin and yang or water and fire is concerned, the one located in the lower body is normal when it ascends; the other located in the upper body is normal when it descends. So, it is thought that heart fire must descend to reach the kidney and the kidney water must ascend to aid the heart. Only then can the physiological functions of the heart and kidney be harmonious. If heart fire fails to descend to reach the kidney, but flares up isolatedly and kidney water fails to ascend to support the heart, but stagnates, the functions of the heart and kidney will not be harmonious. For example, palpitation of vigorous heart,[8] anxiety, sore and weak loin and knees or nocturnal emission are the chief clinical symptoms of "disharmony between the heart and kidney."

In addition, as the yin and yang of the heart and kidney are closely related, they can influence each other when the heart or kidney is affected. For example, overflowing water due to deficient kidney yang can upwardly affect the heart with edema, palpitation with fright, etc. Deficient heart yin can also downwardly affect the kidney yin, causing symptoms of blazing fire[9] due to yin deficiency.

3-4-1-5 Relation between the lung and spleen

The close relation between the lung and spleen is chiefly manifest in the formation of qi in the body mainly depending on the respiratory function of the lung and the transporting and digesting functions of the spleen. Clear qi (air) absorbed by the lung and essential qi from food transported and digested by the spleen and stomach are the basic materials that constitute qi. Whether the respiratory function of the lung and transporting and digesting functions of the spleen are normal or not is closely linked with the flourishing and decline of qi.

The distribution and metabolism of body fluids are chiefly constituted by the lung's clearance and distribution of body fluids, so that endogenous pathogenic damp may be prevented. The spleen's transport of body fluids and distribution of jing (vital principle) of food to the lung is not only the primary condition of the lung's clearing function and regulating the water passage, but actually supply necessary nutrients for the physiological activities of the lung. Hence, there exists an intersupporting relation between the two for the distribution and metabolism of body fluids.

The mutual influence of the lung and spleen in pathology chiefly lies in insufficient qi formation and abnormal water metabolism. For instance, when splenic qi is weak and impaired, deficient lung qi often results. When the spleen fails to carry on its transporting function and the body fluid metabolism is obstructed and watery fluids stagnate, tan-yin (phlegm and excess exudates) will form, which usually influence the lung's clearing and distribution functions, producing conditions such as asthmatic breath, cough, profuse phlegm, etc. When lung trouble is prolonged, the spleen may also be influenced, causing the abnormal function of the spleen or deficient spleen qi, with pathological symptoms, such as dyspnea, abdominal distension, loose stools, even edema, etc.

3-4-1-6 Relation between the lung and liver

The lung and the liver affect the regulation of qi metabolism. Qi is normal when descending, while liver qi is normal when ascending. The harmony between them is a key link for normal qi metabolism. If liver qi is overactive in ascendance or lung qi is inactive in descendance, regurgitation of fire may result, with symptoms such as cough, regurgitation of qi, hemoptysis, etc. called "liver fire invading the lung." If the lung fails to perform its clearing and purifying functions and pernicious dryness and heat are in excess, the liver will fail to flourish and perform its dispersing and discharging functions, causing contracting pain, distension and fullness of the chest and hypochondrium, dizziness, headache, flushed face, congestive eyes, etc. accompanied by cough.

3-4-1-7 Relation between the lung and kidney

It affects water metabolism and respiratory movement. Since the kidney is the yin viscus that mainly controls water, the lung's purifying and descending functions and regulation of the water passage depends upon kidney *qi*. The kidney's control of water depends upon the lung's purifying and descending functions and its regulation of the water passage. If the lung fails to perform its functions, the kidney is affected, causing oliguria, even edema. If kidney *qi* is inactive and the kidney fails to control water, overflowing water may result in edema, asthmatic breath, cough and anxiety.

The lung governs respiration, while the kidney absorbs *qi* (air). The respiratory function of the lung needs to be assisted by the action of the kidney to absorb *qi*. Only if kidney *qi* is enriched can air be inspired by the lung and absorbed by the kidney through the lung's purifying and ascending functions. Therefore, there is the saying that "the lung is the master of *qi*, and the kidney, the root of *qi*." When essential *qi* in the kidney is insufficient and the kidney fails to absorb *qi*, so that *qi* floats or lung *qi* becomes weak or when a long illness affects the kidney, the kidney's failure to absorb *qi* will cause asthmatic breath immediately after exertion, etc. In addition, yin fluids of the lung and kidney are related. Kidney yin is the foundation of yin fluids and deficient kidney yin may affect lung yin. On the contrary, deficient kidney yin cannot replenish lung yin upwardly. So, deficiencies of both lung yin and kidney yin are often seen simultaneously, with malar flush, "steaming of bone"[10] tidal fever, night sweat, dry cough, aphonia, and weak loins and knees, etc. appearing.

3-4-1-8 Relation between the liver and spleen

The liver stores blood and has dispersing and discharging functions, while the spleen governs blood and has transporting and digesting functions as well as being the source of *qi* and blood. The relation between the liver and spleen is in the mutual influence between the liver's dispersing and discharging functions and the spleen's transporting and digesting functions. If the liver fails to perform its functions, the splenic functions would be affected, causing symptoms, such as mental depression, distension and fullness of the chest and hypochondria, abdominal distension and pain, diarrhea or loose stools, etc. Secondly, the liver and spleen are also related in the formation, storage and transportation of blood. If the spleen transports normally and generates blood which does not escape from the vessels, the liver will have enough blood to store. If the spleen is too weak to generate *qi* and blood or the spleen fails to control blood or excessive blood is lost, insufficient liver blood will result. In addition, if pathogenic damp and heat affect the spleen and stomach, the gallbladder is affected by harmful heat and body fluids are excreted and jaundice may appear. It is therefore seen that liver trouble can affect the spleen, and spleen trouble can also affect the liver pathologically.

3-4-1-9 Relation between the liver and kidney

As a close relation exists between the liver and kidney, it is said that "the liver and kidney have the same source." The reaction between the liver's storage of blood and the kidney's storage of *jing* (vital principle) is the generating and transporting relations between *jing* (vital principle) and blood. The generation of blood is based on the *qi* activities of *jing* (vital principle) in the kidney, while the enrichment of vital principle depends upon well-nourished blood. It is therefore said that *jing* (vital principle) and blood often influence each other. For instance, impaired kidney yin may lead to insufficient liver blood and vice versa.

In addition, there is the complementary relationship between the liver's dispersing and discharging functions and the kidney's discharging and storing functions. These are chiefly manifest in physiological functions, such as menstruation in women and ejaculation in males. If they are not harmonious, irregular menstruation, oligomenorrhea or amenorrhea in women or nocturnal emission and failure to ejaculate due to overactive yang, etc. in men may appear.

Since the liver and kidney have the same source, the yin and yang of the liver and kidney are closely related and often influence each other. For example, insufficient kidney yin may lead to insufficient liver yin and inability of yin to restrain yang, resulting in overactive liver yang, called "inadequate water to nourish wood (liver)"; insufficient liver yin may lead to impaired kidney yin, resulting in overactive "premier fire," (referring to heart fire). On the other hand, overactive fire may also affect kidney yin, forming pathological changes of insufficient kidney yin.

3-4-1-10 Relation between the spleen and kidney

The spleen is the postnatal foundation, while the kidney is the prenatal one. Since normal transportation and transformation of *jing* (vital principle) by the spleen must be assisted by the warming of kidney yang, it is said that "spleen yang originates from kidney yang." Only if the vital principle in the kidney is nourished by food, will it be enriched and stable. If kidney yang is too deficient to warm spleen yang, cold and painful abdomen, diarrhea with aqueous-grainy diarrhea or diarrhea before dawn and edema will occur. If the spleen yang becomes weak for long and impairs the kidney yang, diseases or syndromes of deficiencies of both may result.

3-4-2 Relation of the six yang viscera

The six yang viscera transport and digest food. Their functions of digesting, absorbing and excreting food are related.

After entering the stomach and being preliminarily digested by the stomach, food is transmitted to the small intestine. After the small intestine further digests and separates the food into pure and turbid material, the pure nutrients are transported by the spleen to nourish the body, while the remainder is exuded through the bladder and is then changed into urine by the bladder and the turbid material is sent to the large intestine. Urine exuding through the bladder is discharged from the body by the kidney *qi*. The residues that have entered the large intestine are excreted through the anus after being transmitted and dried. The digestion, absorption and excretion of food also depends upon excretion of bile which aids food digestion. The triple energizer is not only the passage through which food is transmitted. What is more important is that the *qi* activities of the triple energizer promote and normalize the transmitting and digesting functions. The six yang viscera must continuously receive, digest, transmit and excrete food, and should be unobstructed rather than blocked. Food must be transmitted and digested, but not retained for a long period of time. Hence, it is said that "the six yang viscera are normal when unobstructed" and "troubles of the six yang viscera are treated by unobstructing them with tonics."

The six yang viscera also influence one another. For example, substantive heat in the stomach that consumes body fluids can cause the large intestine some difficulties in transmitting food residues, thus causing constipation. The dried and inactive large intestine due to constipation may also influence the descendance of stomach *qi*, causing regurgitation of stomach *qi* with nausea, vomiting, etc. Another example is blazing gallbladder fire (heat) which may frequently affect the stomach, leading to failure of stomach *qi* to descend normally in the spleen, and stomach which fumigates and steams the liver, while the gallbladder may have insufficient bile, and cause jaundice.

3-4-3 Relation between the five yin and six yang viscera

This is the relation of yin and yang, and the exterior and interior of the body. The yin viscera are deep and the yang ones superficial. They are interconnected by the meridians pertaining to each of them, so a close relation exists between the five yin and six yang viscera.

3-4-3-1 Relation between the heart and small intestine

The Heart Meridian pertains to the heart and connects with the small intestine, while the Small Intestine Meridian pertains to the small intestine and connects with the heart. Their close relation is established mainly through the interconnection of the meridians, which manifests when the heart transmits its excessive fire to the small intestine, causing oliguria, hot and dark-red urine, dysuria, etc. Pathogenic heat occurring in the small intestine may upwardly affect the heart along the meridians with anxiety, congestive tongue, sore mouth and tongue, etc.

3-4-3-2 Relation between the lung and large intestine

The close relation between the lung and large intestine is mainly established through the interconnection of the meridians. The lung's purifying and descending functions aid the large intestine's transporting function and vice versa. If the large intestine is affected by substantive fire, and the *qi* of yang viscera is obstructed, the lung's function may be affected, causing full chest, asthmatic breath and cough, etc. The other way round, if the lung fails to perform its purifying function and body fluids fail to descend, difficult defecation may occur; if lung *qi* is too weak to promote bowel movements, constipation may occur. If *qi* is too weak, stools may be loose.

3-4-3-3 Relation between the spleen and stomach

The spleen and stomach are closely connected by their meridians. The stomach receives food and the spleen transports and digests it so that food is digested, absorbed and *jing* (vital principle) is distributed by their common function and the body nourished. It is therefore said that the spleen is the "acquired foundation of life."

The spleen sends pure nutrients upward and the stomach sends the turbid matter downward. They oppose and complement each other. The ascending spleen *qi* distributes the refined principle derived from food; descending stomach *qi* makes food and its wastes descend. The stomach should be moist and not too dry, while the spleen should not be too moist. Only if they complement each other can food be completely transported and digested.

Since the spleen and stomach are interconnecting, if the spleen is affected by pathogenic damp and fails to perform its transporting and digesting functions so that the purified *qi* fails to ascend, the stomach's receiving and descending functions may be influenced, resulting in poor appetite, vomiting, nausea, distension and fullness of the epigastrium, etc. If food is taken excessively and retained in the epigastric region and the stomach fails to carry on its descending function, the splenic function of sending purified *qi* upwardly and transporting and digesting food may be influenced, resulting in abdominal distension, diarrhea, etc.

3-4-3-4 Relation between the liver and gallbladder

The gallbladder appends to and is connected with the liver through their meridians. Bile originates from liver *qi*. It can be normally excreted and fully discharged only by passing through the liver's dispersing and discharging functions. If the liver's functions are abnormal, the secretion and excretion of bile will be affected. On the other hand, if the bile is not excreted smoothly, the liver function will be influenced. Thus, the liver and gallbladder are closely related and liver trouble often affects the gallbladder, and gallbladder trouble also often affects the liver, resulting in simultaneous liver and gallbladder trouble, such as blazing fire of the liver and gallbladder[11] and substantial heat in the liver and gallbladder.[12]

3-4-3-5 Relation between the kidney and bladder

The kidney and bladder are closely related through the interconnection of the meridians. Storage and discharge of urine by the bladder depends upon kidney *qi*. If kidney *qi* is sufficient, it will function normally and the bladder is well controlled, so that normal water metabolism is maintained. If not, the bladder will be dysfunctional, resulting in dysuria, or incontinence of urine, or enuresis, frequent urination, etc. For example, incontinence of urine, and polyuria frequently seen in the aged are usually caused by deficient kidney *qi*.

Notes

[1.] Including the bone marrow, spinal cord and brains.

[2.] *Qi* stored in the thorax. It is formed by a combination of respiratory gases and essence from water and food.

[3.] A collective term for substaneous fruit-stone shaped masses.

[4.] Marked by alternate contraction and relaxation of muscle.

[5.] The structure connecting the eyeball with the brain.

[6.] The upper part of the triple energizer.

[7.] A symptom complex of real cold in the lower part of the body and false heat in the upper body. It is caused by weakness and cold in the lower energizer with refluent floating yang. The chief manifestations are shortness of breath, tachypnea, fatigue, dizziness, palpitation, cold clammy limbs, flushed face, copious pale urine, loose stools, etc.

[8.] The sensation of vigorous heart throbbing, frequently seen in organic heart disease.

[9.] The yin liquid becomes insubstantial and leads to overactive consumptive fire with such pathological manifestations as malar flush, dry mouth, hot palms, sores, irritability, quick temper, increased sexual libido, rapid faint pulse, etc.

[10.] Fever due to deficiency of yin, as pernicious heat spreads from the inside of the bone to the outside of the skin. It is usually accompanied by night sweating, frequently seen in pulmonary tuberculosis.

[11.] The pathological manifestations such as dry and bitter mouth, hypochondriac pain, rapid and wiry pulse, yellow tongue coating, etc.

[12.] The pathological change due to stagnation of pathogenic damp and heat in the liver and the gallbladder. The main symptoms are jaundice, fever, bitter taste, hypochondriac pain, nausea and vomiting, anorexia, aversion to fatty food, abdominal distension and pain, yellow urine, loose stools, yellow glossy tongue coating, stringy and rapid pulse.

4. *QI* (VITAL ENERGY), *XUE* (BLOOD) AND *JIN-YE* (BODY FLUIDS)

Qi is the vital principle that continuously moves in the body. Body fluids is a general term for normal aqueous liquids within the body. When classified according to their respective properties into yin and yang, *qi* has promoting and warming actions, pertaining to yang, while blood and body fluids are liquid, nourishing and moistening, and pertain to yin.

The energy that tissues and organs, such as the viscera, meridians, etc. need for their physiological activities originates from *qi*, blood and body fluids. Metabolism depends upon the normal physiological functions of the tissues and organs, such as the viscera, meridians, etc. Therefore, a close relation exists between the tissues and organs in physiopathology. Moreover there is also the basic matter consisting of the body.

4-1 *Qi* (vital energy)

4-1-1 Basic concept

Qi was a concept of Chinese ancients about energy and natural phenomena. As early as the Spring and Autumn and the Warring States Periods (770-221 B.C.), philosophers thought that *qi* was a fundamental substance constituting the world, and everything in the universe is produced by its movement and changes. The basic concept thus gradually developed after it was introduced to the medical field.

The body needs to absorb nutrients from "*qi* between the heaven and earth," so as to nourish *qi* of the five yin viscera and maintain the physiological activities of the body. *Qi* is the most fundamental substance for maintaining life. Based on this viewpoint, TCM explains physiological activities by the movement and changes of *qi*.

4-1-2 Formation

The *qi* of the body originates from prenatal *jing* (vital principle) inherited from the parents, nutrients in the thorax (i.e., refined food called grainy *qi*) and clear *qi* (air). It is formed by combining the three by the functions of internal organs, such as the lung, spleen, stomach, kidney, etc.

Prenatal *jing* (vital principle) can be fully effective only by depending upon the function of *jing* in the kidney; the refined nutrients in water and cereals (diet) can be ingested and derived from food only with the help of the transporting and digesting functions of the spleen and stomach. Clear *qi* (air) can be inspired by depending on the lung. *Qi* is thus formed by the physiological functions of the kidney, spleen, stomach and lung. Only if the physiological functions of the kidney, spleen and stomach, lung, etc. are normal and harmonious can *qi* be properly created. If these functions become abnormal, pathological changes occur, such as deficient *qi*, etc.

For the formation of *qi*, the transporting and digesting function of the spleen and stomach are important. This is because after birth the body depends upon food to maintain its activities. The body's capacity to ingest nutrients from food depends upon the receiving, transporting and digesting functions of the spleen and stomach, so that food can be digested and absorbed. *Jing* is dependent upon the nutrients in food.

4-1-3 Physiological functions

Qi is the most basic material to maintain the body. It controls important physiological functions in the body.

The physiological functions of *qi* are chiefly:

4-1-3-1 The promoting action

As the vital energy, *qi* can promote the growth and development of the body and physiological activities of various tissues and organs, such as the viscera, meridians, etc. as well as the formation and circulation of blood, and the formation, distribution and excretion of body fluids, etc. When *qi* is deficient or declines, its promoting and invigorating actions are reduced, tissues and organs will be weakened and not enough blood and body fluids will be formed and they will circulate more slowly, resulting in deficient blood, slower blood circulation and stagnant liquid, etc.

4-1-3-2 The warming action

Qi is the body's source of heat. Body temperature is kept permanent by the warming action of *qi*. Various tissues and organs carry on their normal functions supported by the warming action of *qi*. Blood and body fluids also maintain their normal circulation by the continuous warming action of *qi*. If the action becomes abnormal, symptoms such as creeping chills, preference for heat, cold limbs, lowered body temperature, slower movement of blood and body fluids, etc. may appear, as well as accumulated and stagnant *qi*, transformation of stagnant *qi* into pathogenic heat, resulting in aversion to heat, preference for cold, fever, etc.

4-1-3-3 The protecting action

The protecting action of the body is complex. It includes various synthetic actions of *qi*, blood and body fluids, tissues and organs, such as the viscera, meridians, etc. The protecting action of *qi* is chiefly manifest in protecting the body surface as well as resisting the invasion of exogenous pathogenic factors. *Plain Questions* states, "The reason why an exogenous pathogenic factor succeeds in invading the body is that *qi* must be weak." The weakened protecting action of *qi* causes weakened body resistance and susceptibility of the body to be affected.

4-1-3-4 The controlling action

This means that *qi* prevents blood and body fluids from flowing away. The manifestations are: controlling blood to make the blood circulate along the blood vessels preventing extravasation; controlling sweat, urine, saliva, gastric fluid, intestinal fluid and semen, etc. checking the volume of their secretion and excretion. If the action is weakened, there is the danger that some of the liquid substances within the body may flow away. If *qi* fails to restrain blood, hemorrhage may result. Inability of *qi* to control body fluids may lead to perspiration, polyuria, or incontinence of urine, salivation, vomiting thin water, diarrhea and prolapse of the rectum. Inability of *qi* to control *jing* may result in nocturnal emission, spermatorrhea, prospermia, etc.

The controlling and promoting actions of *qi* are complementary. *Qi* promotes blood circulation and transportation, as well as distribution and excretion of body fluids. The harmony between these two actions regulates and controls normal circulation, secretion and excretion of liquids within the body. This is a key link to keep blood circulation and water metabolism in a normal balanced state.

4-1-3-5 Activities of *Qi*

This refers to metabolism and transformation of *jing, qi*, blood and body fluids. Various changes occur due to *qi* movement, which determines metabolism and transformation of nutrients, *qi*, blood and body fluids. For example the formation of *qi*, blood and body fluids first needs to transform food into nutrients and then into *qi*, blood and body fluids, etc. *Qi* transforms body fluids into sweat and urine through metabolism and food residues into wastes after the food is digested and absorbed. If *qi* functions abnormally, metabolism of *qi*, blood and body fluids, digestion and absorption of food, and excretion of sweat, urine and stool, etc. will be negatively influenced. Thus *qi* governs the metabolism.

4-1-4 Movement of Qi

Qi is refined matter and energy that moves continuously through tissues and organs, such as the viscera, meridians, etc. stimulating physiological activities.

The movement of *qi* is termed "*qi* mechanism." Although its movement varies, it can be divided into the ascending, descending, entering and leaving classifications.

The tissues and organs, such as the viscera, meridians, etc. are the places where *qi* ascends, descends, goes out and comes in. The movement of *qi* is the foundation of life.

The movement of *qi* not only stimulates the metabolism, but also maintains physiological activities of the tissues and organs. For example, the respiratory function of the lung includes expiration and inspiration as well as the spreading function which clears and sends the turbid matter downward. The digestive function of the spleen, stomach and intestines is considered as a whole; the digestion, absorption, distribution and excretion of food and the stomach sending the turbid matter downward. Water metabolism is considered as a whole from the lung's spreading, clearing and descending functions, to the spleen and stomach's transporting and digesting functions and the kidney's spreading and absorbing the purified vital essence and excreting the turbid matter.

The ascending and descending, going-out and coming-in movements of *qi* are complementary movements. Not every physiological activity must be ascending, descending, leaving and entering. For instance, the liver and spleen are concerned only with ascendance, the lung and stomach are concerned only with descendance. The body is normal only when *qi* movement is harmonious. So, the movement of *qi* is also a key link to maintaining the balance of various physiological functions.

The harmony or balance of *qi* movements is called the harmonious *qi* mechanism and the disharmony or imbalance, disharmonious *qi* mechanism, which is a pathological state. Disharmonious *qi* mechanism varies in its manifestations; obstruction of the movements of *qi* in certain areas. Stagnant *qi* is when *qi* ascends excessively or descends weakly, or when *qi* ascends weakly or descends excessively. "Exhausted *qi*" is the inability of *qi* to move out, so it accumulates. "Obstructed *qi*" or "depressed *qi*," etc. are also symptoms of the disharmonious *qi* mechanism.

4-1-5 Distribution and classification of Qi

As a whole, *qi* consists of the *jing* of the kidney, refined food transported and digested by the spleen and stomach, and the clear *qi* (air) taken in by the lung, which are all formed by the functions of the kidney, spleen and stomach, lung, etc. and which reach and enrich every part of the body. *Qi* has different names because its components location and functions differ. They are mainly:

4-1-5-1 Primordial *qi*

a. Composition and distribution: Primordial *qi* mainly consists of and is derived from *jing* (vital principle) stored in the kidney. *Classic on Difficult Medical Problems* clearly points out that primordial *qi* originates from the kidney, i.e. "The vital portal... is the root of primordial *qi*." The *jing* in the kidney is based on the prenatal *jing* inherited from the parents and the cultivation of the refined principle from food. Consequently it can be seen that whether primordial *qi* flourishes or not is not entirely decided by the prenatal endowment, but is closely related to the gastrosplenic functions of transporting and digesting refined matter from food.

Primordial *qi* flows throughout the body via the triple energizer. It runs inward to reach the viscera and goes outward to reach *couli*[1] on all parts of the body.

b. Main functions: Its main task is to promote the growth and development of the body, warm and stimulate various tissues and organs, such as the viscera and meridians, etc. Various tissues and organs, such as the viscera and meridians, etc. will be vigorous and the constitution strong if the body is full of primordial *qi*. When primordial *qi* is insufficient or is excessively consumed due to prenatal deficiency or postnatal malnutrition or impairment by prolonged illness, it will become weak and decline.

4-1-5-2 Chest *qi*

It is stored in the thorax. The place where it accumulates is termed the "sea of *qi*" as well as "*tanzhong*."

a. Composition and distribution: It is composed of a combination of clear *qi* (air) absorbed by the lung and the refined matter from food transported and digested by the spleen and stomach. So whether the lung's respiratory function and the spleen's transporting and digesting functions are normal or not directly influences its growth or decline.

b. Main functions: One is to promote respiration by passing through the respiratory tract. Whether speech and breath are normal is related to whether chest *qi* flourishes or declines. Another function is to promote *qi* and blood circulation by pouring *qi* into the Heart Meridian. *Qi* and blood circulation, warmth and ability to move the limbs, vision and hearing, heartbeat and heart rhythm, etc. are all related to the flourishing or decline of *qi*.

4-1-5-3 Nutritional *qi*

Nutritional *qi* flows within the meridians together with blood. As it is closely related to blood, they are both jointly called *ying* (nutrients) and *xue* (blood). As an opposite to defensive *qi*, it pertains to yin. Hence it is also called nutritional yin.

a. Composition and distribution: Nutritional *qi* mainly originates from food transported and digested by the spleen and stomach and is derived from the essential part of the refined food. Distributed in the vessels, it becomes part of blood and ascends and descends in the vessels so as to nourish and circulate in the body.

b. Main function: To nourish the body and generate blood. The essential part of food is its main ingredient. The nutrients are needed for the physiological activities of the viscera, meridians, etc.

4-1-5-4 Defensive *qi*

This is the *qi* which flows outside the meridians. Opposite to nutritional *qi*, it pertains to yang. Hence it is also called "defensive yang."

a. Composition and distribution: Defensive *qi* is mainly derived from the refined principle of food, and is strong, active and moves rapidly. So, it is not controlled by the meridians, but runs between the skin and *fenru*[2] fumigates *huangmo*[3] and spreads over the chest and abdomen.

b. Main functions: To protect the body surface and prevent the invasion of exogenous pathogenic factors to nourish the viscera, muscles, skin and hair, etc. to regulate and control the opening and closing of the junction between the skin and muscle and excretion of sweat so as to keep a relatively permanent body temperature.

There is also "visceral *qi*," "meridian *qi*," etc. besides the four kinds of *qi* mentioned above. "Visceral *qi*" and "meridian *qi*" are derived from primordial *qi*. They are the most fundamental substances constituting various viscera and meridians, as well as the material basis that promotes and maintains physiological activities of various viscera and meridians.

There are many names of *qi* in TCM. For instance, the nutritional substance absorbed by the body from food is called the *qi* of water and cereals or grainy *qi*; the pathogenic factor is called evil *qi*; abnormal fluid within the body is termed aqueous *qi*; the physiological function and anti-pathogenic factor of the body are said to be anti-evil *qi*; cold, hot, warm and cold properties and actions of Chinese herbal medicines are called four *qi*, etc. From the above description it may be seen that *qi* has many meanings. It implies features, function, weather, etc. These are different from the *qi* that has been described in this chapter.

4-2 Blood

4-2-1 Basic concept

Blood is one of the fundamental substances that constitutes the body. By circulating within the vessels blood brings nutrition to the cells. If it is extravasated, hemorrhage will occur, called extravasated blood. As the vessel carries on its function of preventing blood from being extravasated, it is called the "residence of blood."

4-2-2 Formation

Blood is chiefly.composed of nutritional *qi* and body fluids. Since the nutritional principle and body fluids originate from the refined matter from food that has been digested and absorbed by the spleen and stomach, the spleen and stomach are the source of *qi* and blood. Blood can be generated through the actions of nutritional *qi* and the lung.

As a whole, nutritional *qi* and body fluids are the main basis for the formation of blood. Since both nutritional *qi* and body fluids originate from the refined matter from food, whether dietary nutrients are rich or not and whether the transporting and digesting functions of the spleen and stomach are strong or not directly influence the formation of blood. A prolonged insufficiency of nutrients or prolonged disharmony of the transporting and digesting functions of the spleen and stomach may lead to insufficient blood.

In addition, there is a relationship between *jing* and blood. *Jing* is stored in the kidney and blood in the liver. If the vital principle in the kidney is full, the liver will be well nourished and blood enriched; if the liver stores enough blood, the kidney will have enough vital principle. Hence, "*jing* and blood originate from the same source."

4-2-3 Function

Blood nourishes and moistens the entire body. It circulates in the vessels and reaches the viscera and skin, muscles, tendons and bone and continuously nourishes and moistens the viscera, tissues and organs to keep physiological activities normal.

The nourishing and moistening action of blood is manifest in a lustrous and fresh complexion, thick and robust muscles, moist and brilliant skin and hair, keen sensation and flexible movement, etc. When blood is deficient or is severely impaired or its nourishing or moistening actions are weakened, pathological changes of systemic or local deficient blood may result, with dizziness, blurred vision, dull complexion, dry and withered hair, dry skin, withered and numb limbs, etc. usually seen in clinic.

4-2-4 Circulation

Blood circulates in the vessels and spreads over the entire body continuously. When it circulates, it supplies rich nutrients to the viscera, tissues and organs of the body.

Blood is yin in nature and is concerned with calmness. It circulates mainly by depending upon the promoting action of *qi*. It is also due to the controlling action of *qi* that blood is not extravasated. If the vessels carry on their function of accumulating and controlling nutritional *qi*, blood will not extravasate and hemorrhages will not occur under normal circumstances.

Normal blood circulation is decided by the harmony or balance between the promoting and controlling actions of *qi*. It is the heartbeat that promotes blood circulation. Normal blood circulation is also closely related to the harmony or balance between the physiological function of certain viscera. For example, the function of the lung and the dispersing function of the liver, etc. are the important factors governing blood. In addition, whether the vessels are open or not and blood is cold or not, etc. directly influences the speed of blood circulation. *Plain Questions* states, "blood likes warmth and dislikes cold. Cold would lead to stagnation of blood while warmth clears blood." Therefore, normal blood circulation not only depends upon whether the physiological functions of the heart are normal or not, but also on whether the physiological functions of the viscera, such as the lung, liver, spleen, etc. are harmonious. If the factors which promote blood circulation increase or the action of blood decreases, the speed of blood circulation will change, and blood may even extravasate, leading to hemorrhage. Otherwise, blood circulation will be slower or obstructed, leading to pathological problems, such as congealed blood, etc.

4-3 Body fluids

4-3-1 Basic concept

Body fluids include fluids within various viscera, tissues and organs and normal secretions, e.g., gastric fluid, intestinal fluid, nasal discharge, tears, etc. Body fluids are fundamental to life.

Jin (clear and thin fluid) and *ye* (turbid and thick fluid) are the two main body fluids, originating from diet and dependent upon the transporting and digesting functions of the spleen and stomach. Their viscosity, features, functions and location vary. Clear and thin fluid that moves easily, spreads to the skin, muscles and pores in the body surface and exudes through and moistens the vessel is termed *jin*; fluid that is creamy and thick, hardly moves, pours into the tissues, such as joints, viscera, brains and marrow, etc. and has the nourishing action is called *ye*. Both of them can transform themselves into each other, and are often referred to jointly. When pathological changes, such as "injured *jin*" and "exhausted *ye*" occur, they must be distinguished in *bianzheng* and *lunzhi* (planning treatment according to diagnosis).

4-3-2 Formation, distribution and excretion

The formation, distribution and excretion of body fluids is a complex physiological process involving a series of physiological functions of several viscera.

Body fluids originate from diet. They are formed in the stomach from the refined matter from food and the small intestine differentiating the purified nutrients from the turbid material and upwardly transporting the nutrients to the spleen. They are distributed and excreted chiefly through the transportation of the spleen and by the spreading and descending actions of the lung and the kidney, and the distributing function of the triple energizer.

The action of the spleen and stomach is to distribute body fluids over the trunk and four extremities via the meridians on the one hand and on the other, to send body fluids upward to reach the lung. All of these actions pertain to the spleen spreading *jin*.

The action of the lung to distribute and excrete body fluids is also called "unobstructing the water passage." The lung distributes *jin-ye* (body fluids) to the body surface by its spreading action in order to bring the nourishing and moistening actions of body fluids to the tissues. In addition, the lung discharges a large amount of moisture during respiration. The lung's spreading, clearing and descending action and clearance of the water passage plays an important role in distributing and excreting body fluids.

The kidney also plays an important role in distributing and excreting body fluids. The vital principle stored in the kidney is the force for the physiological functions as well as that of *qi* activities. Therefore, the stomach's *jing*, the lung's "clearing the water passage" and the small intestine's "differentiating pure nutrients from the turbid material" all depend upon the kidney. Body fluids are distributed throughout the body by the kidney *qi* which sends the clear matter upward and the turbid matter downward to reach the bladder. The amount of urine excreted regulates the metabolism and balance of body fluid.

4-3-3 Function

Body fluids are moistening and nourishing. Those distributed over the body surface moisten the hair and muscles; those pouring into the sense organs moisten and protect the eyes, nose, mouth, etc.; those permeating blood have the action of nourishing and smoothing blood; those pouring into tissues and organs of the viscera nourish and moisten the tissues and organs of various viscera; those exuding into bones nourish and moisten the marrow, spinal cord and brain.

4-4 Interrelation of *qi*, blood and body fluids

Qi, blood and body fluids have their own characteristics and functions. They are fundamental substances constituting the body and maintaining its activities. Their composition is determined by the refined matter from food which is transported and digested by the spleen and stomach and their physiological functions are interdependent.

4-4-1 Relation between *qi* and blood

Qi pertains to yang and blood to yin, and there are four aspects of their relation: *qi* can produce blood, promote blood circulation and control blood, while blood is the carrier of *qi*.

4-4-1-1 *Qi* can generate blood

In the course of its composition and generation, blood never departs from the movement and change of *qi*. Nutritional *qi* and body fluids are the main components of blood, coming from the refined matter from food. Vigorous *qi* would lead to a strong function of producing blood, while deficient *qi* would lead to a weak function of producing blood, even resulting in deficient blood. For this reason, in the treatment of deficient blood in clinic, *qi*-tonifying drugs are commonly used. This is a clinical application of the theory that *qi* can generate blood.

4-4-1-2 *Qi* can promote blood circulation

Blood pertains to yin and is concerned with calmness. It cannot circulate by itself, but must be promoted by *qi*; blood circulates along with *qi* and stagnant *qi* can lead to congealed blood. The blood circulates by depending upon the circulating action of heart *qi*, the spreading and distribution of lung *qi* and the dispersion, discharge and flourishing actions of liver *qi*. So, if deficient *qi* cannot promote blood circulation, *qi* would stagnate and cause obstruction and slow down circulation of blood, forming congealed blood, even blocking collateral meridians, resulting in blood stasis. Disorders in the movement of *qi* would result in abnormal blood circulation. If blood ascends along with *qi*, flushed face, congestive eyes, headache or even hematemesis may occur. If it is exhausted together with *qi*, dropping and distended abdomen, even bloody stool, metrorrhagia, etc. may result. When treating abnormal blood circulation in clinic, drugs for tonifying *qi*, promoting *qi* flow, and checking *qi* regurgitation are frequently used together. This is a practical application of the theory that *qi* can promote blood circulation.

4-4-1-3 Blood as the carrier of *qi*

Blood is the carrier of *qi* and the supplier of nutrients. Since *qi* is full of energy and moves easily, it must rely on blood and body fluids to exist within the body. If it fails to rely on blood and body fluids, it will lose its root, floating and scattering, causing it to become exhausted. Similarly in the case of deficient blood, *qi* will be exhausted. In treatment of hemorrhoea, a therapy of nourishing *qi* and checking exhausted blood is usually used.

4-4-2 Relation between *qi* and body fluids

Qi pertains to yang and body fluids to yin. The relation between *qi* and body fluids is just the same as that between *qi* and blood. The formation, distribution and excretion of body fluids fully depend upon *qi*'s movements and its warming, promoting and controlling actions. As the existence of *qi* within the body not only depends upon blood, but also on body fluids, the latter is said to be the carrier of *qi*.

4-4-2-1 *Qi* can generate body fluids

Body fluids originate from ingested food and rely on the stomach's dissociating essential *qi* and the spleen's transporting and digesting essential *qi*. If gastrosplenic *qi* is normal, body fluids will be rich; if not, formation of body fluids will be affected, causing insufficient body fluids. Thus, the syndrome of deficient *qi* and body fluids may be frequently seen in clinic.

4-4-2-2 *Qi* can transform body fluids

Distribution and transformation of body fluids into sweat and urine, etc. that are excreted from the body depend upon the movement of *qi*. It is due to the spleen spreading and transporting *jing* (vital principle), the lung's functions and kidney *qi* which distributes body fluids throughout the body. Body fluids become sweat and urine after being metabolized. When *qi* movements are unsmooth, the distribution and excretion of body fluids are blocked. When the distribution and excretion of body fluids are blocked and stagnant, *qi* movement will be difficult. Hence, deficient and stagnant *qi* may result in stagnant body fluids, called inability of *qi* to transform water; if stagnant body fluids cause difficulty in the *qi* mechanism, it will be called stagnation of water and blockage of *qi*. These two conditions form endogenous pathogenic damp, phlegm, *yin* (excess exudates) and edema. In clinical treatment, therapies promoting the flow of *qi* and diuresis are used in coordination.

4-4-2-3   *Qi* controls body fluids and body fluids, in turn, carry *qi*

Excretion of body fluids depends upon the promoting action of *qi*. Maintenance of the normal balance of body fluid metabolism also depends upon the controlling action of *qi*. So, deficient or weakened *qi* would lead to a random flow of *qi* from the body fluids, leading to pathological symptoms, such as hyperhidrosis, leakage of sweat[4] polyurine, enuresis, etc. As body fluids can carry *qi*, the disease or syndrome of "*qi* is exhausted together with body fluids" may also appear when a considerable amount of body fluids, such as hyperhidrosis, polyuria, vomiting, diarrhea, etc. are lost.

4-4-3 Relation between blood and body fluids

Both blood and body fluids are moistening and nourishing, and yin in nature. They are closely related.

Both blood and body fluids originate from the refined matter of food. Body fluids become a component of blood after they permeate the vessels.

Blood and body fluids influence each other. For example, when blood is insufficient, body fluids in the exterior or vessels may enter the vessels to compensate for insufficient blood. At the same time, body fluids may form, with pathological problems, such as thirst, dysuria, dry skin, etc. appearing. When body fluids are insufficient, the fluids within the vessels may exude outside, forming pathological conditions, such as empty vessels, insufficient body fluids and dried blood, etc. Hence, for patients with blood loss, it is advisable not to use diaphoresis in clinic. For those with body fluids exhausted by hyperhidrosis or severely consumed body fluids, strong drugs of breaking and expelling congealed blood must not be used at random. This is a practical application of the theory of "body fluids and blood have the same source" in clinic.

Notes

[1] Usually referring to the junction between the muscle and skin.

[2] The location where two pieces of muscles are demarcated. It is so called because they are distinct in layers and boundaries.

[3] The adipose membrane located above the diaphragm and below the heart.

[4] Persistent sweating due to damage of yang *qi* by using too much diaphoresis.

5. MERIDIANS AND THEIR COLLATERALS

The meridian theory, an important component of TCM, includes the physiological functions, pathological changes and interrelationships of the viscera. It was formulated by Chinese ancients during their practice of acupuncture, moxibustion, massage, *qigong*,[1] etc. in combination with anatomical knowledge.

5-1 The concept of the meridian and the formation of its system

5-1-1 Concept of the meridian system

The meridians are the pathways in which the *qi* and blood circulate in the body and through which the viscera and limbs are connected.

The meridians and their collateral meridians is a term for *jing* (meridians) and *luo* (collateral meridians). Most of the meridians run in the deep portion of the body, while their collateral meridians are in the superficial part of the body, some of which are exposed on the body surface. Deeper meridians have certain courses and the superficial meridians run transversely, linking all the viscera, organs, openings and tissues, such as skin, muscles, tendons, bones, etc., in a fine-meshed network.

5-1-2 Formation of the meridian system

The meridian system is composed of the meridians and their collateral meridians.

The meridians can be divided into regular and extraordinary. There are twelve regular ones, i.e., three pairs of yin meridians and three pairs of yang meridians of the hand and foot, collectively called the "twelve regular meridians" that are the main passages in which *qi* and blood circulate. The twelve meridians originate from and terminate at certain areas, lie in certain places and have a certain sequence in circulation. There is a definite rule for their distribution over and passing through the body. Each connects directly with the viscera. The extraordinary meridians, viz., Governor Vessel Meridian, Conception Vessel Meridian, Strategic Vessel Meridian, Girdle Vessel Meridian, Mobility Vessel Meridian of Yin, Mobility Vessel Meridian of Yang, Regulating Vessel Meridian of Yin and Regulating Vessel Meridian of Yang, are collectively termed the "eight extra meridians." They regulate the twelve meridians.

The branches of the twelve meridians spread from the twelve meridians, starting from the four extremities, traversing the deep portion of the viscera, emerging from the superficial portions of the neck and nape. After splitting and running through the interior of the body, the branches of the yang meridians return to yang meridians. After splitting from and running through the interior of the body, those of yin meridians meet those of the yang meridians which are closely related to them. The action of the twelve branches of meridians are chiefly to make the relation between the twelve meridians closer. They make up the regular meridians as they reach the organs and body areas that some regular meridians do not traverse.

The collateral meridians are the small branches of meridians, classified into the large collateral meridians, floating collateral meridians and smaller collateral meridians. The twelve meridians and Governor Vessel Meridian and Conception Vessel Meridians have a large collateral meridian each. With the large collateral meridian of the spleen, they are the "fifteen large collateral meridians." Their main function is to connect with the two related meridians closer on the level of the body surface. The floating collateral meridians are those that traverse the superficial part of the body. The minute ones are the smallest.

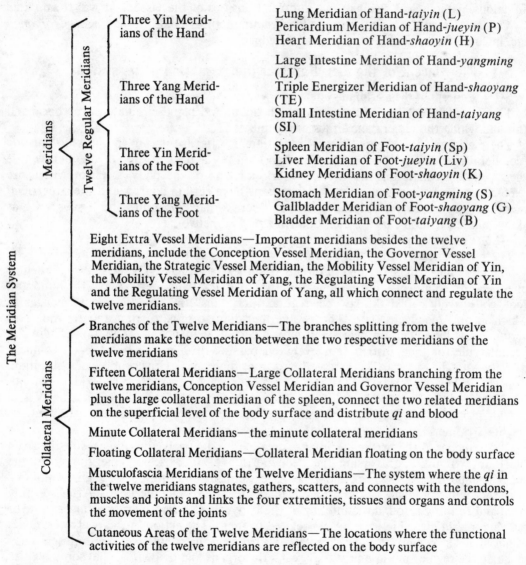

The musculofascia (or musculotendinous) meridians and the cutaneous areas of the meridian connect the twelve meridians with the tendons fascia and muscles respectively with the body surface. The meridian theory holds that the musculofascia meridians are a system, where *qi* "stagnates, gathers, scatters and links" with tendons, fascia, muscles and joints as well as the affiliated part of the twelve meridians, hence called the "musculofascia meridians." They connect the four extremities and various tissues and control the activities of the twelve meridians on the body surface and where meridian *qi* is distributed. The skin is divided into twelve parts corresponding to the twelve meridians, called the "twelve cutaneous areas of meridians." (See above table.)

5-2 Twelve regular meridians

5-2-1 Names

The twelve meridians are symmetrically distributed over both sides of the body, and run respectively through the medial or lateral side of the upper or lower limb. Each meridian respectively pertains to a *zang* or *fu* organ. Hence, the name of each meridian among the twelve meridians includes the hand or foot, yin or yang and *zang* (yin viscera) or *fu* (yang viscera). The meridians of the hands run through the upper limbs and the meridians of the feet run through the medial aspects of the four extremities, pertain to *zang*; those of yang the lateral aspects, pertaining to *fu*. (See the following table.)

Classification of the Names of the Twelve Meridians

	Yin Meridians pertaining to *zang*	Yang Meridians pertaining to *fu*		Location (Yin meridians run through the medial aspect, yang meridians run through the lateral aspect)
Hands	Lung Meridian of *taiyin*	Large Intestine Meridian of *yangming*	**Upper Limbs**	Anterior aspect
	Pericardium Meridian of *jueyin*	Triple Energizer Meridian of *shaoyang*		Midline
	Heart Meridian of *shaoyin*	Small Intestine Meridian of *taiyang*		Posterior aspect
Feet	Spleen Meridian of *taiyin*	Stomach Meridian of *yangming*	**Lower Limbs**	Anterior aspect
	Liver Meridian of *jueyin*	Gallbladder Meridian of *shaoyang*		Midline
	Kidney Meridian of *shaoyin*	Bladder Meridian of *taiyang*		Posterior aspect

5-2-2 Direction, connection, distribution, relation and sequence

5-2-2-1 Direction and connection

There is a rule for the direction and connection of the twelve meridians. "Three yin meridians of the hand and foot from the viscera to the hands; three yang meridians of the hand, from the hand to the head; three yang meridians of the foot, from the head to the foot; three yin meridians of the foot, from the foot to the abdomen." (*Miraculous Pivot*). The three yin meridians of the hand run from the chest cavity to the fingertips. The three yang meridians of the hand run from the fingertips to the head and face where they link with three yang meridians of the foot. The three yang meridians of the foot run from the head and face to the tips of the toes, connecting the three yin meridians of the foot; the three yin meridians of the foot run from the toes to the abdominal and thoraxic cavities, where they join the three yin meridians of the hand. (See the following figure). In such a way, a circulating pathway is established.

The three yang meridians of the hand end at the foot and start from the head, and all of them cross at the head "all yang meridians meet at the head."

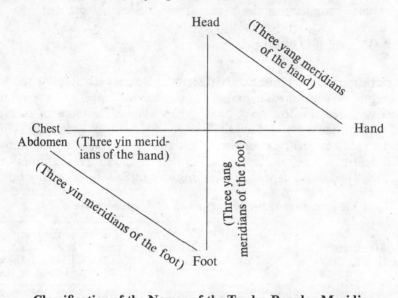

Classification of the Names of the Twelve Regular Meridians

	Yin Meridians (pertaining to yang)	Yang Meridians (pertaining to yin)		Course (The yin meridians run along the medial aspect, the yang meridians run along the lateral aspect)
Hand	Lung Meridian of *taiyin*	Large Intestine Meridian of *yangming*	Upper Limb	Anterior Border (i.e., medial)
	Pericardium Meridian of *jueyin*	Triple Energizer Meridian of *shaoyang*		Midline
	Heart Meridian of *shaoyin*	Small Intestine Meridian of *taiyang*		Posterior Border (i.e., ulnar)
Foot	Spleen Meridian of *taiyin**	Stomach Meridian of *yangming*	Lower Limb	Anterior Border
	Liver Meridian of *jueyin**	Gallbladder Meridian of *shaoyang*		Midline
	Kidney Meridian of *shaoyin*	Bladder Meridian of *taiyang*		Posterior Border

* At the lower leg and dorsal foot, the Liver Meridian lies on the anterior border, but the Spleen Meridian at the midline. After crossing at a location 8 *cun* above the medial malleolus, the Spleen Meridian is on the anterior border whereas the Liver Meridian is in the middle.

5-2-2-2 Distribution

There is a rule for the distribution of the twelve meridians on the surface, i.e., in the four extremities, a yin meridian is distributed over the medial aspect and a yang meridian over the lateral; the *taiyin* and *yangming* meridians are anterior, the *shaoyin* and *taiyang* meridians posterior, and the *jueyin* and *shaoyang* meridians are in the middle. In the head and face, the *yangming* meridian runs through the face and forehead, the *taiyang* meridian crosses the cheek, vertex and back of the head, while the *shaoyang* meridian travels along the lateral side of the head. On the trunk, the three yang meridians of the hand, run through the scapular region; among the three yang meridians of the foot, the *yangming* meridian runs anteriorly (the chest and abdomen), the *taiyang* meridian, posteriorly (the back) and the *shaoyang* meridian, laterally. The three yin meridians of the hand all emerge from the area below the axilla, whereas the three yin meridians of the foot run through the abdominal surface. The sequence of the meridians running through the abdominal surface from the interior of the body to the exterior is: the Meridian of Foot-*shaoyin*, the Meridian of Foot-*yangming*, the Meridian of Foot-*taiyin* and the Meridian of Foot-*jueyin*.

5-2-2-3 Relationship between the meridians

The six pairs of meridians, the three yin meridians and the three yang meridians of the hand and foot are connected by the branches of their meridians and their large collateral meridians. The meridians of Foot-*taiyang* and Foot-*shaoyin*, the meridians of Foot-*shaoyang* and Foot-*jueyin* and the meridians of Foot-*yangming* and Foot-*taiyin* are closely related. The meridians of Hand-*taiyang* and Hand-*shaoyin*, the meridians of Hand-*shaoyang* and Hand-*jueyin* and the meridians of Hand-*yangming* and Hand-*taiyin* are closely related. "The two meridians that are closely connected at the tips of the four extremities run through the two aspects of the four extremities (after crossing at a location 8 *cun* above the medial malleolus, the Liver Meridian of Foot-*jueyin* and the Spleen Meridian of Foot-*taiyin* exchange their locations. The Spleen Meridian of Foot-*taiyin* is situated on the anterior border and the Liver Meridian of Foot-*jueyin*, in the middle) and respectively connect with the viscera that are closely related. The Bladder Meridian of Foot-*taiyang* pertains to the bladder and connects with the kidney and the Kidney Meridian of Foot-*shaoyin*, pertaining to the kidney, links with the bladder."

The yin and yang viscera that are closely related cooperate in their physiological functions and influence each other in their pathology since each of the twelve meridians pertains to and connects with its yin or yang viscus. For example, the spleen transports and digests food and sends the pure nutrients upward, the stomach receives ingested food and sends the turbid matter downward; heart fire may be transferred downward to the small intestine, etc. In treatment, acupoints of the twelve meridians that are closely related may be used alternately, e.g., those of the Lung Meridian may be applied to treat troubles of the large intestine instead of puncturing the Large Intestine Meridian.

5-2-2-4 Sequence of flow of *qi* and blood in the meridian

Qi and blood in the meridians circulate by starting from the Lung Meridian of Hand-*taiyin* to the Liver Meridian of Foot-*jueyin*. The sequence is as follows:

Lung Meridian of Hand-*taiyin* → Tip of the index finger → Large Intestine Meridian of Hand-*yangming*　Near ala nasi

Stomach Meridian of Foot-*yangming* → Tip of the big toe → Spleen Meridian of Foot-*taiyin*   In the heart

Heart Meridian of Hand-*shaoyin* → Tip of the small finger → Small Intestine Meridian of Hand-*taiyang*   Inner canthus

Bladder Meridian of Foot-*taiyang* →Tips of the small toe →Kidney Meridian of Foot-*shaoyin* In the chest

Pericardium Meridian of Hand-*jueyin* → Tip of the ring finger →Triple Energizer Meridian of Hand-*shaoyang*   Outer canthus

Gallbladder Meridian of Foot-*shaoyang* →The big toe →Liver Meridian of Foot-*jueyin*   In the lung

5-2-3 Course
5-2-3-1 Lung Meridian of Hand-*taiyin* (L)
It originates from the middle energizer (the middle portion of the body) and runs downward to connect with the large intestine. Turning back, it goes along the orifice of the stomach (the lower orifice, pylorus and the upper orifice, cardia), and passes through the diaphragm to enter the lung. From the internal zone between the lung and throat, it runs transversely to the supralateral chest area, (*Zhongfu* L 1) and emerges from the surface of the body under the clavicle. Descending along the anterior border of the medial aspect of the upper arm, it reaches the cubital fossa. Then, it runs continuously downward along the medial aspect of the forearm and arrives at the medial aspect of the styloid process of the radius above the wrist, where it enters the *cunkou* section.[2] Passing through the thenar eminence, it traverses the radial border, merging into or ending at the medial aspect of the tip of the thumb (*Shaoshang* L 11). (Fig. 3)

Another section proximal to the wrist emerges from *Lieque* (L 7) and runs directly to the radial side of the tip of the index finger (*Shangyang* LI 1) to connect with the Large Intestine Meridian of Hand-*yangming*.

5-2-3-2 Large Intestine Meridian of Hand-*yangming* (LI)
It starts from the tip of the radial side of the index finger (*Shangyang*, LI 1) runs upward along the radial side of the index finger between the tendons of the thumb, and then continues to ascend along the lateral aspect of the forearm to the lateral border of the extensor side of the upper arm, and to the anterior border of the scapular joint. Then, along the anterior border of the acromion, it goes up to the 7th cervical vertebra (*Dazhui*, GV 14) and then descends anteriorly to the supraclavicular fossa to enter the thoracic cavity and connects with the lung. It runs downward to pass through the diaphragm and finally merges into the large intestine, its pertaining organ. (Fig. 4)

Another section runs upwards from the supraclavicular fossa, passes through the neck to reach the cheek and enters the gum of the lower teeth. Then, it curves around the lip and crosses to the opposite meridian at the philtrum. From there, the left one goes to the right and the right one to the left, on both sides of the nose (*Yingxiang*, LI 20), where it links with the Stomach Meridian of Foot-*yangming*.

5-2-3-3 Stomach Meridian of Foot-*yangming* (S)
It originates from the lateral side of ala nasi (*Yingxiang*, LI 20). It ascends to the bridge of the nose, where it meets the Bladder Meridian of Foot-*taiyang* (*Jingming*, B 1). Turning downward along the lateral side of the nose (*Chengqi*, S 1), it enters the upper gum. Then it curves around the lips and runs downward to meet the Conception Vessel

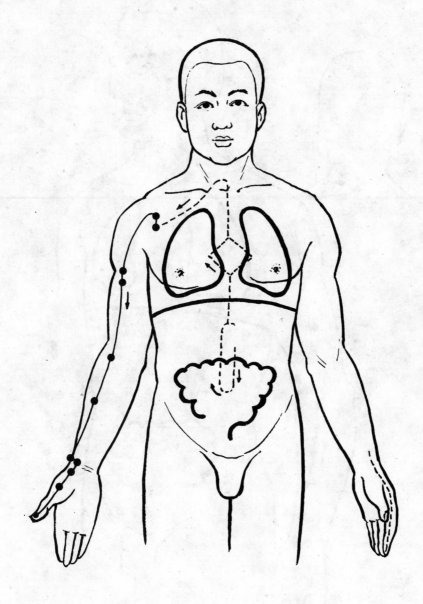

Fig. 3.　Lung Meridian of Hand-*taiyin* (L)

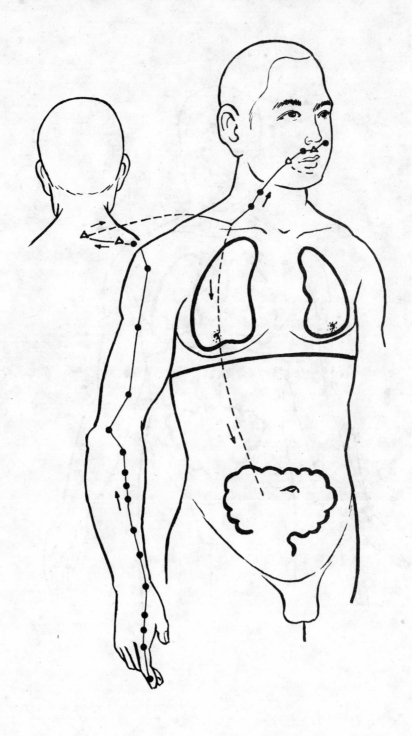

Fig. 4.   Large Intestine Meridian of Hand-*yangming* (LI)

Meridian at the mentolabial groove (*Chengjiang*, CV 24). Then it goes posteriorly across the lower portion of the cheek at *Daying* (S 5). Winding along the angle of the mandibular region (*Jiache*, S 6), it ascends in front of the ear and traverses *Shangguan* (G 3) of the Gallbladder Meridian of Foot-*shaoyang*. Then it follows the anterior hairline and reaches the forehead (*Touwei*, S 8).

The neck section: Emerges in front of *Daying* (S 5), and runs downward to *Renying* (S 9). From there it goes along the throat and enters the supraclavicular fossa to connect with the spleen, its pertaining organ.

The straight section: Arises from the supraclavicular fossa. It passes downward through the nipple. It descends along the umbilicus and enters *Qichong* (S 30) on the lateral side of the lower abdomen.

The section from the lower orifice of the stomach: Descends inside the abdomen and joins the previous section of the meridian at *Qichong* (S 30). Running downward, it traverses *Biguan* (S 31), and then through Femur-*Futu* (S 32), and reaches the knee. From there, it continues downward along the anterior border of the lateral aspect of the tip of the second toe (*Lidui*, S 45).

The tibial section: Emerges from *Zusanli* (S 36), 3 *cun* below the knee, and enters the lateral side of the middle toe.

The section from the dorsal foot: Arises from *Chongyang* (S 42) and terminates at the medial side of the tip of the big toe (*Yinbai*, Sp 1), where it links with the Spleen Meridian of Foot-*taiyin*. (Fig. 5)

5-2-3-4 Spleen Meridian of Foot-*taiyin* (Sp)

It starts from the tip of the big toe (*Yinbai*, Sp 1). It runs along the medial aspect of the foot at the junction of the "pinkish and pale skin," and ascends in front of the medial malleolus up to the leg. It follows the posterior aspect of the tibia, crosses and goes in front of the Liver Meridian of Foot-*jueyin*. Passing through the antero-medial aspect of the knee and thigh, it enters the abdomen, then the spleen, its pertaining organ and connects with the stomach. From there, it ascends, traversing the diaphragm and running alongside the esophagus. When it reaches the root of the tongue, it spreads over its lower surface.

The section from the stomach: Goes upward through the diaphragm and flows into the heart to link with the Heart Meridian of Hand-*shaoyin*. (Fig. 6)

5-2-3-5 Heart Meridian of Hand-*shaoyin* (H)

It originates from the heart. Emerging, it spreads over the "cardiac connection."[4] It passes through the diaphragm to connect to the small intestine.

The ascending section from the "cardiac connection": Runs alongside the esophagus to connect with the "ocular connection."[5]

The straight section from the cardiac connection: Goes upward to the lung, then runs downward and emerges from the axilla. From there it goes along the posterior border of the medial aspect of the upper arm behind the Lung Meridian of Hand-*taiyin* and the Pericardium Meridian of Hand-*jueyin* down to the cubital fossa of the forearm to the pisiform region proximal to the palm and enters the palm. Then, it follows the medial aspect of the little finger to its tip (*Shaochong*, H 9) and links with the Small Intestine Meridian of Hand-*taiyang*. (Fig. 7)

5-2-3-6 Small Intestine Meridian of Hand-*taiyang* (SI)

It starts from the ulnar side of the tip of the baby finger (*Shaoze*, SI 1). Following the

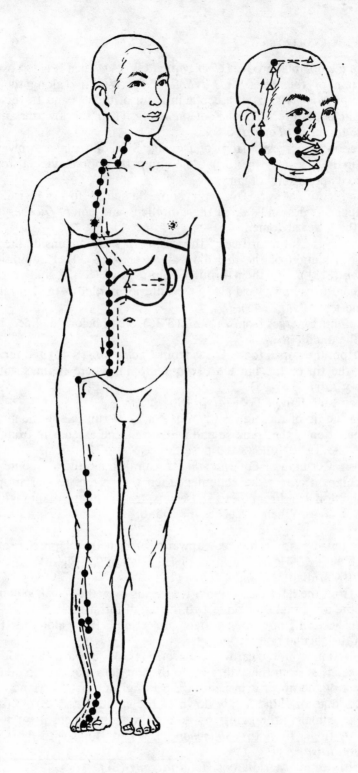

Fig. 5.   Stomach Meridian of Foot-*yangming* (S)

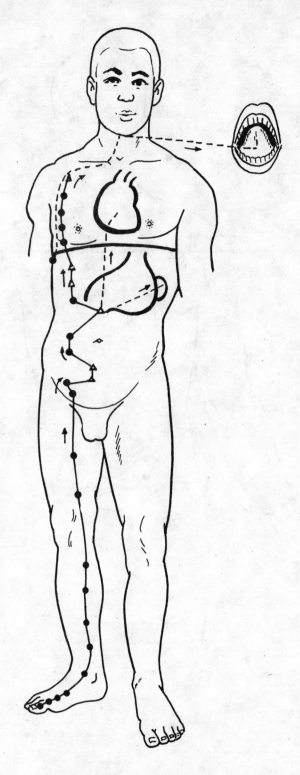

Fig. 6.　Spleen Meridian of Foot-*taiyin* (Sp)

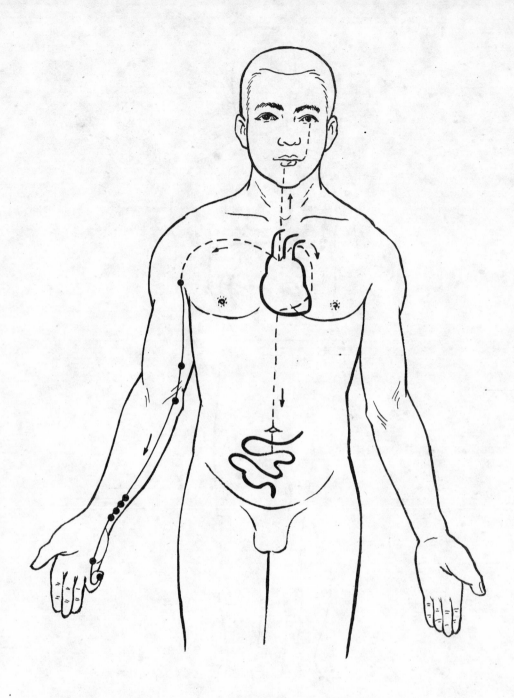

Fig. 7.   Heart Meridian of Hand-*shaoyin* (H)

ulnar side of the dorsal hand, it reaches the wrist where it emerges from the styloid process of the ulna. From there between the olecranion of the ulna and medial epicondyle of the humerus, it runs along the posterior border of the lateral aspect of the upper arm to the shoulder joint. Circling the scapular region, it meets the Conception Vessel Meridian on the superior aspect of the shoulder at *Dazhui* (GV 14). Then, turning downward to the supraclavicular fossa, it connects with the heart. From there it descends along the esophagus, passes through the diaphragm, reaches the stomach, and finally enters the small intestine, its pertaining organ.

The section from the supraclavicular fossa: Ascends to the neck and further to the chest. It enters the ear (*Tinggong*, SI 19) via the outer canthus.

The second section from the cheek runs upward to the infraorbital region (*Quanliao*, SI 18) and further to the lateral side of the nose. It then reaches the inner canthus (*Jingming*, B 1) to link with the Bladder Meridian of Foot-*taiyang*. (Fig. 8)

5-2-3-7 Bladder Meridian of Foot-*taiyang* (B)

It originates from the inner canthus (*Jingming*, B 1). Ascending to the forehead, it joins the Governor Vessel Meridian at the vertex (*Baihui*, GV 20) where a section arises, running to the temple.

The straight section enters and communicates with the brain from the vertex. It then emerges and bifurcates into two lines, descending along the posterior aspect of the neck. Running downward alongside the medial aspect of the scapular and parallel to the vertebral column, it reaches the lumbar region, where it enters the body cavity via the paravertebral muscle to connect with the kidney and joins its pertaining organ, the bladder.

The section of the lumbar region: Descends through the gluteal region and ends in the popliteal fossa.

The section from the posterior aspect of the neck: Runs straight downward along the medial border of the scapula. Passing through the gluteal region (*Huantiao*, G 30), downward along the posterior aspect of the thigh on the lateral side, it meets the preceding section descending from the lumbar region in the popliteal fossa. From there it descends to the leg and further to the posterior aspect of the 5th metatarsal bone. Then it reaches the lateral side of the tip of the little toe (*Zhiyin*, B 67), where it links with the Kidney Meridian of Foot-*shaoyin*. (Fig. 9)

5-2-3-8 Kidney Meridian of Foot-*shaoyin* (K)

It starts from the inferior aspect of the small toe and runs obliquely towards the sole (*Yongquan*, K 1). Emerging from the lower aspect of the tuberosity of the navicular bone and running behind the medial malleolus, it enters the heel. Then it ascends along the medial side of the leg upward along the posteromedial aspect of the thigh towards the vertebral column (*Changqiang*, GV 1), where it enters the kidney, its pertaining organ, and connects to the gallbladder. Ascending and passing through the liver and diaphragm, it enters the lung, running along the throat and terminates at the root of the tongue.

Another section springs from the lung, joins the heart and flows into the chest to link with the Pericardium Meridian of Hand-*jueyin*. (Fig. 10)

5-2-3-9 Pericardium Meridian of Hand-*jueyin* (P)

It originates from the chest, and enters its pertaining organ, the pericardium. Then, it descends through the diaphragm to the abdomen, connecting with the triple energizer.

The section arising from the chest: Runs inside the chest, emerges from the costal

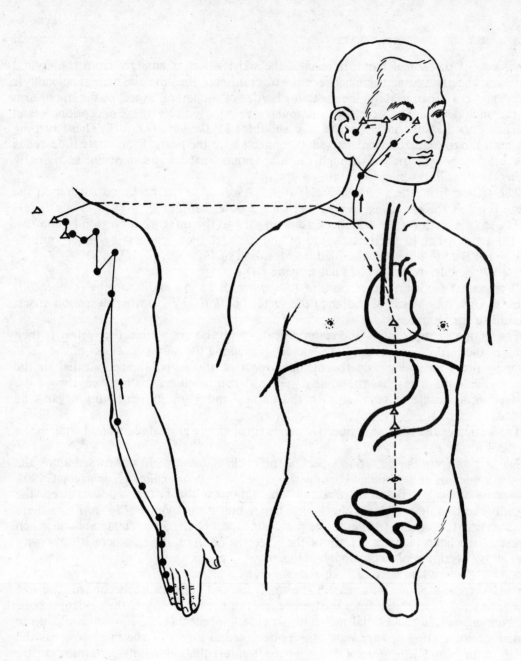

Fig. 8.   Small Intestine Meridian of Hand-*taiyang* (SI)

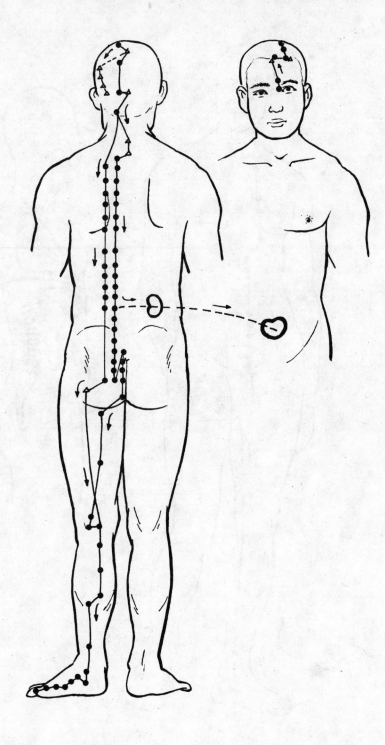

Fig. 9.　Bladder Meridian of Foot-*taiyang* (B)

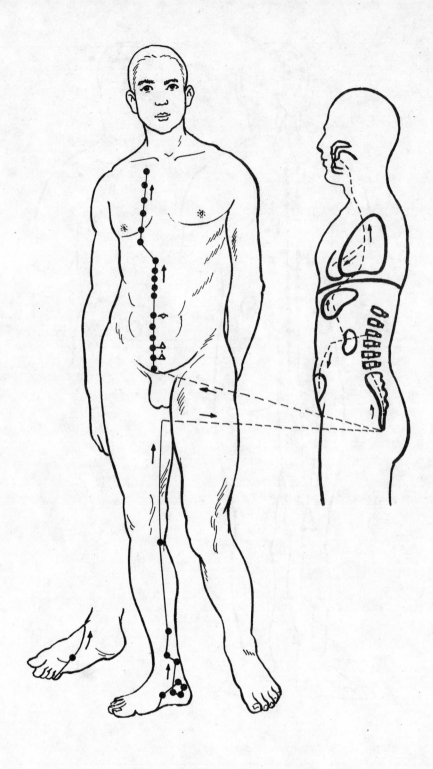

Fig. 10.   Kidney Meridian of Foot-*shaoyin* (K)

region at the point 3 *cun* below the anterior axillary fold (*Tianchi*, P 1) and ascends to the axilla. Following the medial aspect of the upper arm, it runs downward between the Lung Meridian of Hand-*taiyin* and the Heart Meridian of Hand-*shaoyin* to the cubital fossa, further downward to the forearm between the tendons of m. palmaris longus and m. flexor carpi radialis, to the palm. From there it passes along the middle finger right down to its tip (*Zhongchong*, P 9).

Another section arises from the palm at *Laogong* (P 8): Runs along the right finger to its tip (*Guanchong*, TE 1), and links with the Triple Energizer Meridian of Hand-*shaoyang*. (Fig. 11)

5-2-3-10 Triple Energizer Meridian of Hand-*shaoyang* (TE)

It starts from the ulnar side of the tip of the ring finger (*Guanchong*, TE 1), running upward between the fourth and fifth metacarpal bones along the dorsal aspect of the wrist to the lateral aspect of the forearm between the radius and ulna. Passing through the olecranion and along the lateral aspect of the upper arm, it reaches the shoulder region, where it crosses and passes behind the Gallbladder Meridian of Foot-*shaoyang*. Winding over to the supraclavicular fossa, it spreads in the chest to connect with the pericardium. Then, it descends through the diaphragm down to the abdomen and joins its pertaining organ, the triple energizer.

A section originates from the chest. Running upward, it emerges from the supraclavicular fossa. From there it descends to the neck, running along the posterior border of the ear, and further to the superior aspect of the ear. It then turns downward to the cheek and terminates in the infraorbital region.

The auricular section: Arises from the retroauricular region and enters the ear. Then, it emerges in front of the ear, crosses the previous section at the cheek and reaches the outer canthus (*Sizhukong*, TE 23) to link with the Gallbladder Meridian of Foot-*shaoyang*. (Fig. 12)

5-2-3-11 Gallbladder Meridian of Foot-*shaoyang* (G)

It originates from the outer canthus (*Tongziliao*, G 1), ascends to the corner of the forehead (*Hanyan*, G 4), then curves downward to the retroauricular region and runs along the side of the neck in front of the Triple Energizer Meridian of Hand-*shaoyang* to the shoulder. Turning back, it traverses and passes behind the Triple Energizer Meridian of Hand-*shaoyang* to the supraclavicular fossa.

The retroauricular section: Arises from the retroauricular region and enters the ear. It then comes out and passes through the preauricular region to the posterior aspect of the outer canthus.

The section arising from the outer canthus: Runs downward to *Daying* (S 5) and meets the Triple Energizer Meridian of Hand-*shaoyang* in the infra-orbital region. Then, passing through *Jiache* (S 6), it descends to the neck and enters the supraclavicular fossa where it meets the main meridian. From there it further descends into the chest, passes through the diaphragm to connect with the liver and enters its pertaining organ, the gallbladder. Then it runs inside the hypochondriac region, comes out from the lateral side of the lower abdomen near the femoral artery at the inguinal region. From there it runs superficially along the margin of the pubic region. From there it transversely goes into the hip region (*Huantiao*, G 30).

The straight section: Runs downward from the supraclavicular fossa, passes in front of the axilla along the lateral aspect of the chest and through the free end of the floating

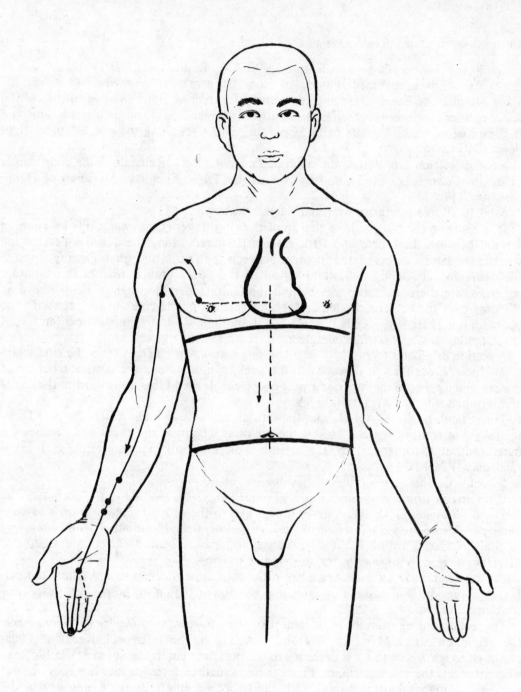

Fig. 11. Pericardium Meridian of Hand-*jueyin* (P)

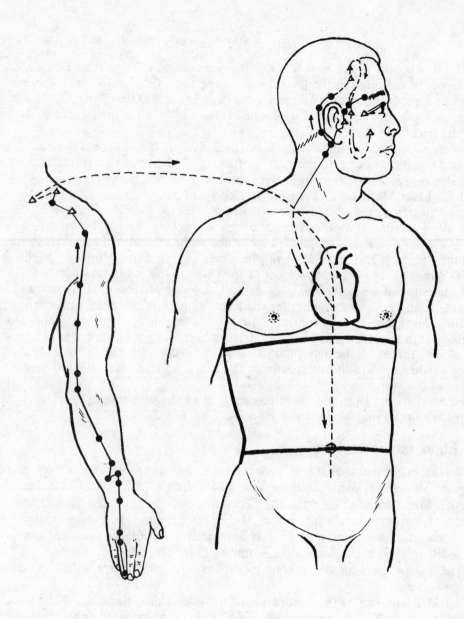

Fig. 12. Triple Energizer Meridian of Hand-*shaoyang* (TE)

rib to the hip region where it meets the previous section. Then it descends along the lateral aspect of the thigh to the lateral side of the knee. Going further downward along the anterior aspect of the fibula all the way to its lower end (*Xuanzhong*, G 39), it reaches the anterior aspect of the external malleolus. It then follows the dorsal foot to the lateral side of the tip of the 4th toe.

The section of the dorsal foot: Springs from *Zulinqi* (G 41), runs between the first and second metatarsal bones to the distal portion of the big toe and terminates at its hairy region (*Dadun*, Liv 1) where it links with the Liver Meridian of Foot-*jueyin*. (Fig. 13)

5-2-3-12 Liver Meridian of Foot-*jueyin* (Liv)

It originates from the dorsal hairy region of the big toe (*Dadun*, Liv 1). Running upward along the dorsal foot, passing through *Zhongfeng* (Liv 4) 1 *cun* in front of the medial malleolus, it ascends to the area 8 *cun* above the medial malleolus where it crosses behind the Spleen Meridian of Foot-*taiyin*. Then, it runs further upward to the medial side of the knee along the medial aspect of the thigh to the pubic region, where it curves around the external genitalia and goes up to the lower abdomen. It then runs upward and curves round the stomach to enter the liver, its pertaining organ, and connects with the gallbladder. From there it continues to ascend, passing through the diaphragm, and branching out in the costal and hypochondriac region. Then it ascends along the posterior aspect of the throat to the nasopharynx and connects with the "ocular connection." Running further upward, it emerges from the forehead and meets the Governor Vessel Meridian at the vertex.

The section arising from the liver: Passes through the diaphragm, flows into the lung and links with the Lung Meridian of Hand-*taiyin*. (Fig. 14)

5-3 Eight extra meridians

The eight extra meridians is a general term for the Governor Vessel Meridian, Conception Vessel Meridian, Strategic Vessel Meridian, Girdle Vessel Meridian, Mobility Vessel Meridian of Yin, Mobility Vessel Meridian of Yang, Regulating Vessel Meridian of Yin and Regulating Vessel Meridian of Yang. They are so called because they are not distributed as regularly as the twelve meridians, they are not directly connected with the viscera, and differ from the twelve meridians.

Intersecting or crossing the twelve meridians, the eight extra meridians have the following actions:

a. Further strengthening the connection of the twelve meridians, e.g., "The Regulating Vessel Meridian of Yang connects with yang" and combines all the yang meridians and "The Regulating Vessel Meridian of Yin connects with yin" and combines all the yin meridians. "The Girdle Vessel Meridian controls all the meridians" and connects the meridians in the lumbar and abdominal regions. The Strategic Vessel Meridian unobstructs the upper and lower parts of the body, and irrigates the three yin meridians and the three yang meridians. The Governor Vessel Meridian is the "sea of all the yin meridians."

b. Regulating *qi* and blood in the twelve meridians. When *qi* and blood are in excess, they flow into and are stored in the eight extra meridians. When the twelve meridians lack *qi* and blood, they can be recharged from the eight extra meridians.

c. They are closely related with the yin viscera, such as the liver, kidney, etc. and the

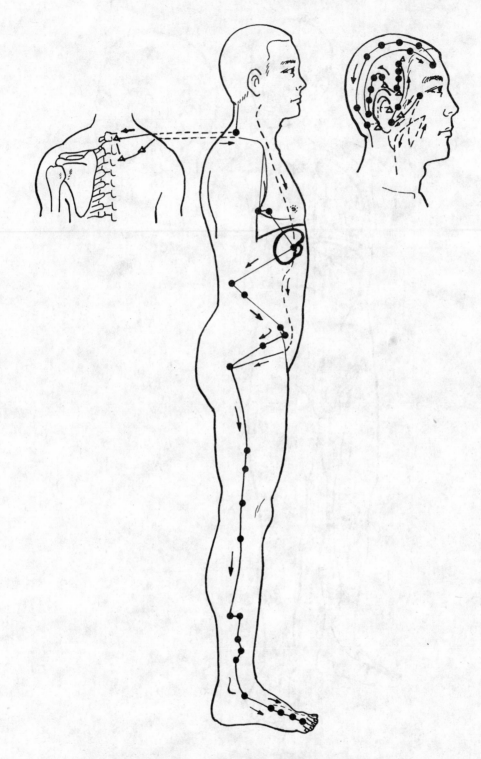

Fig. 13.   Gallbladder Meridian of Foot-*shaoyang* (G)

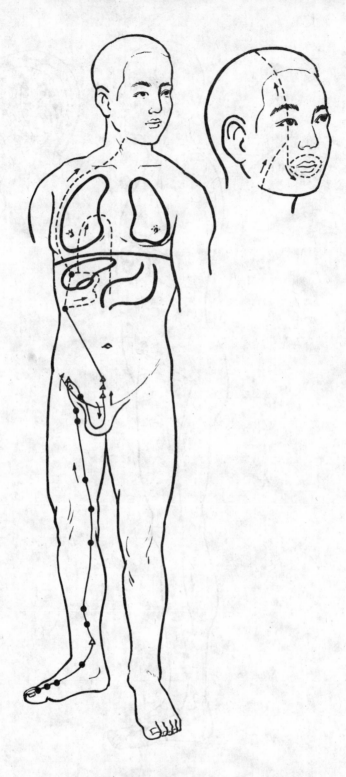

Fig. 14.   Liver Meridian of Foot-*jueyin* (Liv)

unusual organs, such as the uterus, brain, marrow, etc. and connect with one another to a certain extent.

5-3-1 Governor Vessel Meridian (GV)

5-3-1-1 The Course

The Governor Vessel Meridian starts from the uterus. Descending, it merges at the perineum. Then it ascends posteriorly along the interior of the spinal column to *Fengfu* (GV 16) at the nape, where it enters the brain. It further ascends to the vertex and winds along the midline of the forehead to the columella of the nose.

The first section: Splits from the inside of the spinal column and merges into the kidney.

The second section: Ascends directly from the inner abdomen and passes through the umbilicus and then through the heart to the throat. Then it ascends to reach the central region below the eyes (Fig. 15).

5-3-1-2 Main function

Since it runs along the posterior midline of the back and frequently joins the three yang meridians of the hand and foot and the Regulating Vessel Meridian of Yang, it can control all the yang meridians of the body. Thus, it is also called the "sea of yang meridians." As it traverses the spinal column, runs upward to enter the brain and merges into the kidneys after splitting from the spinal column, it is related to the brain, spinal cord and kidneys.

5-3-2 Conception Vessel Meridian (CV)

5-3-2-1 The course

The conception Vessel Meridian starts from the uterus and emerges from the perineum. It runs anteriorly to the pubic region and ascends along the interior of the abdomen, passing through *Guanyuan* (CV 4) and other acupoints along the frontal middle to the throat. Running further upward, it curves around the lips, passes through the chest and enters the infraorbital regions (*Chengqi*, S 1). (Fig. 16)

5-3-2-2 Main function

As the Conception Vessel Meridian runs along the anterior middle of the abdomen, frequently crosses the three yin meridians of the hand and foot and the Regulating Vessel Meridian of Yin and can receive *qi* from the yin meridian, it is thus called the "sea of yin meridians." It originates from the uterus and is concerned with the uterus and fetus.

5-3-3 Strategic Vessel Meridian

5-3-3-1 The course

The strategic Vessel Meridian originates from the lower abdomen and descends and emerges from the perineum. It then ascends and runs inside the vertebral column, while its superficial portion passes through the *qichong* region where it splits into two sections which coincide with the Kidney Meridian of Foot-*shaoyin*, running along both sides of the abdomen up to the throat and curving around the lip.

The first section: Originates from the kidney together with the Kidney Meridian of Foot-*shaoyin*, descends and emerges from the *qichong* region, enters the popliteal fossa along the medial aspect of the thigh, then travels downward to the sole along the medial border of the tibia. Another section from the posterior and medial malleolus runs anteriorly and enters the dorsal foot and big toe.

The second section: Starts from the uterus, runs backward to communicate with the Governor Vessel Meridian and then ascends inside the vertebral column.

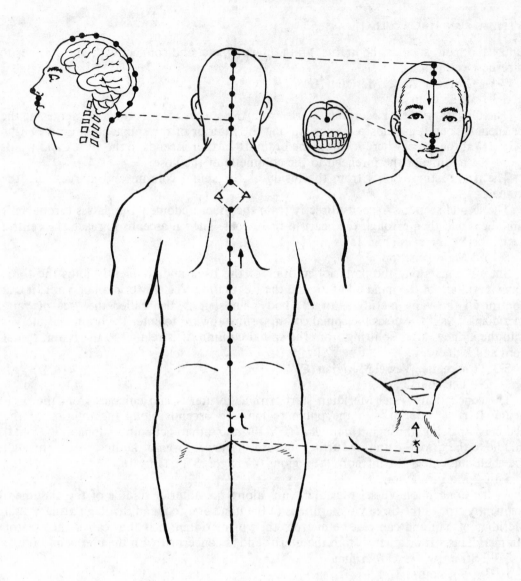

Fig. 15.　Governor Vessel Meridian (GV)

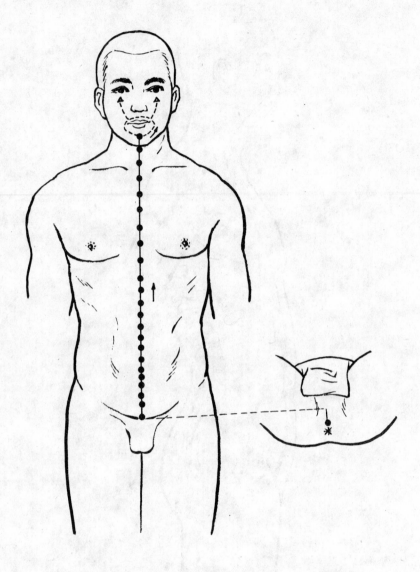

Fig. 16.   Conception Vessel Meridian (CV)

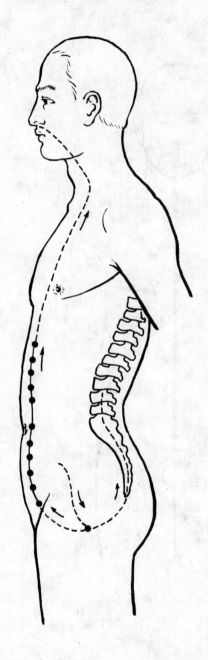

Fig. 17.   Strategic Vessel Meridian

5-3-3-2 Main function

As it ascends to reach the head, descends to reach the foot, traverses the body, becomes the strategic keypass of *qi* and blood and regulates them in the twelve meridians, it is called the "sea of blood" and is closely related to menstruation.

5-3-4 Girdle Vessel Meridian

5-3-4-1 The course

Girdle Vessel Meridian starts from the hypochondrium, descends obliquely to reach *Weidao* (G 28), then surrounds the body in a circle. The section in the abdominal surface descends to the lower abdomen (Fig. 18).

5-3-4-2 Main function

It curves around the waist like a belt and can control all the meridians traversing vertically.

5-3-5 Mobility Vessel Meridians of Yin and Yang

5-3-5-1 The course

The Mobility Vessel Meridians are a pair of meridians, situated on the left and right sides of the body. Both of them start from the area below the malleolus.

The Mobility Vessel Meridian of Yin splits from *Zhaohai* (K 6) below the malleolus, directly ascends along the posteriomedial malleolus along the medial aspect of the lower limb, then enters the supraclavicular fossa via the external genitalia, abdomen and chest, and then emerges anteriorly from *Renying* (S. 9) to reach the inner canthus via the side of the nose, joining the *taiyang* meridians of the hand and foot and the Mobility Vessel Meridian of Yang (Fig. 19).

After splitting from *Shenmai* (B. 62) below the lateral malleolus, the Mobility Vessel Meridian of Yang ascends along the posterolateral malleolus, passes through the abdomen, continuously ascends along the posterolateral chest, scapular region, lateral aspect of the neck to the corner of the mouth, then reaches the inner canthus to connect with the *taiyang* meridians of the hand and foot and the Mobility Vessel Meridian of Yin. Then it runs further upward to the hairline, runs downward to the posterior ear and meets with the Gallbladder Meridian of Foot-*shaoyang* at *Fenchi*. (Fig. 20)

5-3-5-2 Main function

They have the action of nourishing the eye, controlling the movement of the eyelids and lower limbs. The Mobility Vessel Meridians of Yin and Yang "respectively govern the left and right yin and yang of the body."

5-3-6 Regulating Vessel Meridians of Yin and Yang

5-3-6-1 The course

The Regulating Vessel Meridian of Yin originates from the medial aspect of the leg where the three yin meridians join, then ascends along the medial aspect of the lower limb to the abdomen. Ascending together with the Spleen Meridian of Foot-*taiyin* to reach the hypochondriac region, it meets the meridian of foot-*jueyin* and then runs upward to reach the throat, connecting with the Conception Vessel Meridian (Fig. 21).

The Regulating Vessel Meridian of Yang starts from the area below the lateral malleolus, runs upward parallel to the Gallbladder Meridian of Foot-*shaoyang*, then ascends along the lateral aspect of the lower limb, passes through the posterior aspect of the trunk, and then goes upward to reach the shoulder, runs anteriorly to the forehead via the neck and joins the Governor Vessel Meridian. (Fig. 22)

5-3-6-2 Main function

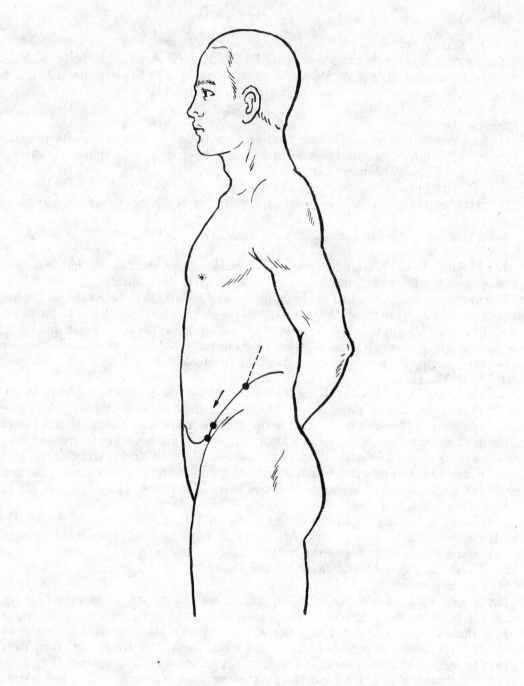

Fig. 18.　Girdle Vessel Meridian

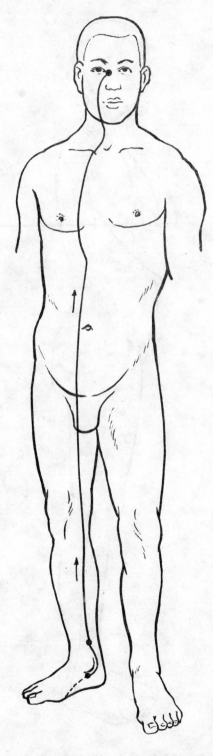

Fig. 19.   Mobility Vessel Meridian of Yin

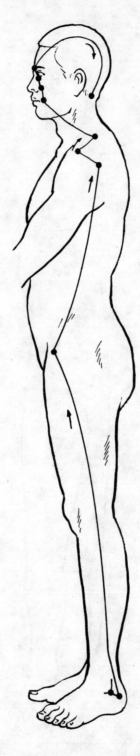

Fig. 20.　Mobility Vessel Meridian of Yang

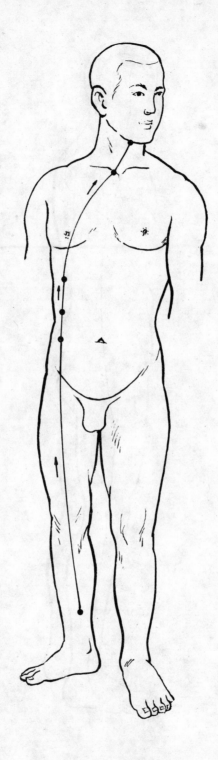

Fig. 21.   Regulating Vessel Meridian of Yin

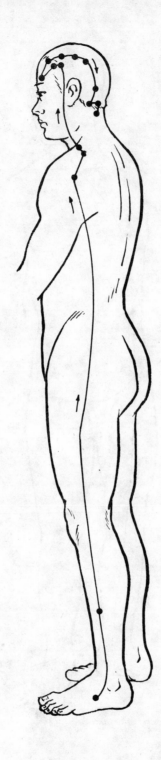

Fig. 22.   Regulating Vessel Meridian of Yang

The function of the Mobility Vessel Meridian of Yin is "to hold all the yin meridians together" that of the Mobility Vessel Meridian of Yang, "to hold all the yang meridians together."

5-4 Branches of the twelve meridians, large collateral meridians, musculo-fascia (or musculotendinous) meridians and cutaneous areas of meridians

5-4-1 Branches of the twelve meridians

The twelve branches of meridians are the important ones that split from the twelve meridians and pass through the chest, abdomen and head. All of them split from the four extremities where the twelve meridians traverse (usually the portion above the elbow and knee) and enter the deep part of the viscus, then emerge from the body surface to run upward to the head and face, finally those of the yin meridians meet those of the yang meridians and respectively merge into the three yang meridians.

5-4-1-1 Physiological function

Since certain areas where the twelve branches of meridians traverse at points the twelve meridians do not traverse, they have an important action in physiology as well as treatment.

Their chief actions are as follows:

a. Strengthening the connection between the two closely related meridians among the twelve meridians within the body. After the twelve branches of meridians enter the body cavity, the two meridians that are closely related coincide with each other and pass through the viscera that are also closely related, and when they emerge from the body surface, the branch of the yin meridian connects with that of the yang meridian on the body surface.

b. Strengthening the centripetal connection between the superficial and deep parts of the body and the four extremities and trunk. It plays an important role in widening the body's connection with the meridians and the transmission from the exterior to the interior of the body where the branches of the twelve meridians split from the sections of the twelve meridians in the four extremities and traverse centripetally after entering the body.

c. Strengthening the connection between the twelve meridians to the head and face. This mainly refers to the six yang meridians, but not only the branches of the six yang meridians traverse the head and face, but also those of the six yin meridians too. After meeting those of the yang meridians, the branches of the three yin meridians of the hand meet at the head and face via the throat. This is the foundation for the theory that "*qi* and blood in the twelve meridians and their 365 collateral meridians run upward to reach the face and pass through sense organs." (*Miraculous Pivot*)

d. Widening the range of indications of the twelve meridians: As the branches of the twelve meridians distribute themselves over the area where the twelve meridians do not reach, the range of indications of the acupoints are widened correspondingly. For example, although the meridian of foot-*taiyang* does not reach the anus, its branch enters the anus so that acupoints, such as *Chengshan* (B 57) and *Chengjin* (B 56) of the meridian may be chosen for treating anus trouble.

e. Strengthening the connection between the three yin and yang meridians of the foot and the heart. As the branches of the three yin and yang meridians of the foot ascend to pass through the abdomen and chest, they are connected with the heart in the chest cavity and make the connection of the viscera in the abdominal cavity closer. Therefore, the branches of the twelve meridians are important to the connection between the viscera and the heart in the abdominal cavity and lay the foundation for the theory that "the heart is the Chief of the five yin and six yang viscera."

5-4-1-2 The course

a. The branches of the meridians of foot-*taiyang* and foot-*shaoyin* (the first correspondence)

The branch of the meridian of foot-*taiyang* splits from the popliteal fossa where the meridian of foot-*taiyang* traverses, a section of it splits from the area 5 *cun* below the sacrum, enters the anus, runs upward to connect with the bladder, reaches the posterior heart along the paravertebral muscles and merges into the heart; the vertebral section continues to ascend along the paravertebral muscles, emerges from the nape and finally meets the meridians of foot-*taiyang*.

The branch of the meridian of foot-*shaoyin* also splits from the popliteal fossa where the meridian of foot-*shaoyin* traverses, and coincides with that of the meridian of foot-*taiyang* to reach the kidney, then splits from the second lumbar vertebra and merges into the Girdle Vessel Meridian. The vertebral section continues to run upward, connects with the root of the tongue, then merges from the neck and meets that of the meridian of foot-*taiyang*. (Fig. 23)

b. The branches of the meridians of foot-*shaoyang* and foot-*jueyin* (the second correspondence)

The branch of the meridian of foot-*shaoyang* splits from the lateral thigh where the meridian of foot-*shaoyang* traverses, curves around the anterior thigh, enters the pubic region, meets that of the meridian of foot-*jueyin*, ascends to enter the hypochondriac region, connects with the gallbladder along the inside of the chest cavity, spreads over and ascends to reach the liver, passes through the heart, runs upward along the esophagus, emerges from the mandibular region and the corner of the mouth, spreads over the face, connects with the "ocular connection," the outer canthus and finally merges into the meridian of foot-*shaoyang*.

The branch of the meridian of foot-*jueyin* splits from the dorsal foot where the meridian of foot-*jueyin* traverses, runs upward to the pubic region and coincides with the meridian of foot-*shaoyang*. (Fig. 24)

c. The branches of the meridians of foot-*yangming* and foot-*taiyin* (the third correspondence)

The branch of the meridian of foot-*yangming* splits from the anterior thigh where the meridian of foot-*yangming* passes through, enters the abdominal cavity, connects with the stomach, spreads over the spleen, runs upward to pass through the heart, emerges from the mouth, ascends to the root of the nose and infraorbital region, runs back to connect with the "ocular connection" and finally merges into the meridian of foot-*yangming*.

The branch of the meridian of foot-*taiyin* splits from the medial aspect of the hip where the meridian of foot-*taiyin* traverses, reaches the frontal thigh, coincides with that of the meridian of foot-*yangming*, runs upward to the throat and passes through the tongue (Fig. 25).

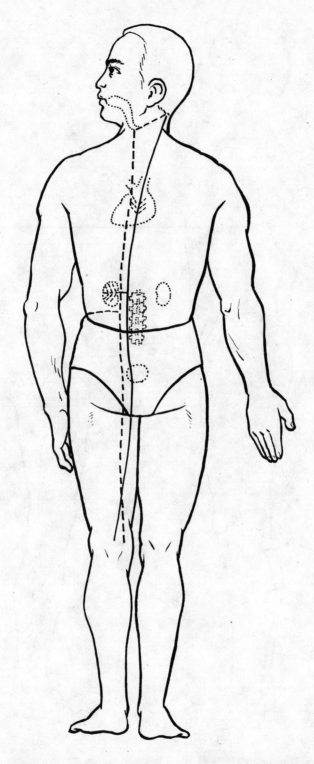

Fig. 23.   The Branches of the Meridians of Foot-*taiyang* and Foot-*shaoyin*

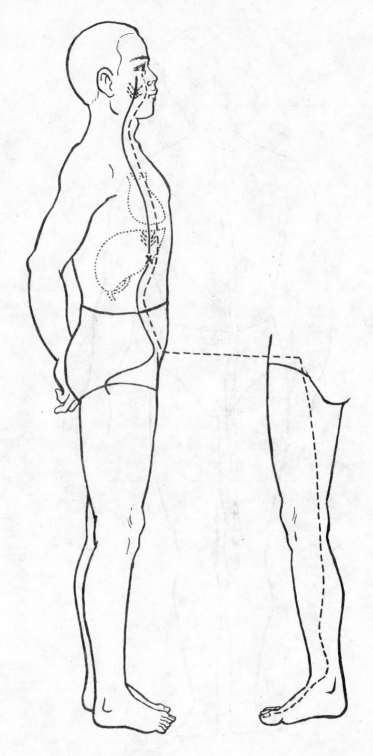

Fig. 24. The Branches of the Meridians of Foot-*shaoyang* and Foot-*jueyin*

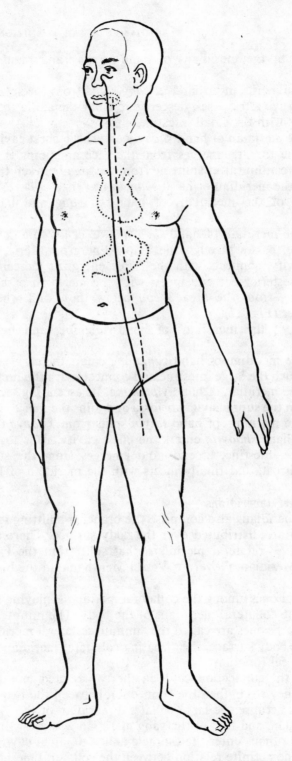

Fig. 25.   The Branches of the Meridians of Foot-*yangming* and Foot-*taiyin*

d. The branches of the meridians of hand-*taiyang* and hand-*shaoyin* (the fourth correspondence)

The branch of the meridian of hand-*taiyang* splits from the scapular joint where the meridian of hand-*taiyang* traverses, descends to enter the axilla fossa, runs to the heart and finally connects with the small intestine.

The branch of the meridian of hand-*shaoyin* enters the chest cavity, connects with the heart, ascends to the throat, emerges from the face and joins the meridian of hand-*taiyang* at the inner canthus after splitting from the area between the two tendons in the axillar fossa where the meridian of hand-*shaoyin* traverses (Fig. 26).

e. The branches of the meridians of hand-*shaoyang* and hand-*jueyin* (the fifth correspondence)

The branch of the meridian of hand-*shaoyang* descends to enter the supraclavicular fossa of the clavicle, passes through the Triple Energizer Meridian of Hand-*shaoyin*, enters the chest cavity, connects with the triple energizer, descends along the throat, emerges from the posterior ear and meets with the meridian of hand-*shaoyang* at the nipple after splitting from the area 3 *cun* below the axilla where the meridian of hand-*jueyin* traverses (Fig. 27).

f. The branches of the meridians of hand-*yangming* and hand-*taiyin* (the sixth correspondence)

The branch of the meridian of hand-*yangming* enters the cervical vertebra below the nape, descends to reach the large intestine and connects with the lung after splitting from *Jianyu* (LI 15) of the meridian of hand-*yangming*. Its ascending section passes along the throat, emerges from the supraclavicular fossa and joins the meridian of hand-*yangming*.

The branch of the meridian of hand-*taiyin* splits from *Yuanye* (G 22), runs in front of the meridian of hand-*shaoyin*, enters the chest cavity, runs to the lung, distributes itself over the large intestine, ascends and emerges from the supraclavicular fossa, ascends along the throat, and finally meets with the meridian of hand-*yangming* (Fig. 28).

5-4-2 Large collateral meridians

Large collateral meridians also comprise the branches splitting from the main meridians, most of which are distributed over the body surface. There are fifteen collateral meridians; the twelve collateral meridians that split from the twelve meridians, the Conception Vessel Meridian, Governor Vessel Meridian and the big collateral meridian of the spleen.

They are the major ones among the collateral meridians, playing a leading role among the numerous minute collateral meridians of the body. The minute collateral meridians that split from the large ones are called the "minute collateral meridians"; those that are distributed over the body surface, the "floating collateral meridians."

5-4-2-1 Physiological function

a. Strengthening the connection between the two related meridians which link the twelve meridians. They strengthen the connection between the two related meridians in the trunk and limbs because the large collateral meridian of the yin meridian connects with the yang meridian, and that of the yang meridian with the yin meridian. Although certain collateral meridians enter the thoracic and abdominal cavities and connect with the viscera, there is no definite relation between the collateral meridians and the viscera.

b. Controlling other collateral meridians and strengthening the connection between the

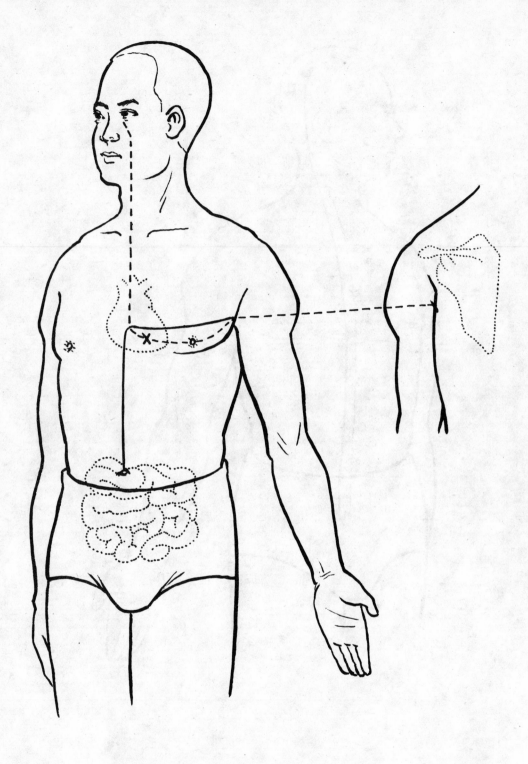

Fig. 26.   The Branches of the Meridians of Hand-*taiyang* and Hand-*shaoyin*

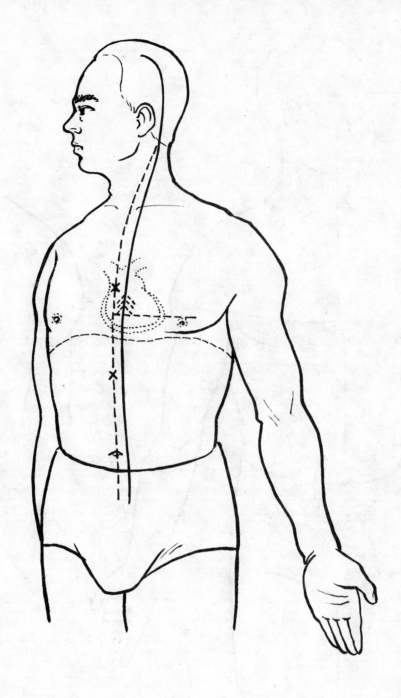

Fig. 27.   The Branches of the Meridians of Hand-*shaoyang* and Hand-*jueyin*

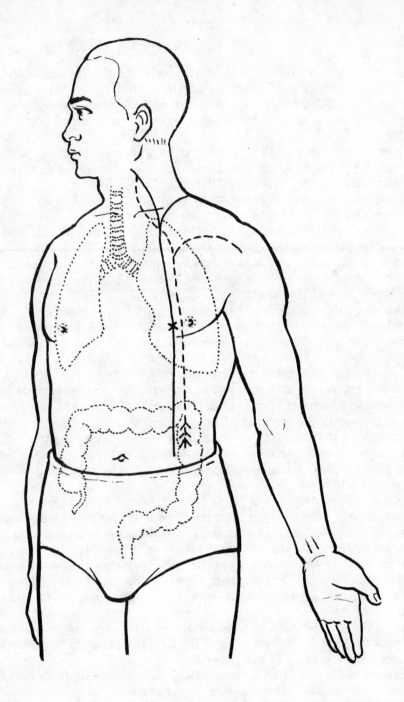

Fig. 28.   The Branches of the Meridians of Hand-*yangming* and Hand-*taiyin*.

anterior, posterior and lateral portions of the body. As the branch of the Conception Vessel Meridian is distributed over the abdomen and that of the Governor Vessel Meridian, the back, and the collateral meridian of the spleen, the chest, and hypochondriac region, the integral unity of the anterior, posterior and lateral portions of the body are strengthened.

c. Nourishing the body with *qi* and blood: The minute and floating collateral meridians split from the large collateral meridians and are spread over the body like a network which mesh with the tissues of the entire body. *Qi* and blood flow in the main in a linear way and then spread to every direction so as to nourish the body.

5-4-2-2 Locations

The location of the fifteen collateral meridians is that those of the twelve meridians split from the area distal to the elbow and knee and those of the external and internal meridians are interconnected; those of the Conception Vessel Meridian are distributed over the abdomen and those of the Governor Vessel Meridian, the back; those of the spleen, the lateral side of the body.

a. The branch of the meridian of hand-*taiyin* splits from *Lieque* (L 7), runs from the superior aspect of the wrist, then goes to the meridian of hand-*yangming* at the point 0.5 *cun* posterior to the wrist; its section coincides with the meridian of hand-*taiyin*, directly enters the palm and distributes itself over the thenar prominence.

b. The branch of the meridian of hand-*taiyang* splits from *Tongli* (H 5), runs to the meridian of hand-*taiyang* 1 *cun* posterior to the wrist; its section ascends from the area 1.5 *cun* posterior to the wrist, enters the heart along the meridian of hand-*shaoyin*, ascends to connect with the tongue and finally merges into the "ocular connection."

c. The branch of the meridian of hand-*jueyin*, after splitting from *Neiguan* (P 6), emerges from the place between the two tendons, 2 *cun* posterior to the wrist, ascends along the main meridian of hand-*jueyin*, connects with the pericardium and links with the "cardiac connection."

d. The branch of the meridian of hand-*taiyang*, after splitting from *Zhizheng* (S 17), enters the meridian of hand-*shaoyin* 5 *cun* posterior to the wrist; its minor section ascends to pass through the elbow and then connects with the scapular region.

e. The branch of the meridian of hand-*yangming*, after splitting from *Pianli* (LI 6), runs to the meridian of hand-*taiyin* from the spot 3 *cun* posterior to the wrist; its minor section runs upward along the arm, passes through *Jianyu* (LI 15), ascends to reach the mandibular region and spreads over the teeth. Its minor section enters the ear and meets with the meridian.

f. The branch of the meridian of hand-*shaoyang*, after splitting from *Waiguan* (TE 5) 2 *cun* posterior to the wrist, curves around the lateral side of the upper arm, enters the chest and meets the meridian of hand-*jueyin*.

g. The branch of the meridian of foot-*taiyang*, after splitting from *Feiyang* (B 58) 7 *cun* posterior to the lateral malleolus, runs to the meridian of foot-*shaoyin*.

h. The branch of the meridian of foot-*shaoyang*, after splitting from *Guangming* (G 37) 5 *cun* posterior to the lateral malleolus, runs to the meridian of foot-*jueyin* and then descends to connect with the dorsal foot.

i. The branch of the meridian of foot-*yangming*, after splitting from *Fenglong* (S 40) 8 *cun* posterior to the lateral malleolus, runs to the meridian of foot-*taiyin*; its minor section ascends along the lateral side of the tibia to connect with the vertex, where it meets various meridians and then connects with the throat.

j. The branch of the meridian of foot-*taiyin*, after splitting from *Gongsun* (Sp 4), runs to the meridian of foot-*yangming* 1 *cun* posterior to the first metatarso-phalangeal bone. Its minor section enters the abdominal cavity and connects with the stomach.

k. The branch of the meridian of foot-*shaoyin*, after splitting from *Dazhong* (K 4), curves around the heel in the posteriomedial malleolus; its minor section coincides with the meridian of foot-*shaoyin*, runs downward to communicate with the lumbar vertebra.

l. The branch of the meridian of foot-*jueyin*, after splitting from *Ligou* (Liv 5), runs to the meridian of foot-*shaoyang* 5 *cun* above the medial aspect of the malleolus; its minor section passes through the tibia, ascends to the testes and gathers at the penis.

m. The branch of the Conception Vessel Meridian, after splitting from *Jiuwei* (CV 15), runs downward from the xyphoid and merges into the abdomen.

n. The branch of the Governor Vessel Meridian, after splitting from *Changqiang* (GV 1) ascends along the paravertebral region to reach the nape and merges into the heat; its descending section starts from the scapular region, deviates to reach the foot-*taiyang* meridian to the left and right, and enters the paravertebral muscles.

o. The collateral meridian of the spleen, after splitting from *Dabao* (So 21), emerges from the spot 3 *cun* below *Yuanye* (G 22) and emerges into the thoracic and hypochondriac regions.

5-4-3 Musculofascia (or musculotendinous) meridians

"The musculofascia meridians" are the branches of the twelve meridians that connect with tendons and muscles. Their functions are based on *qi* and blood in the meridian and regulated by the twelve meridians. Therefore, they are also classified into a twelve-meridian system, called the "twelve musculofascia meridians."

5-4-3-1 Physiological function

Their main function is to control the bone and promote the flexion and extension of joints.

5-4-3-2 Distribution

In general, they are distributed from the tips of the four extremities to the head and body superficially and usually gather near the joints and bones, some of which enter the chest cavity, but do not connect with the viscera. Their distribution is almost the same as that of the twelve meridians on the body surface, but their trends are not entirely the same. The three yang meridians of the hand and foot are distributed over the lateral aspect of the trunk; those of the three yin meridians of the hand and foot, the medial aspect of the trunk, some of them even enter the thoracic and abdominal cavities.

The following describes their distribution:

a. The musculofascia meridian of foot-*taiyang* starts from the small toe, ascends to the external malleolus, and descends obliquely to gather at the knee. Its lower section runs along the external malleolus and gathers at the heel, and runs upwardly along the Achilles bursa tendon to the popliteal fossa. Its minor section gathers at the calf, ascends along the medial aspect of the popliteal fossa, coincides with another branch, gathers at the buttock and ascends along the vertebral column to reach the nape; its vertical section gathers at the occipital bone, ascends to reach the vertex, descends from the forehead and gathers at the nose; the branch forms in the upper eyelids and descends to gather near the nose. Its branch at the back gathers at acromin from the lateral aspect of the posterior axilla; another branch enters into the area below the axilla then upwardly runs out of the supraclavica and then gathers at the mastoid process of the temporal bone. A tertiary branch splits from the above-mentioned branch from the supraclavicular fossa, ascends obliquely to gather near the nose (Fig. 29).

Symptoms: Swelling and pain radiating from the small toe; spasm in the hollow of the knee; tension and spasm of the muscles of the back and neck; inability to lift the arm; boring pain between the axilla and the supraclavicular fossa that prevents the patient from moving the arm.

b. The musculofascia meridian of foot-*shaoyang* starts from the fourth toe, ascends to gather at the external malleolus, runs upward along the lateral border of the tibia and gathers at the lateral aspect of the knee. Its section starts from the fibula and runs upward along the lateral aspect of the thigh, the frontal section of which ends at *futu*[6] and the posterior section of which connects with the sacral region. The vertical section passes through the hypochondriar region, runs upward along the anterior border of the axilla, connects with the lateral chest and breast and ties with the supraclavicular fossa. The vertical section emerges upwardly from the axilla, passes through the supraclavicular fossa, runs in front of the musculofascia meridian of *taiyang*, ascends to reach the corner of the forehead along the posterior ear, joins at the vertex, then runs back to descend to the mandibular region and then descends to end near the nose. The section gathers at the outer canthus (Fig. 30).

Symptoms: Clonic spasm, tenseness, or stiffness in the muscle regions touched by the meridians, especially in the fourth toe, the knee, the upper leg, the glutei, the bow of the ribs, the pectoral muscles and the neck. The chiasma of the musculofascia meridian on the parietal bone is responsible for a crosswise combination of symptoms of the parallel meridians, e.g., paresis of the left eyelid and pain in the right musculofascia meridian.

c. The musculofascia meridian of foot-*yangming*: Starts from the second and third toes and spreads at the dorsal foot, turns obliquely to cover the fibula, ascends to join the lateral aspect of the knee and the great trochanter region and then descends along the hypochondriac region to connect with the vertebral column. The vertical section ascends along the tibia and knots at the knee. Its section reaches the fibula region and coincides with that of foot-*shaoyang*. The vertical section ascends along *futu*, spreads in front of the femur, gathers at the pubic region, ascends to distribute itself over the abdomen, distributes near the nose, while the lower section knots at the nose, the upper portion of which coincides with that of the foot-*yangming* meridians, connects with the lower eyelids (Fig. 31). The section runs through the cheek and gathers in front of the ear.

Symptoms: Spasmotic pain, twitchings, pareses and paralysis in the region touched by the musculofascia meridian, especially radiating from the third toe in the direction of the tibia, on the dorsum of the foot, in the anterior femeral region, on the gluteus maximus and from the abdominal wall through the supraclavicular fossa up to the cheek. If the muscles of the cheek are implicated, distorted mouth and inability to open or to close the eyes; oozing tumours on the genitals may be seen.

d. The musculofascia meridian of foot-*taiyin*: Starts from the tip of the medial aspect of the big toe and ascends to gather at the malleolus; the vertical portion connects with the medial aspect of the malleolus of the tibia, ascends along the medial aspect of the thigh, gathers in front of the femur, gathers at the pubic region ascends to reach the abdomen, to the umbilicus, passes through the abdomen, the rib and merges into the chest. The section inside the body appends to the vertebral column (Fig. 32).

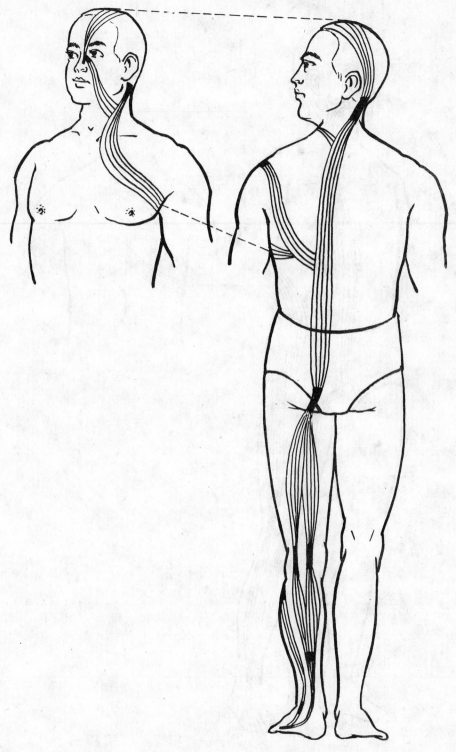

Fig. 29.   Musculofascia Meridian of Foot-*taiyang*

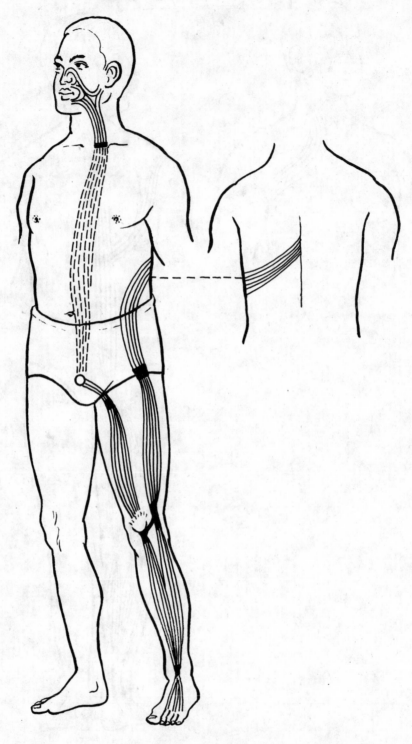

Fig. 30.　The Musculofascia Meridian of Foot-*shaoyang*

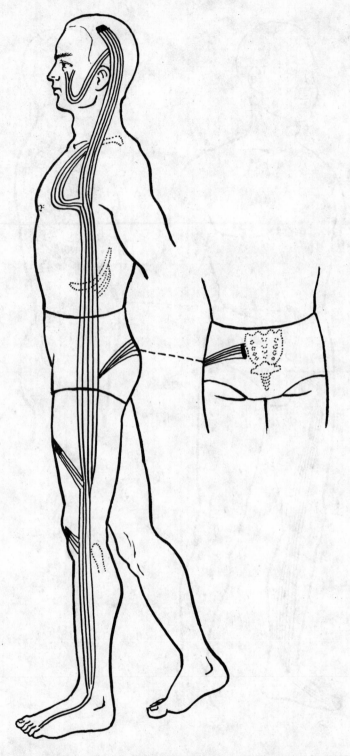

Fig. 31.   The Musculofascia Meridian of Foot-*yangming*

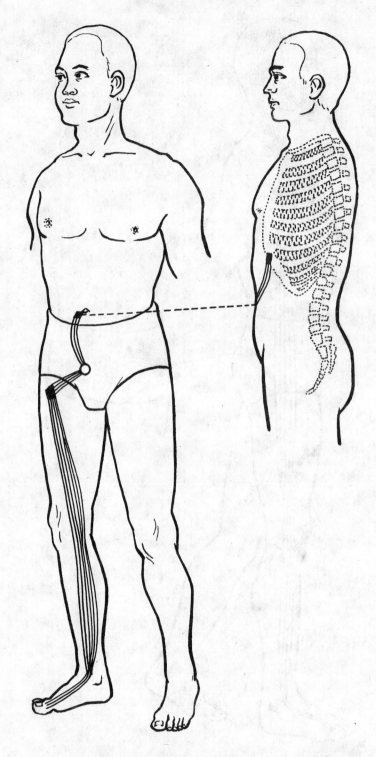

Fig. 32.   The Musculofascia Meridian of Foot-*taiyin*

Symptoms: Pain and spasm radiating from the big toe towards the malleolus; pain in the condyle of the medial tibia; pain radiating forward and upward from the internal femeral region; pain in the genitals radiating upward toward the navel; cutaneous pain in the thorax and spine.

e. The musculofascia meridian of foot-*shaoyin*: Starts from the interior aspect of the small toe, coincides with and runs obliquely along that of the foot-*taiyin* meridian along the area below the lateral aspect of malleolus, gathers at the root of the foot, joins that of the foot-*taiyang* meridian, ascends to the area below the medial aspect of the malleolus, runs along the medial aspect of the thigh, gathers at the pubic region, runs inside and along the vertebral column, ascends to reach the vertex, gathers at the occipital bone and meets foot-*taiyang* (Fig. 33).

Symptoms: Spasms and twitching in all regions (especially the lower extremities) touched by the musculofascia meridian. Spasmotic paralysis, contortions, atrophy and general symptoms associated with this meridian are that the extremity or the body cannot bend forward on the side opposite the one affected. There is an unfavourable prognosis if the recurrence of spasm in the region touched by this meridian is too violent or too frequent.

f. The musculofascia meridian of foot-*jueyin*: Starts dorsally from the tip of the big toe, ascends and spreads out before the internal malleolus, ascends along the tibia and below the internal malleolus of the tibia, runs upward along the tibia, then to the hypochondyle of the tibia, to the pubic region and finally connects with various musculofascia meridians (Fig. 34).

Symptoms: Pain radiating from the big toe towards the medial malleolus, pain in the condyle of the medial tibia; pain and spasm in the internal femeral region; impotence.

g. The musculofascia meridian of hand-*taiyang* originates dorsally on the tip of the small finger, gathers at the arm, spreads behind the epicondyle of the humerus, enters and combines with the inferior aspect of the axilla. One of its sections runs back to pass through the posterolateral axilla, ascends to curve around the scapula and merges obliquely from the anterior musculofascia meridian of *taiyang* and to the mastoid process of the temporal bone (Fig. 35).

Symptoms: Pain in parts of the arm supplied by the musculofascia meridian; ringing and pain in the ear, pain radiating from the ear towards the mandible; dim eyesight remedied only by closing the eyes for a while; tensions in the muscles of the neck; carbuncle on the neck.

h. The musculofascia meridian of hand-*shaoyang*: Starts from the tip of the ring finger, distributes at the dorsal wrist, ascends along the forearm to spread around the elbow, ascends and curves around the lateral forearm to reach the shoulder, runs to the neck and finally meets that of hand-*taiyang*. One of its sections enters the corner of the mandibular region and connects with the root of the tongue. The other ascends from the corner of the mandible, runs in front of the ear to connect with the outer canthus, ascends to reach the forehead and knots at the corner of the forehead (Fig. 36).

Symptoms: Tension and spasm in the regions served by this musculofascia meridian; spastic rolling of the tongue.

i. The musculofascia meridian of hand-*yangming*: Starts from the tip of the index finger, connects with the dorsal wrist, ascends along the forearm and joins the lateral aspect of the elbow, runs up the forearm and joins the lateral aspect of the upper arm,

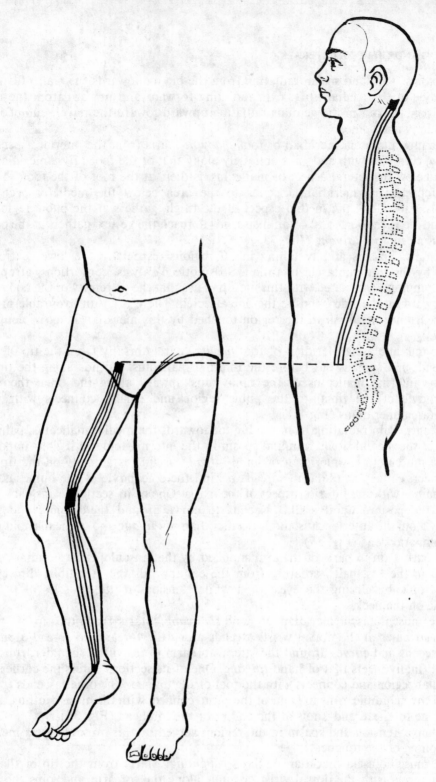

Fig. 33.   The Musculofascia Meridian of Foot-*shaoyin*

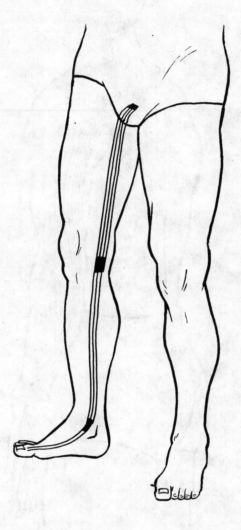

Fig. 34.   The Musculofascia Meridian of Foot-*jueyin*

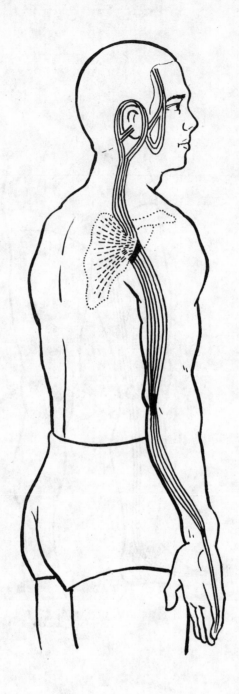

Fig. 35.　The Musculofascia Meridian of Hand-*taiyang*

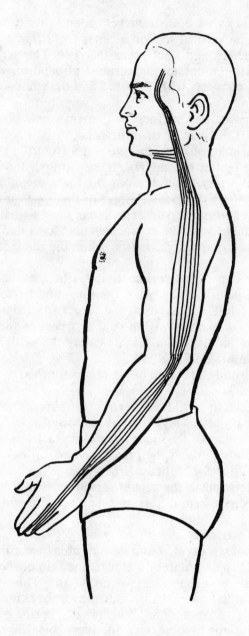

Fig. 36.　The Musculofascia Meridian of Hand-*shaoyang*

finally entering *Jianyu* (LI 15). Its branch curves around the scapular region and runs along the spinous column, the vertical section ascends from *Jianyu* (LI 15) to the neck; the branch ascends to the cheek and knots near the nose. The vertical branch ascends and emerges from the anterio-musculofascia meridian of hand-*taiyang*, ascends to reach the corner of the forehead, connects with the head and descends to the mandible on its opposite side (Fig. 37).

Symptoms: Twitching, spasm, and stiffness in the region touched by this musculofascia meridian. Inability to lift the arm or turn the head.

j. The musculofascia meridian of hand-*taiyin*: Starts from the superior aspect of the thumb, runs upward along it, ties behind *yiji*,[7] runs through the lateral aspect of the *cunkou* section of the radial artery, ascends along the forearm and gathers at the elbow; then it continues to ascend along the medial aspect of the upper arm, enters the inferior aspect of the axilla, emerges from the supraclavicular fossa and links with *Jianyu* (LI 15). Its upper portion combines with the supraclavicular fossa and its lower portion, in the chest, passes through the diaphragm, meets below the diaphragm and reaches the hypochondrium. (Fig. 38)

Symptoms: Pain and tension in the regions touched by the musculofascia meridian. In the case of violent pain, pleuritis, abscess of the lung, and hemoptysis may occur.

k. The musculofascia meridian of hand-*jueyin*: Starts from the middle finger, coincides with that of hand-*taiyin*, gathers at the medial aspect of the elbow, ascends and merges into the anteroposterior hypochondrium; enters the axilla, distributes over the chest and gathers at the diaphragm. (Fig. 39)

Symptoms: Feeling of tension and spasm of the region touched as pleuritis and phthisis must be expected.

l. The musculofascia meridian of hand-*shaoyin*: Starts from the medial aspect of the small finger, links with the processus styloidus ulnae posterior to the wrist, ascends and distributes over the medial aspect of the elbow, continues to ascend and enters the axilla, joins that of hand-*taiyin*, runs through the breast, gathers at the chest, descends to the diaphragm and connects with the umbilicus. (Fig. 40)

Symptoms: Tension and spasm in the region served by this musculofascia meridian; in severe cases, organic changes, hemoptysis, purulent sputum and poor prognosis must be expected.

5-4-4 Cutaneous areas of meridian

The skin surface of the body is divided into various areas according to the distribution of the twelve meridians and their collaterals. Hence, the skin of the body is divided into twelve areas, called twelve cutaneous areas of meridians. These areas are where the twelve meridians and their collaterals are distributed over the skin surface and where the *qi* in the twelve meridians is distributed. So, it aids in diagnosing pathological symptoms of certain viscera and meridians by observing the morphological change of the skin of the different locations. Pathological changes of the viscera are treated by administering such therapies as warming moxibustion, hot ironing, etc. at a certain place. This is the application of the theory of cutaneous areas of the meridians in diagnosis and treatment.

5-5 Physiology of meridians and application of the meridian theory

5-5-1 Physiological functions

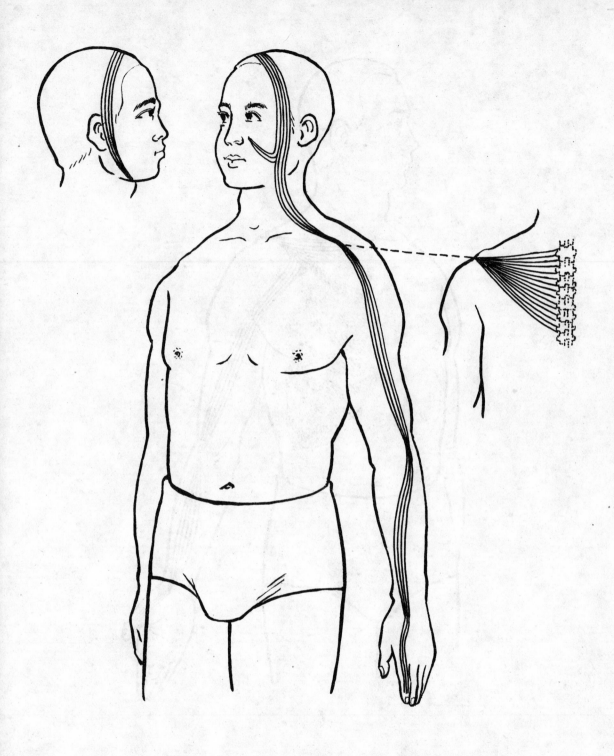

Fig. 37. The Musculofascia Meridian of Hand-*yangming*

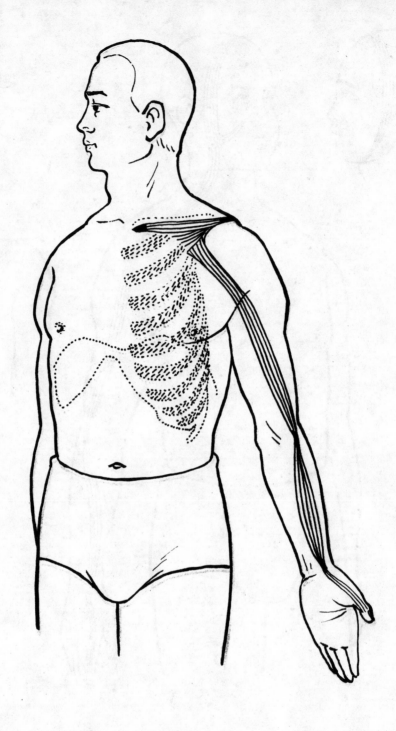

Fig. 38.　The Musculofascia Meridian of Hand-*taiyin*

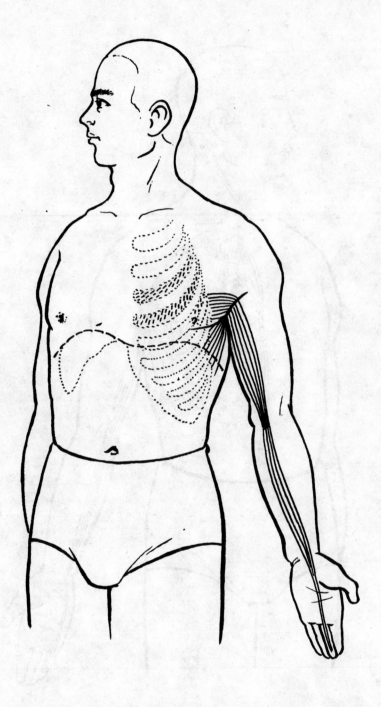

Fig. 39.   The Musculofascia Meridian of Hand-*jueyin*

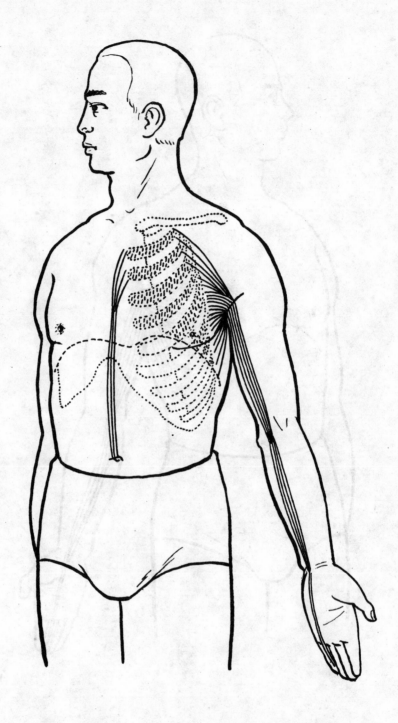

Fig. 40.   The Musculofascia Meridian of Hand-*shaoyin*

The functions of the meridians are called "meridian *qi*." Their physiological functions are chiefly to communicate the exterior of the body with the interior, the upper with the lower, to connect the viscera and organs, to promote *qi* and blood circulation, to nourish the viscera and tissues and to regulate the functions of various parts of the body.

5-5-1-1 Communicating the exterior of the body with the interior, the upper with the lower and connecting with the viscera and organs

The body consists of the five yin and six yang viscera, the four extremities, tissues, five sense organs[8] and nine openings, skin, muscles, vessels, tendons and bones. Although the meridians have different physiological functions, they jointly carry on their functions to keep the harmony of different parts of the body. This coordination is achieved by the communicating action of the meridians. Various viscera, tissues and organs are linked to form a unity of which the exterior and interior, upper and lower portions of the body are closely connected and intersupporting because the twelve meridians and their collateral meridians form a network that merges at the interior of the body and emerges from the exterior. It communicates the upper portion of the body with the lower and connects the viscera through the eight extra meridians and the twelve meridians, and the musculofascia and cutaneous areas of the twelve meridians connect tendons, vessels, skin and muscles. Here are the following connections through which the meridians connect the viscera, tissues and organs.

a. The connection between the viscera and limbs is established through the twelve meridians. Since the twelve meridians are connected with the five yin and six yang viscera, and their *qi* spreads to and accumulates in the musculofascia of the twelve meridians and distributes itself over the cutaneous areas of meridians, the skin, tendons, muscles and tissues connect with the viscera through the meridians.

b. The connection between the viscera, the five sense organs and nine openings: The eyes, ears, nose, mouth, tongue, external genital organs and anus are the areas where the meridians traverse, while the meridian connects internally with the viscera. The five sense organs and nine openings are thus connected with the viscera through the meridians. For example, the Heart Meridian of Hand-*shaoyin* pertains to the heart, connects with the small intestine and upwardly links with the "ocular connection," ascending to reach the tongue. The Liver Meridian of Foot-*jueyin* pertains to the liver, connects with the gallbladder and upwardly links with the "ocular connection." The Stomach Meridian of Foot-*yangming* pertains to the stomach, connects with the spleen and curves around the lips, etc.

c. The connection between the five yin and the six yang viscera: Each of the twelve meridians connects with and pertains to a yin or yang viscus respectively so that the connection between a related yin viscus or a yang viscus is strengthened. Some of the meridians connect with several viscera, e.g., the branch of the Stomach Meridian upwardly communicates with the heart; the Spleen Meridian merges into the heart; the branch of the Gallbladder Meridian passes through the heart; the Kidney Meridian merges from and connects with the heart; the Heart Meridian ascends to reach the lung; the Small Intestine Meridian reaches the stomach, the Liver Meridian runs along the stomach, the Lung Meridian passes through and runs along the openings of the stomach; the Kidney Meridian passes through the liver.

d. The connection between the meridians: The twelve meridians have a certain link and sequence of the flow of *qi* and blood. The criss-cross network of the twelve regular

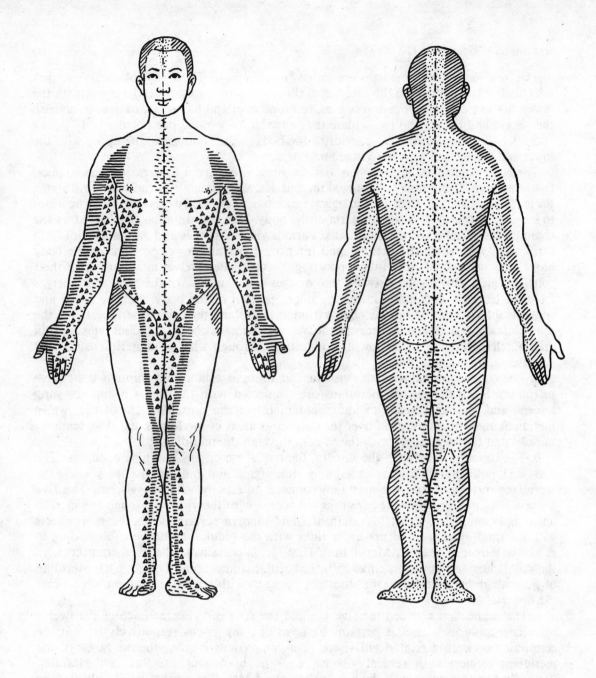

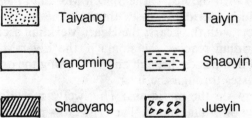

Taiyang   Taiyin

Yangming   Shaoyin

Shaoyang   Jueyin

Fig. 41.   The Subcutaneous Areas of the Six Meridians

meridians and eight extra meridians, and the interconnection of the eight extra meridians, form multiple connections among the meridians. For example, as the three yang meridians of the hand and foot all join at *Dazhui* (GV 14) of the Governor Vessel Meridian and the Mobility Vessel Meridian of Yang and the Governor Vessel Meridian meet at *Fengfu* (GV 16), the Governor Vessel Meridian is termed the "sea of yang Meridians." The three yin meridians of the foot and the Regulating Meridian of Yin and the Strategic Vessel Meridian among the eight extra meridians all meet at the Conception Vessel Meridian and the three yin meridians of the foot ascend to link with the three yin meridians of the hand. The Conception Vessel Meridian is said to be the "sea of yin meridians." As the Strategic Vessel Meridian coincides with the Conception Vessel Meridian in the chest, and the posterior branch communicates with the Governor Vessel Meridian and connects with the twelve meridians, it is called the "sea of the twelve meridians"; the Governor Vessel Meridian, the Conception Vessel Meridian and the Strategic Vessel Meridian all originate from the uterus.

5-5-1-2 Promoting *qi* and blood circulation and nourishing the viscera and tissues

All the tissues and organs of the body can maintain their normal physiological activities when nourished by *qi* and blood. But *qi* and blood rely on the meridians for their circulation in the body, so as to nourish the viscera, tissues and organs, and resist exogenous pathogenic factors and protect the body.

5-5-1-3 The inducing and conducting actions

The meridian system has the transmitting and conducting actions of sensation induced by acupuncture of other stimuli. The *deqi*[10] and *xingqi*[11] phenomena are manifestations of the transmitting and conducting actions of the meridians.

5-5-1-4 Regulating the balance

The meridian promotes *qi* and blood circulation and harmonizes yin and yang to keep a kinetic equilibrium in the body. When the person is ill, with symptoms of disharmony between *qi* and blood and a relative flourishing and decline of yin and yang, acupuncture and moxibustion may be applied to stimulate the meridian and bring its regulating action into play. In this way it can "purge the excess, tonify the deficiency and balance yin and yang." Experimental studies prove that puncturing certain acupoints of the meridian can regulate the functions of various viscera, i.e., the hyperfunctional one can be restrained and the hypofunctional one can be activated.

5-5-2 Application of the meridian theory

5-5-2-1 Pathological processes

Under normal physiological conditions, the meridian promotes *qi* and blood circulation through its transmitting and conducting actions. If disease occurs, it will become the pathway to transmit the pathogenic factor. As the five yin and six yang viscera communicate through the meridian, the meridian may become the pathway through which pathological processes of the viscera influence one another. For example, as the Liver Meridian of Foot-*jueyin* runs along the stomach and merges into the lung, liver trouble may invade the stomach and lung; because the Kidney Meridian of Foot-*shaoyin* enters the lung and connects with the heart, overflowing water due to a weak kidney may injure the heart and lung. In another example heart fire affecting the large intestine and *qi* obstruction in the yang viscera may disturb pulmonary *qi*, resulting in asthmatic breath, cough, fullness in the chest, etc.

The meridian is not only a pathway through which an exogenous pathogenic factor invades the body and pathological processes of the five yin and six yang viscera influence one another, but one through which the pathological processes of the viscera and tissues on the body surface influence each other. The pathological change of the viscera may reflect itself on the body surface and manifest itself at certain locations or at its corresponding sense organs. For instance, distension and pain in the hypochondria and lower abdomen are frequently seen in the pattern of stagnant liver *qi* because the Liver Meridian of Foot-*jueyin* reaches the lower abdomen and distributes itself over the hypochondria; real cardiac pain (angina pectoris) is not only manifest in a precordia pain, but frequently radiates to the ulnar border of the medial aspect of the limbs because the Heart Meridian of Hand-*shaoyin* runs through the posterior border of the medial aspect of the upper limb. In another example, swollen eyes are ascribed to blazing liver fire. All are reactions conducted by the meridian.

5-5-2-2 Guiding diagnosis and treatment

a. Guiding diagnosis: Since a meridian has a certain course, connects with and pertains to a certain viscus and reflects diseases or syndromes of the viscus it pertains to, it may be regarded as the evidence for diagnosis of disease according to the area where the symptoms of disease appear in combination with the area it traverses and the viscus it connects with. For example, pain in the supraclavicular fossa is often ascribed to a pathological process of the lung. Again, as for headache, pain in the forehead is usually concerned with the *yangming* meridian; bilateral headache, the *shaoyang* meridian; pain in the occipital region and nape, the *taiyang* meridian; pain in the vertex, the *jueyin* meridian. Identification of syndromes with the names of the six meridians in *Treatise on Febrile Diseases* is a syndrome-identification system that developed on the basis of the meridian theory. Marked tenderness or certain morphological changes in the skin can be found in the area where the meridian traverses or in certain acupoints where *qi* in the meridian gathers. This also aids in diagnosing a disease. For instance, when the lung is affected, a nodule may appear at *Feishu* (B 13). With an intestinal carbuncle[12] tenderness may be found in the acupoint *Lanwei*; in patients with prolonged dyspnea, abnormal changes may be seen at *Pishu* (B 20), etc.

b. Guiding clinical treatment: The meridian theory has been widely applied in the treatment of various clinical specialities, particularly those of acupuncture, moxibustion, massage and drugs.

Acupuncture and massage treatments chiefly include the selection of acupoints from the area proximal to the pathological changes and distal along the course of the meridian. In this way the pathological change of a certain meridian or viscus can be treated, and the functions of the meridian, *qi* and blood regulated. But, before the selection of the acupoint, the syndromes must first of all, be identified according to the meridian theory, and acupoints selected according to the course of the meridian after ascertaining which meridian the disease pertains to. This is the selection of acupoints of the corresponding meridian.

As for drug treatment, drugs can reach the affected area only via the meridian that transports them. Medical experts in ancient times established the theory of "meridian-tropism[13] of a drug" according to the special action of certain drugs to certain viscera. Zhang Jiegu and Li Gao, medical specialists of the Jin and Yuan dynasties (1115-1368) put forward the "drug-guidance" theory, e.g., for headache due to the affected meridian of *yangming*. Notopterygium incisium may be prescribed, for that due to the affected meridian of *yangming*, radix angelicae, for that due to the affected meridian of *shaoyang*, radix bupleuri.

In addition, therapies, such as acupuncture anesthesia, ear acupuncture, electro-acupuncture, suture-embedment and suture therapy which are popularly used in clinic at present were developed under the guidance of the meridian theory with success. These therapies, in turn, further develop the meridian theory.

Notes

[1.] Chinese deep-breathing exercises: a system of exercises for physical fitness and the treatment of diseases by deep-breathing and conscious mind control in order to tranquillize mental activities, in combination with the harmonious and slow movements of the limbs and trunk.

[2.] The location at both wrists, medial to the head of the radius, where pulse diagnosis is performed.

[3.] The boundary between whitish and pinkish coloured skin.

[4.] The large blood vessels directly connected to the heart.

[5.] The structure connecting the eyeball with the brain.

[6.] The most prominent portion of the muscles on the anterior aspect of the thigh when the knee is extended. It is so called because it looks like a rabbit in the sitting position; the name of the acupoint, located in the centre of *futu*.

[7.] The edge of the prominence of the palm proximal to the thumb or that of the sole proximal to the big toe; the name of the acupoint situated at the midpoint of the boundary between the skin of darker colour and that of lighter colour of the thenar eminence of the hand.

[8.] A collective term for eyes, ears, nose, tongue and mouth.

[9.] Eyes, ears, nostril, mouth, urethral meatus and anus.

[10.] Needling sensation During acupuncture, the patient may feel soreness, numbness, distension, heaviness, etc. and the acupuncture doctor may feel a heavy and tense reaction while needling. It is also called "acquiring *qi*."

[11.] Promoting the circulation of *qi* in the meridian.

[12.] Acute suppurative inflammation of the intestines.

[13.] The theory which explains the action of drugs to the viscera, meridians and various parts of the body.

6. THE CAUSE OF DISEASE

There are various pathological factors such as abnormal weather change, pestilential infection, mental irritation, improper diet, fatigue and lack of physical exercise, injuries from falls and heavy lifting, fractures, sprains and strains, wounds, insect or animal bites, etc. All of these may lead to disease. The effect of a certain pathological stage may become the cause of another, e.g., *tan-yin* (phlegm and excess exudates) and congealed blood are not only formed due to the dysfunction of the viscera, *qi* and blood but are also pathogenic factors of a pathological process.

6-1 The cause of disease

Disease is mainly caused by the "six excesses",[1] pestilence, the "seven emotions,"[2] improper diet, fatigue and lack of physical exercise, traumatic wound, insect or animal bites, etc. Ancient medical experts classified them to explain their characteristics. For example, *Internal Classic* classified them into yin and yang categories. In his *Synopsis of the Golden Bookcase*, Zhang Zhongjing of the Han Dynasty (206 to 220) pointed out that there were several ways for disease to occur, i.e., when a pathogenic factor invades the meridian and further invades the viscera, infection of the skin, and injuries from excess sexual activity, wounds, insect or animal bites.

TCM holds that there is no pathological symptom without any cause. TCM diagnosis mainly depends upon analysing the symptoms to determine the application of drugs in treatment, and understand pathogenic factors.

6-1-1 The six excesses

"Six excesses" is a general term for six exogenous pathogenic factors; wind, cold, summer-heat, damp, dryness and fire (heat). They are called the "six *qi*," and represent climatic changes. They are the conditions for general growth and normally do not harm the body. Man lives by relying on air, water and food, and adapts according to seasonal changes. When people recognize the changes in their life and adapt to them, the six climatic factors do not affect them so much. When weather changes abnormally (e.g., abnormal cold in warm spring, abnormal heat in cool autumn, etc.) or too rapidly and the body resistance is weak, weather can become a pathogenic factor and invade the body, causing disease. Under such circumstances, climatic factors are called the "six excesses," and are also termed the "six evils," which belong to the category of exogenous pathogenic factors.

The characteristics of the six excesses in causing disease:

a. Disease is often related to the weather, seasons and geographical environment. For example wind disease usually occurs in the spring; summer-heat disease, in the summer; damp disease, in the late summer and early autumn; dryness, in the late autumn; cold disease in the winter, etc. Pathogenic damp usually causes disease due to prolonged living in a humid place, and dry heat or fire (heat) usually causes disease due to working or living at a place with a high temperature, etc.

b. The six excesses may invade the body and cause disease, for example, wind-cold, cold, damp-heat, diarrhea or *bi* (block) syndrome due to pathogenic wind-cold-damp, etc.

c. The six excesses not only influence one another, but also change into each other under certain conditions, e.g., pathogenic cold may invade the deep part of the body and transform itself into pernicious heat; prolonged pathogenic summer-heat and damp may injure the yin of the body after transforming into pathogenic dryness, etc.

d. In the course of disease caused by the six excesses, the body surface, or mouth and nose may be invaded. The six exogenous pathogenic factors include pathological reactions caused by a variety of pathogenic factors, such as bacteria, and viruses, physical and chemical factors and climatic factors.

In addition, there are other pathological reactions which generate wind, cold, damp, heat and fire that are not caused by the six excesses, but by the dysfunction of the viscera. They do not belong to the category of exogenous pathogenic factors, but to production of the five endogenous pathogenic factors, although their symptoms may resemble the symptoms of the six exogenous pathogenic factors.

6-1-1-1 Wind occurs chiefly in spring but may appear in every season

Diseases caused by pathogenic wind occur more frequently, and are not limited to the spring. TCM asserts that pathogenic wind is an important pathogen which leads to exogenous febrile diseases.

Pathogenic wind usually invades the body from its surface and the junction between the skin and muscle, causing an exogenous wind disease.

The features of pathogenic wind and how it causes disease are as follows:

a. Pathogenic wind is yang in nature and is characterized by an upward and outgoing dispersion, usually invading the yang (upper portion of the body). As it is moving and ascending, spreading, outgoing and dispersing, it belongs to the yang pathogen, and often injures the upper portion (head and face) of the body, yang meridians, and body surface, and opens the junction between the skin and muscles. Headache, perspiration, aversion to wind, etc. are often seen.

b. Occurring in gusts and characterized by an indefinite disease location and tending to move incessantly. For example, in the *bi* syndrome caused by pathogenic wind-cold-damp, wandering arthralgia is a manifestation of pathogenic wind. Repeated rashes characterized by itching has similar features. Exogenous febrile diseases caused mainly by pathogenic wind usually attack the body suddenly and progress rapidly.

c. Wind is the chief pathogen that causes hundreds of diseases: Pathogenic wind is the major factor among the six climatic factors. Pathogenic cold, damp, dryness and heat usually invade the body in association with pathogenic wind, e.g., exogenous wind-cold, wind-heat and wind-damp, etc. The ancients even regarded pathogenic wind as a general term for all exogenous factors.

6-1-1-2 Cold

In winter, the body is likely to be invaded by cold as the temperature falls rapidly. In addition, getting drenched by rain, wading, or exposure to wind when sweating can also cause a cold.

Cold affection is divided into exogenous cold and endogenous cold. The former refers to the external invasion of pathogenic cold and the disease caused by it is subdivided into "cold injury" and "pathogenic cold attack." It is called cold injury because pathogenic cold injures the body surface and obstructs defensive yang *qi*, pathogenic cold attack means that the pathogenic factor attacks the interior of the body directly and injures the yang *qi* of the viscera. Endogenous cold is a pathological reaction of insufficient yang *qi* leading to hypofunction of the body. Although exogenous cold differs from endogenous cold, they influence each other. A body with deficient yang *qi* and endogenous cold is easily affected by exogenous cold, while exogenous cold stagnating for a long time often impairs yang *qi* and produces endogenous cold.

The features of pathogenic cold and how it causes disease are as follows:

a. Pathogenic cold, which is a yin pathogen, easily consumes yang *qi*. As cold is a manifestation of excess yin *qi*, it is yin in nature, i.e., "an excess of yin causing cold." Originally yang *qi* may restrain yin. If yin cold is in relative excess, the yang *qi* not only fails to expel pathogenic yin cold, but it is counteracted by yin cold. It is therefore called "an excess of yin causing yang disease." If yang *qi* is consumed and its warming action lost, the cold syndrome of hypofunction may appear. If exogenous cold invades the body surface and defensive yang *qi* is blocked, creeping chills would be seen. If pathogenic cold directly attacks the spleen, chills would be seen. If pathogenic cold directly attacks the spleen and stomach and spleen yang is consumed, cold and pain in the epigastrium and abdomen, vomiting and diarrhea may occur. If heart yang and kidney yang are deficient and pathogenic cold attacks the *shaoyin* meridian, creeping chills, cold clammy extremities, diarrhea with undigested food, profuse watery urine, restlessness, faint minute pulse, etc. may appear.

b. Cold is characterized by stagnation: Normal circulation of *qi* and blood in the body fully depends upon the warmth and promotion of yang *qi*. Whenever pathogenic yin cold is in relative excess and yang *qi* is consumed, *qi* and blood will be blocked, resulting in pain. Thus, pain will frequently occur when pathogenic cold affects the body.

c. Cold is characterized by contraction: The invasion of pathogenic cold may cause stagnation of the *qi* mechanism with contraction and spasm of the junction between the skin and muscle, meridians, fascia and vessels. If pathogenic cold invades the body surface, the pores and the junction will be blocked, and if defensive yang *qi* fails to spread, chills and fever may occur. If pathogenic cold stagnates in the meridians and joints and the meridians are rigid and contracted, difficulty extending and flexing the trunk and limbs or cold clammy limbs and trunk may result.

6-1-1-3 Summer-heat

It is generated by fire (intense heat). Summer heat mainly occurs between the Summer Solstice[3] and the Beginning of Autumn[4]. Pathogenic summer-heat is an exogenous pathogenic factor and there is no endogenous summer-heat.

The features of pathogenic summer-heat and how it causes disease are as follows:

a. Summer-heat is a yang pathogen. Summer-heat is generated from summer fire (intense heat). As fire pertains to yang, summer-heat is yang in nature. A series of yang heat symptoms, such as strong fever,[5] anxiety, flushed face and full, large pulse, etc. appear when summer-heat injures the body.

b. Summer-heat is characterized by ascendance and dispersion, and consumes *qi* and body fluids. Pathogenic summer-heat is ascending and flourishing and can cause the junction between the skin and muscle to open and hyperhidrosis. Hyperhidrosis can lead to consumption of body fluids causing thirst, scanty dark-red urine, etc. If pathogenic summer-heat disturbs the Mind, it can cause anxiety and restlessness. *Qi* is likely to be excreted together with body fluids when hyperhidrosis occurs, resulting in *qi* deficiency. So, patients affected by pathogenic summer-heat usually suffer from short breath and general weakness, even sudden fainting and unconsciousness.

c. Summer-heat is often associated with damp: In summer it is hot, rainy and wet. Hence, pathogenic summer-heat frequently causes diseases involving pathogenic damp, characterized by symptoms of damp obstruction at the four extremities, chest distress, vomiting, loose stools or difficulty in bowel movements, etc. besides symptoms of summer-heat, such as fever, polydipsia, etc.

6-1-1-4 Damp

Pathogenic damp is prevalent in late summer. At the junction between the summer and autumn, yang heat decreases, aqueous *qi* increases and damp prevails. It is the time of the year when damp flourishes most. Pathogenic damp that causes disease is divided into exogenous invasion of damp, such as humid weather, wading or being rain-drenched, or prolonged living in a damp place, etc. The latter is a pathological function which leads to stagnant aqueous damp. Both of them influence each other in the course of disease although they are different. Injury by exogenous damp, obstruction of the spleen by pathogenic damp and the spleen's failure to perform its transporting function are likely to form endogenous damp make the body vulnerable to the invasion of exogenous damp.

The features of pathogenic damp and how it causes disease are as follows:

a. Damp is characterized by heaviness and turbidity. Damp affection may often cause a sensation of heaviness and distension of the head, systemic lassitude, sores and heaviness of the four extremities. Retention of pathogenic damp in the meridians and joints can lead to the obstruction of yang *qi* in its distribution, with numb skin, pain and heaviness in the joints, etc. It is also known as "damp *bi*"[6] or "stagnant *bi*"[7] syndrome. Pathogenic damp can also cause the disease manifested by ocular excreta, loose stools, diarrhea with mucoid fluid and purulent blood, cloudy urine, profuse leukorrhea and eczema that diffuses with escaping liquids, etc. All of them are pathological reactions of pathogenic damp characterized by turbidity.

b. Pathogenic damp, a yin pathogen is likely to obstruct *qi* and consume yang *qi*. As damp is heavy and turbid, and similar to water in nature, it is a yin pathogen. When pathogenic damp is retained in the viscera and meridians, it is most likely to obstruct *qi*, so that the *qi* ascends and descends abnormally and the meridian is blocked with chest distress, distension of the epigastrium, scanty urine, difficult bowel movements, etc. As damp is a yin pathogen and exogenous yin causes a yang disease, it is most likely to consume yang *qi* when invading the body. Since the spleen corresponds to yin earth, it is the chief yin viscus in transporting aqueous damp. Furthermore, it likes dryness, but not humidity. Exogenous pathogenic damp retained within the body often first obstructs the spleen and makes it inactive in transporting and digesting food so that aqueous damp stagnates, resulting in diarrhea, oliguria, edema, ascites, etc.

c. Damp characterized by viscosity and stagnation is chiefly manifested in: a) The symptom of damp disease is usually viscous and stagnant, e.g., the excreta are usually stagnant and obstructed; b) a damp disease is usually prolonged and difficult to cure, with a prolonged course or recurrent onset, e.g., damp *bi* syndrome, eczema, damp-warm disease,[8] etc.

d. Damp tends to descend and invade the yin portion of the body. The symptoms of damp disease commonly occur in the lower limbs. In addition, gonorrhea, leukorrhea and diarrhea are frequently caused by a downward attack of pathogenic damp.

6-1-1-5 Dryness

Pathogenic dryness prevails in the autumn. Exogenous dryness usually invades the lung via the mouth and nose. It is divided into warm dry and cool dry. Summer *qi* remains hot and pathogenic dryness and warmth (mild heat) invade the body jointly in early autumn. Therefore, a dry-warm disease (or syndrome)[9] is frequently seen in that season. As there is pathogenic cold in late autumn and early winter, pathogenic dryness and cold combine to invade the body, and a dry-cool disease sometimes appears.

The features of pathogenic dryness and how it causes disease are as follows:

a. Pathogenic dryness consumes body fluids, forming the pathological state of deficient body fluids, with dry mouth and nose, dry throat and thirst, dry or even chapped skin, withered hair, scanty urine, constipation, etc.

b. Pathogenic dryness is likely to injure the lung because the lung is a delicate viscus and tends to favour moisture not dryness. It controls respiration and communicates directly with the atmosphere.

Since it corresponds externally to skin and hair and opens to the nose, pathogenic dryness usually invades the body via the mouth and nose. Thus body fluids are likely to be consumed, and the dispersing, clearing and descending functions affected, resulting in dry cough and less sputum, or mucoid sputum difficult to expectorate or blood streaked sputum, asthmatic breath, thoracalgia, etc.

6-1-1-6 Fire (intense heat)

Fire and heat are produced by excessive yang. However they have somewhat different characteristics. Warmth, heat and fire have different intensities. Warmth is milder than heat, whereas fire is more intense than heat. Pathogenic heat usually involves the body in a combination of factors, such as wind-heat, summer-heat and damp-heat from outside, whereas fire is often generated internally, e.g., pathological changes such as blazing heart fire, overactive liver fire, wild gallbladder fire, etc.

The diseases caused by pathogenic fire (heat) are divided into the external affections usually due to the direct invasion of pathogenic warmth and heat, whereas the internal affections due to the disharmony between the viscera, yin and yang, *qi* and blood and excess yang *qi*. In addition, the so-called affection of pathogenic wind, cold, summer-heat, damp and dryness or mental irritation, i.e., "five extreme emotions"[11] can also be transformed into fire under certain circumstances.

The features of pathogenic fire and how it causes disease are as follows:

a. Fire (heat) is a yang pathogen characterized by flaring up. As yang embodies restlessness and ascendance, and fire is flaring up in nature, when fire (heat) injures the body, it usually causes high fever, aversion to heat, polydipsia, perspiration, full and frequent pulse, etc. As it flares up, it may often disturb the Mind, resulting in anxiety and insomnia, restlessness, mental confusion and even delirium, etc. *Plain Questions* states, "Anxiety and mania are due to pernicious heat." A fire (heat) disease or syndrome is usually manifested in the upper portion of the body and the head and face.

b. Pathogenic fire is likely to consume body fluids. Pathogenic fire (heat) tends to squeeze fluids outside and consumes yin fluid. Therefore, the affection of pathogenic fire (heat) is frequently accompanied by symptoms of consumed body fluids, thirst and indulgence in drinking, dry throat, and tongue, dark-red urine, constipation, as well as other heat signs.

Plain Questions points out: "Strong fever impairs *qi*." Vigorous fire can severely impair the body's anti-pathogenic factors, resulting in systemic hypofunction.

c. Pathogenic fire is likely to generate internal wind and cause hemorrhage. When invading the body, pathogenic fire (heat) usually impairs the Liver Meridian, consumes yin fluid and deprives the tendons and vessels of nourishment. It also causes the internal movement of liver wind, called "extreme heat generating pernicious wind" manifested by high fever, mental confusion, delirium, convulsions of the four extremities, upward fixation of the eye, stiff neck, opisthotonos, etc. *Plain Questions* states, "febrile unconsciousness and convulsions are due to fire." At the same time, pathogenic fire (heat) can accelerate blood circulation, impair the vessels, even make blood extravasate, resulting in various hemorrhages, such as epistaxis, bloody stool, hematuria, skin eruptions, metrorrhagia, menorrhagia, hematemesis, etc.

d. Pathogenic fire is likely to cause skin infections. When pathogenic fire (heat) enters *xue* (blood) it can accumulate locally, and cause skin infections. Syndromes of red, swollen, protruding, burning sores pertain to yang and are ascribed to fire.

In addition, as fire (heat) corresponds to the heart, and the latter controls blood and vessels and stores the Mind, excess fire can result in hot or rapidly moving blood, mental restlessness, polydipsia, or delirium and mania, or coma due to pathogenic fire disturbing the heart.

6-1-2 Pestilential factors

Pestilential factors are highly infectious pathogens. In TCM literature, they are also termed *wen-yu, li-qi, lei-qi, yi-qi, du-qi, gui-lei, zhi-qi*, etc.

Pestilential factors are characterized by a rapid onset of a critical disease, severe infection, and are highly contagious.

They may cause disease in local areas, as well as over large parts of the body, e.g., the grand pestilence of head, swelling cheek, epidemic toxic dysentery, diphtheria, scarlet fever, smallpox, cholera, plague, etc., as well as other infectious diseases.

The occurrence and prevalence of pestilential factors are usually related to the following factors:

a. Climatic factors: Abnormal weather changes, e.g., prolonged drought, hot summer, mountainous plague, etc.

b. Environment and diet, e.g., polluted air, water or food.

c. Delayed prevention and isolation.

d. Social influence: Public health programs have helped control severe infectious diseases, such as plague, smallpox, etc.

6-1-3 Internal injuries by the seven emotions

Joy, anger, melancholy, meditation, grief, fear and fright are seven emotional changes, pertaining to mental pathogenic factors. They are the different reactions of the body to a stimulus. Under normal circumstances, they do not cause disease. Only when a sudden, strong or prolonged mental irritation exceeds the range of normal physiological activities is the *qi* disturbed; the viscera, yin and yang *qi* and blood are in disharmony and disease can occur.

6-1-3-1 Relation between the seven emotions and *qi* and blood in the viscera

The emotions are closely related to the viscera, while the functional activities of the viscera mainly rely on warmth, promotion by *qi* and nourishment by blood. Emotional changes influence different viscera, *qi* and blood. For example, *Plain Questions* states,

"Excess blood leads to anger while deficient blood gives rise to fright." *Miraculous Pivot* states, "deficiency of liver *qi* leads to fear, while excess heart *qi* is followed by persistent laugh."

6-1-3-2 Characteristics of the seven emotions and disease mechanism

The seven emotions differ from the six excesses. The latter invades the body via the skin, mouth and nose, with an external syndrome seen at the initial stage, while the corresponding viscera, cause *qi* and blood to be in disharmony, resulting in pathological problems.

a. Directly injuring the viscera: *Plain Questions* states, "Anger injures the liver," "Overjoy injures the heart," "Prolonged meditation injures the spleen," "Persisting melancholy injures the lung," and "Great fear injures the kidney." Different emotional irritations exert different influences upon various viscera.

A variety of emotional irritations are concerned with the heart. As the heart is the Chief of the five yin and six yang viscera, the impaired Mind (heart) may also affect other viscera. Depressed anger injures the liver and dysfunctional liver *qi* often invades the spleen and stomach, resulting in syndromes, such as disharmony between the liver and spleen and disharmony between the liver and stomach, etc.

The heart controls blood and stores the Mind. The liver stores blood and performs its dispersing and discharging functions and lies in the middle energizer, the pivot for ascendance and descendance of *qi* and blood. For these reasons, the disease or syndrome caused by the seven emotions is frequently seen in the heart, liver and spleen with some disharmony between *qi* and blood. For example, too much meditation often injures the heart and spleen, resulting in mental disorders, and the spleen's failure to function normally, etc. Depressed anger injures the liver and results in regurgitating *qi* accompanied by blood. Moreover, distension and pain in the hypochondria due to stagnant *qi* in the Liver Meridian, etc. may appear or *qi* and blood stagnate, resulting in hypochondriac pain, dysmenorrhea, amenorrhea, or abdominal masses. In addition, internal injuries by emotional factors may produce fire, i.e., "five emotions producing fire," resulting in symptoms, such as excess fire due to deficient yin or diseases of stagnation of pathogenic damp, food and sputum.

b. Influencing the viscera and *qi* mechanism: *Plain Questions* states, "Anger arousing ascending *qi*, joy inducing sluggish *qi*, excess sorrow dissipating *qi*, fear causing descending *qi*... fright causing disturbed *qi*... worry causing stagnant *qi*." "Anger arousing ascending *qi*" means that too much anger can make liver *qi* regurgitate together with blood, flushed face, or hematemesis, even sudden fainting.

"Joy inducing sluggish *qi*" includes tense emotion and sluggish heart *qi*. Under normal circumstances, joy can alleviate mental intensity and unobstruct nutritional *qi* and defensive *qi* and ease the Mind. But, overjoy can also make heart *qi* sluggish, and Spirit absent, resulting in absentmindedness, even loss of spirit, mania, etc.

"Excess sorrow dispersing *qi*" implies that melancholy can consume and depress lung *qi*.

"Fear causing descending *qi*" means that fear can weaken kidney *qi* and disperse *qi* with incontinence of urine and stools, or painful bones, atrophic *jue* syndrome and night emission due to consumed *jing* (vital principle).

"Fright causing disturbed *qi*" means that overthinking can frighten a person quite a lot.

"Worry causing stagnant *qi*" means that overthinking can injure the Mind and affect the spleen, leading to stagnant *qi*. It is thought that since "meditation" originates from the spleen and forms in the heart, too much thinking can not only impair the Mind, but also affect the spleen. Prolonged consumed blood and malnourished heart can lead to palpitation, amnesia, insomnia and dreaminess. A stagnant *qi* mechanism can lead to the spleen's failure to transport and digest food, resulting in dyspepsia, distension and fullness of the epigastrium, loose stool, etc.

c. Abnormal change of mood can aggravate or rapidly worsen the disease.

For example if a patient with a history of hypertension gets angry and liver yang suddenly becomes overactive, his or her blood pressure may rapidly increase and vertigo even sudden fainting, aphonia, hemiplegia and facial paralysis may be seen. Similarly a patient with heart disease can also become aggravated or rapidly worsened due to mood changes.

6-1-4 Improper diet, fatigue and lack of physical exercise

6-1-4-1 Improper diet

Improper diet, contaminated food or preference for certain food, often cause disease. Improper diet mainly injures the spleen and stomach, leading to an abnormal ascent and descent of spleen and stomach *qi*, and causing internal damp to stagnate and generate phlegm or produce pernicious heat or result in other diseases.

a. Overeating and hunger: It is advisable to take food regularly. Overeating or hunger often causes diseases. Hunger can lead to an insufficient *qi* and blood. If prolonged, *qi* and blood will decline and become deficient, resulting in disease. Insufficient *qi* and blood can produce weak anti-pathogenic factors, which are likely to be complicated by a secondary disease. Overeating can result in the inability of the spleen and stomach to digest, absorb and transport, leading to obstruction of food. This can injure the spleen and stomach, and produce epigastric distension and fullness, eructation, acid regurgitation, anorexia, vomiting and diarrhea, etc. Prolonged food retention may produce pernicious heat, while unripened, cold or cool food may injure the spleen and stomach and cause damp accumulation and generate phlegm; prolonged food retention in infants may also cause ganji[13] with hot palms and soles, anxiety and a tendency to cry, abdominal distension and fullness, yellow complexion, emaciation, etc. Constant overeating not only leads to dyspepsia but also affects *qi* and blood circulation and causes tendons and vessels to stagnate, resulting in dysentery or hemorrhoids. Overeating of rich food is likely to produce internal heat, even causing carbuncle, cellulitis, toxic sores, etc.

b. Contaminated food: Taking contaminated food may cause various gastrointestinal disorders, resulting in abdominal pain, vomiting, diarrhea, dysentery, etc. or disease due to parasites with abdominal pain, yellow complexion, emaciation, etc. If roundworm ascends to the bile duct, excruciating pain in the upper abdomen with intermittent attacks may appear, with vomiting, roundworms and cold clammy extremities. If erosive and toxic food is taken, poisoning symptoms, such as excruciating pain in the abdomen, vomiting, diarrhea, etc. may result and even coma or death may occur in severe cases.

c. Preference for certain food: A diet should be sensible so as to obtain the whole range of nutritional needs of the body. When extremely cold or hot food is taken or only certain food eaten, a disharmony between yin and yang due to malnutrition may result.

Preference for extremely cold or hot food: If unripened raw or cold food is overeaten, yang *qi* of the spleen and stomach may be injured, leading to internal cold and damp with pain, diarrhea, etc.; if pungent, warm, dry and hot food is taken excessively, pernicious heat can accumulate in the stomach and intestines, causing thirst, fullness, distension and pain in the abdomen, constipation or even hemorrhoids.

Preference for certain foods: The Spirit, *qi* and blood of the body are generated by the five tastes.[14] The five tastes correspond respectively to the five yin viscera. *Plain Questions* states, "Entering the stomach, the five-taste foods act upon the five yin viscera, i.e., sour food acts upon the liver; bitter food on the heart; sweet food on the spleen; pungent food on the lung; salty food on the kidney." If certain foods are taken for long periods of time, the viscera will become relatively hyperfunctional or even be impaired, causing various pathogenic changes. Thus, *Plain Questions* states, "Too much sour food can lead to excessive liver *qi* and exhausted spleen *qi*; too much salty food can lead to injury of bones, muscle atrophy, and restrained heart *qi*; too much sweet food can lead to asthmatic breath and restlessness, dull complexion and dysfunctional kidney *qi*; too much bitter food can lead to the spleen *qi* becoming dry, and retention of stomach *qi*; too much pungent food can lead to obstruction of the musculofascia meridians and impairment of the Spirit," and too much salty food can lead to dull complexion; too much bitter food to withered skin and dropping hair; too much pungent food to rigid vessels and withered nails; too much sour food to thickened skin and dry and thin lips; too much sweet food to painful bones and alopecia.

6-1-4-2 Fatigue and lack of physical exercise

Normal physical activity and exercise aid in circulating *qi* and blood and keeping healthy. Rest alleviates fatigue and restores mental and physical health. But, overwork, extreme fatigue for a long time, including excess physical labour, mental labour and sexual activity, or lack of physical exercise can cause illness.

a. Fatigue including overexertion, too much thinking and excessive sexual activity.

Overexertion: Prolonged overexertion can cause disease. Overexertion can consume *qi*. If prolonged, *qi* diminishes. This causes mental fatigue and emaciation.

Too much worry or thinking can injure the heart and spleen. Both may consume heart blood and injure spleen *qi*, resulting in palpitation, amnesia, insomnia, dreaminess due to malnourishment of the heart (Mind), dyspepsia, abdominal distension, loose stools, etc. due to the spleen's failure to carry on its transporting and digesting functions.

Excess sexual activity: The kidney stores *jing* (vital principle) which must not be excessively excreted. If sexual activity is too frequent, *jing* can be severely consumed, causing sore and weak loins and knees, vertigo and tinnitus, listlessness, sexual hypofunction or nocturnal emission, prospermia, even impotence, etc.

b. Lack of physical exercise: The body needs proper exercise every day so that *qi* and blood can circulate normally. If one does neither physical labour nor exercise, *qi* and blood will be obstructed, and the spleen and stomach will become hypofunctional, resulting in poor appetite, and general weakness and lassitude, low spirit, weak limbs and trunk, or puffiness, palpitation immediately after exertion, asthmatic breath and perspiration, etc. which may cause a secondary disease.

6-1-5 External injuries

External injuries include gunshot wounds, incised wounds, injuries from falls, fractures, sprains and strains, burns, scalds, frostbite, insect and animal bites, etc. They may cause congealed blood, swelling, pain and hemorrhage of the skin and muscles, or injuries of tendons, fractures and luxation. In severe cases, they may injure the internal organs, or result in hemorrhoae, leading to coma, convulsions, loss of yang and collapse, etc. Three examples are discussed in this section.

In mild cases of burns or scalds, the skin would be injured with congestion, swelling, hotness and pain in the affected areas, or blisters and excruciating pain; in severe cases, muscles, tendons and bones may be injured and analgesic, the vulnerary area may be leather-like or white or carbonized. In the most severe cases, as the vulnerary area is too large, there may appear anxiety, fever, dry mouth and thirst, oliguria, etc., and sometimes death due to excruciating pain, inward attack of toxic fire and evaporation or exudation of body fluids besides local symptoms.

Frostbite refers to injuries caused by cold temperatures, a common disease in north China. The lower the temperature and the longer the cold attack, the more severe the frostbite. In systemic frostbite, as pernicious cold is a yin pathogen and likely to consume yang *qi* and its warming action, and chills may appear, gradually lowering body temperature, pallor, with dark-purplish lips, tongue and nails, numbness, mental fatigue, or lethargy, faint breath and retarded and minute pulse. If not saved in time, the patient may die. Local frostbite usually occurs on the hands, feet, ear, tip of the nose and cheek. At the early stage, as the cold causes contraction in the affected area, the meridians (vessels) become spasmotic and *qi* and blood are obstructed, the warmth and nourishment of the local area are affected, leading to local pallor and numbness of the skin, even swelling, distension and dark-purplish, itching, painful and burning-hot skin, or blisters in varied shapes that are likely to become infected after rupture.

In mild cases of insect, snake and animal bites, the injury occurs locally, arousing swelling, pain and hemorrhage; in severe cases, an internal organ can be injured or death can follow due to hemorrhae. Snakebite may cause systemic poisonous symptoms. If not treated in time, death due to poisoning often results.

6-1-6 *Tan-yin* (phlegm and excess exudates) and congealed blood

Tan-yin and congealed blood are pathological products formed in the course of disease after the body is affected by pathogenic factors.

6-1-6-1 *Tan-yin*

Both *tan* (phlegm) and *yin* (excess exudates) are pathological products formed by abnormal water metabolism. In general, the greasy and turbid material is called *tan* and the thin and clear material, *yin*. The former not only refers to the sputum that is coughed up, but also includes *luo-li*,[15], phlegmatic nodules[16] and fluid that stagnate within the tissues, viscera, meridians etc. that cannot be seen, but determined through its clinical symptoms, therefore called "shapeless phlegm." *Yin* is the aqueous matter retained locally. It has different names because it is retained in different areas and varies with symptoms. For example, in *Synopsis of the Golden Bookcases*, *tan-yin*, *xian-yin*, *yi-yin*, *zhi-yin*, etc. are mentioned.

Formation: *tan-yin* is usually formed by the six excesses, improper diet or the seven emotions, etc. They cause dysfunction of the lung, spleen and kidney and once the water metabolism is obstructed, body fluids are retained. This is because the lung spleen, kidney and the triple energizer are related to water metabolism. The lung carries on its dispersing and descending functions, clears the water tract and distributes body fluids. The spleen transports and digests aqueous liquid, whereas the triple energizer is the passage for liquid. Therefore, a dysfunctional lung, spleen, kidney and triple energizer may cause damp to accumulate and generate *tan-yin*. After the formation of *tan-yin*, *yin* is usually retained and accumulated in the intestine and stomach, hypochondriac region and skin, while *tan* ascends and descends together with *qi*, runs to the viscera inwardly and tendons, bones, skin and muscles outwardly, forming various diseases or symptoms.

The characteristics of *tan-yin* diseases or syndromes: The formation of *tan-yin*. It may obstruct the meridians influencing *qi* and blood circulation and the functions of the meridians, while it may also stagnate in the viscera retarding visceral functions and the ascent and descent of *qi*.

The characteristics of phlegm diseases or syndromes: If phlegm stagnates in the lung, asthmatic breath, cough and sputum may be seen. If it obstructs the heart, heart blood circulation is not smooth and chest distress and palpitation may result. When it disturbs the Mind, mental confusion, idiocy, and mania may be caused. If it stagnates in the stomach so that the stomach fails to propel food downward, nausea, vomiting, epigastric distension and fullness may occur. If it lies in the meridians, tendons and bones, there may be *luo-li*, phlegmatic nodules, numb limbs and trunk, or hemiplegia or yin cellulitis,[17] *liu-zhu*,[18] etc.; if it upwardly invades the head, vertigo and fainting may be seen; if it stagnates in the throat, obstruction of the throat so that the phlegm can neither be swallowed nor coughed up may occur.

Characteristics of *yin* (excess exudates) diseases or syndromes: If excess exudates stagnate in the intestine, borborygma will occur; if stagnation occurs in the chest and hypochondriac region, distension and fullness of the chest and hypochondrium and cough, causing pain will appear. If stagnation occurs in the diaphragm, chest distress, asthmatic breath and cough, difficulty in lying flat and puffiness may result; if it exudes through the skin, edema, no sweating and painful and heavy body may result. *Tan-yin* diseases or syndromes are analysed in association with slippery glossy tongue coating, slippery or stringy pulse, etc. besides their clinical characteristics.

6-1-6-2 Congealed blood

This refers to congealed blood within the body, including the extravasated blood that accumulates within the body or circulates unsmoothly which obstructs meridians and viscera. It is a pathological product formed through a disease process, as well as a pathological factor causing certain diseases itself.

Its formation is chiefly due to *qi* deficiency, *qi* stagnation, cold blood, blood heat, etc. Deficient or stagnant *qi* fails to promote normal circulation of blood; stagnant pathogenic cold in the meridian-vessel makes the meridian-vessel contract and blood circulate unsmoothly; or pathogenic heat to enter *ying* (nutrition) and *xue* (blood) phases and a combination of blood and pathogenic heat, etc. may all form congealed blood. Extravasated blood accumulates within the body and forms congealed blood due to internal and external injuries, hypofunctional *qi* due to weak or wild blood heat, etc.

Characteristics of congealed blood diseases or syndromes:

After its formation, congealed blood cannot be nourished by normal blood, but influences general or local blood circulation causing pain, hemorrhage or blocked meridians and palpable masses as "the new blood cannot be generated when the congealed blood is not eliminated," etc. The diseases or syndromes of congealed blood vary according to the location and cause. If it obstructs the heart, palpitation, chest distress, cardialgia, dark-purplish lips and purplish finger and toenails may appear. If it obstructs the stomach and intestine, hematemesis and bloody stool may result. If it attacks the heart, hypochondriac pain and palpable masses may be seen or mania may occur. If it obstructs the uterus, lower abdominal pain, irregular menstruation, dysmenorrhea, amenorrhea, dark-purplish menstrual flow with clots or metrorrhagia can take place. If it obstructs the tip of the limb, *tuoju*[19] may be seen. If it obstructs the local areas of the limb, local swelling, pain and dark-purplish colour can appear.

Although the disease or syndrome of congealed blood varies, its common clinical characteristics can be classified as follows: stabbing pain, immovable pain and pain relieved by pressure or aggravated at night. There is also the type of masses caused by trauma of local skin and hematoma and ecchymosis with swelling and distension. If congealed blood accumulates within the body and stagnates for long, firm immovable abdominal masses can be formed. Hemorrhage usually with dark-purplish blood is accompanied by clots. During clinical inspection, prolonged skin, dark-purplish lips, nails and tongue proper, or petechia, ecchymosis, hypoglossal varices, etc. and a minute and unsmooth, sunken and stringy, or irregular and regular intermittent pulse may be seen.

6-2 Principles of occurrence and change of disease

"Yin flourishes smoothly and yang vivified steadily" is the normal functioning of viscera and meridians and when *qi* and blood, yin and yang are in balance. When these functions become abnormal and the balance is lost, so that "yin and yang are in disharmony" disease will occur. The occurrence and change of disease is mainly concerned with two aspects; the anti-pathogenic factors and pathogenic factors.

6-2-1 Anti-pathogenic and pathogenic factors and the onset of disease

The anti-pathogenic factor refers to the functions of the viscera, meridians, *qi* and blood, etc., the immune system and the recovery ability of the body. The pathogenic factors are various causative agents. The change of disease is the struggle between anti-pathogenic and pathogenic factors.

6-2-1-1 Deficient anti-pathogenic factor as a cause of disease

TCM emphasizes that the anti-pathogenic factor is important and holds that if the visceral function is normal, the anti-pathogenic factor will flourish, *qi* and blood will be enriched and defensive *qi* will be strong. In this case the pathogenic factors cannot invade the body and disease will be prevented. *Plain Questions* states, "Pathogenic factors cannot succeed in invading the body when one's anti-pathogenic factors are strong enough." Only when the anti-pathogenic factors are relatively weak can the pathogenic factors invade the body and break the balance between yin and yang, and disturb functions of the viscera and meridians, resulting in disease. The reason why the pathogenic factors succeed in invading the body is therefore that the anti-pathogenic factors are weak.

6-2-1-2 The pathogenic factor

TCM does not neglect the importance of pathogenic factors in causing disease. The pathogenic factor is the principal cause of disease. Under certain circumstances, it may even play an independent role. For example, high temperature, an electric shock, chemical toxins, wounds, frostbite, snakebite, etc. will injure the body even if one's anti-pathogenic factors are strong enough.

6-2-1-3 The anti-pathogenic factor

The struggle between the anti-pathogenic and pathogenic factors influences the development and transformation of disease.

a. No disease occurs when the anti-pathogenic factors conquer the pathogenic threat.

When the pathogenic factors invade the body, the anti-pathogenic factors resist them. Various pathogenic factors are always present, but many people who have contact with them do not get sick.

b. In the course of the struggle between anti-pathogenic and pathogenic factors, pathogenic factors may be comparatively strong, whereas anti-pathogenic factors can be weak. In this case the viscera, yin and yang and *qi* and blood lose their harmony and the *qi* mechanism is disturbed and disease can occur.

After the onset of disease, the severity and depth of the infection and the diseases or syndromes vary.

The relation between disease and anti-pathogenic factors: In the case where the anti-pathogenic factors are strong and struggle against the pathogenic factors, an excess syndrome will occur. Whereas when anti-pathogenic factors are weak and ineffectively struggle against the pathogenic factors, an excess-deficiency syndrome will result.

The relation between the disease and the features of the pathogenic factors: In general, the infection of yang pathogens is likely to lead to a relative excess of yang and injury of yin, with an excess-heat syndrome occurring. An infection of yin pathogens can lead to a cold-excess syndrome or cold-damp syndrome due to a relative excess of yin and injury of yang.

c. The pathogenic factor is the underlying cause of disease. Some pathogenic factors can affect tendons, bones and meridians, while others may directly enter the viscera. Different affected areas cause different diseases or syndromes.

6-2-2 The environment and invasion of disease

The invasion of disease is related to the environment. The external environment chiefly refers to the living and working environment, including weather changes, geographical conditions and environmental hygiene, etc. and the internal environment is the anti-pathogenic factor of the body. Whether the anti-pathogenic factor is strong or not is also connected with a person's mental state.

6-2-2-1 The external environment and invasion of disease

Man has gradually adapted to nature, however abnormal weather changes or a polluted environment and bad environmental hygiene may also cause disease.

Climatic factor: The six excesses and pestilential factors relate to climatic factors. Since it is windy in the spring, a wind-warm (mild heat) disease or syndrome often occurs. As it is hot in summer, a febrile disease or sunstroke is often diagnosed. As it is contracting and clearing in the autumn, a dry disease may often appear. As it is cold in the winter, a disease due to exogenous pathogenic cold may occur. Similarly, the occurrence and spreading of infectious diseases are also closely related to weather. Particularly, rapid or delayed weather changes are more likely to lead to infectious diseases. For example, measles, pertussion, epidemic cerebrospinal meningitis usually spread in autumn and spring, whereas dysentery and epidemic encephalitis B usually spread in the summer and autumn, etc. because the weather conditions at those times are suitable for the reproduction and spreading of the bacteria and viruses that cause these diseases.

Geographical factors: As natural conditions vary, diseases often occur under different geographical conditions. For example, carbuncles and sores frequently appear among the people in southeast China because it is located near the sea, is warm and rainy, and the people there eat a lot of fish and salty food. Diseases due to internal injuries often occur in northwest China because it is dry, cold and icy, and people there have a strong constitution because they eat meat, cheese and milk, and thus are not easily affected by exogenous pathogenic factors. In addition, endemic diseases occur in certain regions where certain substances are in shortage, e.g., endemic goiter is commonly seen in the regions far away from the sea due to lack of iodine(I).

The living and working environment: Industrial gases and waste matter usually contain poisonous substances and which can harm the body and cause acute or chronic poisoning. Harmful powder dust can also disrupt normal physiological activities. Wide application of agricultural chemicals may also cause harmful side effects. Certain diseases spread via the respiratory tract, e.g., flu, measles, pertussion, pulmonary tuberculosis, hepatitis, etc. Poor hygenic conditions, mosquitoes and flies, polluted air, water or food may all result in disease. Wounds, insect or animal bites, mental irritation, fatigue, prolonged reading, sitting, standing and walking can cause diseases. *Plain Questions* states, "Prolonged reading injures blood... prolonged sitting injures muscles, prolonged standing injures bones, and prolonged walking injures tendons."

6-2-2-2 The internal environment and invasion of disease

TCM holds that pathogenic factors influence the occurrence of disease and that weak anti-pathogenic factors are the internal causes of disease. People with different constitutions are affected by pathogenic factors in different intensities.

In general, whether the anti-pathogenic factors are strong or not is decided by a person's constitution and mental state.

a. The relation between body constitution and anti-pathogenic factors: If the body constitution is strong, the viscera will function normally, *jing* (vital principle), *qi*, blood and body fluids will be enriched and the anti-pathogenic factor strong; if not, the viscera will be hypofunctional and *jing*, *qi*, blood and body fluids will be weakened.

The constitution is related to natural endowment, diet, personal care and regular physical exercise. Generally speaking, if the natural environment is enriched, the body constitution will be strong; if not, it will usually be weak. Proper diet and nutrition are necessary to insure healthy growth and development. Improper diet and lack of nutrition affect the production of *qi* and blood, and result in a weak constitution. However overeating can also injure the spleen and stomach. Preference for certain foods can also increase certain substances and decrease others within the body, so that the normal functions are imbalanced and the constitution is weakened. Physical exercise and labour promote the circulation of *qi* and blood and help to keep good health. Lack of physical exercise can affect the circulation and cause the spleen and stomach to become hypofunctional, often resulting in a weak constitution.

b. The relation between the mental state and anti-pathogenic factor: The mental state is directly influenced by emotional factors. When one's emotions are normal, the *qi* mechanism will be normal, *qi* and blood regulated, the visceral functions harmonious and the anti-pathogenic factors strong; if one is depressed, yin and yang, *qi*, blood and viscera will become disharmonious, thus the anti-pathogenic factors are weakened. Hence, attention should be paid to checking the emotions, resting the mind and keeping in good spirits to keep *qi* circulating smoothly. Thus mental regulation can strengthen body resistance and prevent disease.

Notes

1. The six excesses refers to weather: wind, cold, summer-heat, dampness, dryness and fire (heat).
2. Seven kinds of emotional reactions: joy, anger, meditation, fear, grief, melancholy and anxiety.
3. The 10th solar term among the Twenty-four Solar Terms. (July, in Chinese calendar).
4. The 13th solar term among the Twenty-four Solar Terms. (August).
5. High fever in the excess symptom complex.
6. 7. A *bi* (black) syndrome caused by excess pathogenic damp and characterized by a feeling of heaviness and numbness in the limbs and body, with well-localized swelling and pain. It impairs the mobility of joint and tendons, and limited movements.
8. A chronic febrile disease caused by exposure to damp and hot pathogens. It is often seen between the summer and autumn, mainly affects the gastro-intestinal tract. It includes such illnesses as abebteris typhoid, etc.
9. Autumn Dryness. A disease caused by exposure to dry pathogens in Autumn. There are two types: Cold Dry and Hot Dry with manifestations such as headache, fever, dry cough, dry throat, nose and lips, anxiety and thirst, etc.
10. It is the Autumn Dry of cool nature, with manifestations such as headache, fever, chills, no sweating and dry nose.
11. Pathogenic wind, cold, summer-heat, damp and dryness go to their extreme.
12. An atrophic debility with atrophy and weakness of cold hands and lips and feet.
13. Infantile malnutrition characterized by emaciation, abdominal distension, and nutritional disorders with chronic indigestion.
14. Referring to the five tastes of drugs; pungent, sweet, sour, bitter and salty.
15. Lymphadenitis scrofulosa of the neck. The smaller one is called *luo* and the larger one, *li*.
16. A collective term for subcutaneous fruit-stone shaped masses.
17. A general term for the suppurative inflammation of subcutaneous or other soft tissues, manifested as diffused flat swelling with the overlying skin a normal colour, no heat, and little pain. It will not subside before suppuration, and resists rupture after suppuration. After rupture, it is slow to heal with persistent discharge of thin pus.
18. Recurrent metastatic abscesses in the deep layer or the muscles.
19. Gangrene of the fingers or toes with excruciating pain at first, and after a long time necrosis and sloughing off of the skin, subcutaneous tissues, muscles and bones, resembling thromboangitis obliteration.

7. PATHOGENESIS

The occurrence, development and change of disease are related to the constitution and the characteristics of the pathogenic factors. When pathogenic factors affect the body, the body's anti-pathogenic factors must react to restore the balance between yin and yang and restore the functions of the viscera and meridians and return *qi* and blood dysfunctions to normal. Each disease or syndrome has its own pathogenesis, such as the flourishing and decline of yin and yang, disharmony between yin and yang, abnormal *qi* and blood, dysfunctional meridians and viscera, etc.

7-1 Flourishing and decline of anti-pathogenic and pathogenic factors

The flourishing and decline of anti-pathogenic and pattogenic factors refers to the changes in the anti-pathogenic and pathogenic factors during a disease. The struggle between them not only relates to the occurrence of disease, but influences the development of a disease, and recovery, corresponding to the change of *xu* (deficiency) and *shi* (excess) of a disease or syndrome.

7-1-1 Flourishing and decline of anti-pathogenic and pathogenic factors and their deficiency and excess

In the course of the development and change of disease, anti-pathogenic and pathogenic factors are not static, but flourishing and declining as they fight against each other. In general, the growing and flourishing anti-pathogenic factors subdue the pathogenic ones; and conversely, the growing and flourishing pathogenic factors impair the anti-pathogenic ones. Along with the flourishing and decline of the anti-pathogenic and pathogenic factors within the body, the change of the disease or syndrome in deficiency or excess takes place.

Plain Questions states, "Excess pathogenic factors can lead to excess, while the deprived essential *qi* is followed by deficiency." The excess syndrome is caused by the six exogenous pathogenic factors such as retention of phlegm, food, water, blood, etc. For instance, pathological processes, such as profuse phlegm and saliva, dyspepsia, overflowing aqueous damp, internal blood stasis will be seen, as well as strong fever, mania, coarse voice, abdominal pain aggravated by pressure, anuria and constipation, full forceful pulse, etc.

Deficiency is an insufficient anti-pathogenic factor with a weak pathological reaction. The deficient anti-pathogenic factor is therefore the major aspect to consider. As the physiological function of *qi*, blood, body fluids, meridians and viscera, etc. are comparatively weak, a strong pathological reaction is hardly possible against the pathogenic factor. Therefore certain signs in the pathogenesis of the excess or deficiency syndrome can be recognized. The occurrence of real excess and an apparent deficiency is often caused by a stagnant pathogenic factor, meridian blockage and inability of *qi* and blood to reach the external part of the body. Real deficiency and false excess are caused by deficient *qi* and blood in the viscera and hypofunctional transportation and digestion by the viscera. Hence, when analysing the deficiency or excess of a pathogenesis, it is possible there will be false signs.

7-1-2 Flourishing and decline of pathogenic and anti-pathogenic factors and transformation of disease

In the course of disease, expansion and decline of the anti-pathogenic and pathogenic factors change continuously. Under ordinary circumstances, when the anti-pathogenic factor is not too weak and can resist the pathogenic factor, the disease can be fought. However, in other circumstances, when the disease has not yet been cured, the pathogenic factor gradually increases and the disease becomes worse sometimes leading to death. Thus, the development of disease actually depends upon how much the two factors flourish and decline.

A series of symptoms may appear, including general weakness and decline of the body condition, i.e., the deficiency syndrome. A deficiency syndrome is commonly seen in a body with a weak constitution or at the late stage of a disease. For example, a severe or prolonged illness can consume the essential *qi* or consume *qi*, blood, body fluids and yin and yang. This can cause such symptoms as hyperhidrosis, vomiting and diarrhea, hemorrhoae, etc., which in turn will further weaken body resistance. General weakness may occur with symptoms such as mental fatigue and general lassitude, withered complexion, palpitation and shortness of breath, and perspiration, or deficient yin signs such as night sweat, heat in the chest, palms and soles or declined yang signs such as chills and cold limbs and a weak forceful pulse, etc.

The flourishing and decline of the anti-pathogenic and pathogenic factors not only cause simple deficiency or excess, but very often pathological reactions where both are intermingled. This is frequently seen in a prolonged and complex illness. Another example of a mixed type is: When a disease is improperly treated, the pathogenic factor remains for a long time and weakens the anti-pathogenic factor so that it cannot expel the pathogen. Meanwhile general weakness causes stagnation and blockage of more pathological products, such as internally generating aqueous damp, *tan-yin*, congealed blood, etc. Later these factors may all lead to the transformation of the disease from an excess to a deficiency type, or inversely, an excess one caused by deficiency.

In summary, in the development of disease, deficiency and excess of pathogenesis are relative. There is also often a natural tendency for diseases to develop from an excess to a deficiency, an excess resulting from a deficiency or a mixture of the two. Therefore, the pathogenic development of deficiency and excess cannot only be regarded from a static and absolute viewpoint.

7-1-2-1 Anti-pathogenic factor conquering pathogenic factor

This is when the disease takes a turn for the better in the flourishing and decline of the anti-pathogenic and pathogenic factors. The condition improves because the patient's anti-pathogenic factor is strong enough to resist the pathogenic factor, or the patient is properly treated in time so that the pathogenic factor cannot develop. In this case the body's pathological manifestations gradually disappear, tissue lesions such as the viscera, meridians, etc. are repaired, consumed *jing* (vital principle), *qi*, blood and body fluids, etc. can also gradually be supplemented, and the balance between yin and yang reestablished so that the disease is cured. For example, in exogenous febrile diseases caused by the six excesses, the pathogenic factor invades the body via the skin, or mouth and nose.

If the anti-pathogenic factor is strong enough, it can stop the development of the disease within the body surface or meridians, and it can expel the pathogenic factor from the body. The anti-pathogenic factor eliminates the pathogen and nutritional and defensive *qi* are regulated and the patient recovers as soon as diaphoresis is used.

7-1-2-2 Pathogenic factor conquering anti-pathogenic factor

This is where the disease worsens and even causes death because the anti-pathogenic factor is comparatively weak or the pathogenic one is stronger and the body resistance gradually weakens so that the development of the pathogenic factor cannot be restrained. Consequently the pathological lesions of the body become more and more severe, resulting in a gradual aggravation of the disease. If the anti-pathogenic factor declines, but the pathogenic one remains strong, the functions of *qi*, blood, viscera, meridians, etc. would decline, yin would divorce from yang and death would result. For example, with exogenous febrile diseases, the signs of "depletion of yin" and "depletion of yang" are typical. Here the pathogenic factor cannot conquer the pathogenic factor and the pathogenic factor flourishes while its counterpart declines.

If both factors are equally strong, or the anti-pathogenic factor is weak and the pathogenic factor persists or the anti-pathogenic factor has difficulty recovering after the pathogen is eliminated, these conditions would often be causes for many diseases turning from acute to chronic.

7-2 Disharmony between yin and yang

Disharmony between yin and yang means that during the development of disease, the balance between yin and yang is lost, forming pathological states of an excess with a decline of either yin or yang and inability of yin to restrain yang or vice versa. At the same time, it includes the disharmony between the viscera, meridians, *qi* and blood, nutritional *qi* and defensive *qi*, etc. as well as the abnormal movements of *qi*. Since the action of various pathogenic factors, such as the six excesses, the seven emotions, improper diet, fatigue and lack of physical exercise, etc. cause disease and create disharmony between yin and yang within the body, the disharmony between yin and yang is also the internal course of disease.

7-2-1 Relative flourishing of yin or yang

The relative flourishing of yin or yang mainly refers to the excess syndrome due to a pathogenic factor causing an excess syndrome. After a yang pathogen invades the body, a relative excess of yang may form; while a yin pathogen entering the body may cause a relative excess of yin.

Yin and yang are interconnected, i.e., excess yang leads to deficient yin and vice versa. This means that overactive yang restrains yin, leading to deficient yin and vice versa. Thus excess yang causes a yin disease and excess yin, a yang one (*Plain Questions*). According to *Plain Questions* excess yang produces a heat syndrome whereas excess yin, a cold one.

7-2-1-1 The absolute excess of yang

This refers to a pathological state of excess yang *qi*, with hyperfunction and excess heat which appear in the course of disease within the body. Generally speaking, it is usually characterized by an excess yang heat syndrome but yin is not deficient. Absolute excess yang is mainly caused by the affection of yang pathogens, like warmth (mild heat) and heat, yin pathogens, and also by internal injuries caused by the five emotional factors, production of fire (intense heat) by the five emotions, or production of heat due to stagnant *qi*, congealed blood, food retention, etc. Yang is characterized by heat, movement, dryness when it is in excess, e.g., strong fever, flushed face, congestive eyes, etc. are all signs of excess yang. An excess of yang leads to deficient yin. In pathogenesis, deficient yin must be divided into relative deficient yin and absolute deficient yin. When a pathogenic factor causes the yang of the body to be excessive, an excess heat syndrome may appear because of deficient yin. When excess yang consumes yin fluids within the body, yin will be deficient. This leads to the transformation of an excess-heat syndrome into a deficient-heat one, or an excess-heat syndrome associated with deficient yin.

7-2-1-2 The absolute excess of yin

This signifies a pathological state of absolute excess yin *qi* with dysfunction or hypofunction, or insufficient warmth and stagnation of pathological metabolic products appearing in the course of disease. It is usually characterized by an excess-cold syndrome due to excess yin with yang remaining static. It is usually caused by the affection of pathogenic cold, damp and yin or overeating unripened and cold food, blockage of the middle energizer by pernicious cold, yang's failure to restrain yin that results in internal cold and excess yin.

Yin is characterized by cold, calmness and dampness. Excess yin produces cold, e.g., cold limbs and trunk, pale tongue, etc. Excess yin leads to deficient yang. Although it can be divided into relative deficient yang and absolute yin because yang is concerned with movement and is likely to be consumed and internal cold excess yin is usually due to deficiency, it is actually accompanied by deficient yang in different degrees and it is very difficult to clearly distinguish a relative deficient yang from an absolute consumed yang.

7-2-2 The absolute decline of yin or yang

A relative decline of yin or yang refers to the deficiency syndrome characterized by general weakness due to exhausted essential *qi*. Here, exhausted essential *qi* stands for deficiencies of *jing* (vital principle), *qi*, blood, body fluids, etc. and their hypofunction as well as the hypofunction and disharmony of the viscera and meridians. The tissues and organs of the body, such as *jing*, *qi*, blood, body fluids, viscera, meridians, etc. and their physiological functions can all be classified into yin and yang. Under normal physiological conditions, they are balanced within the body. In case there is hypofunction of yin or yang for some reason, the restraining principle cannot perform properly, causing a relative excess of its opposite and forming pathological phenomena such as deficient yang produces cold, (cold due to asthenia) deficient yin produces heat (fever due to asthenia). Thus, the deficiency of one leads to the excess of the other.

7-2-2-1 The absolute decline of yang

A pathological state of deficient yang features hypofunction and insufficient warmth in the body. Generally speaking, it is usually characterized by a cold deficiency syndrome due to insufficient yang *qi*, the yang's failure to restrain yin and relative excess of yin. It is mainly caused by insufficient congenital endowment, malnutrition, internal injuries due to fatigue and lack of physical exercise or impaired yang *qi* caused by a prolonged illness, or too much sexual activity.

Deficiency of yang *qi* usually refers to deficiencies of spleen yang and kidney yang. A decline of kidney yang (insufficiency of mingmen fire) is important in the pathogenesis of the relative decline of yang. As yang *qi* is too weak to restrain yin and its warming function is weakened, cold dominates and the functions of tissues and organs, such as viscera and meridians decrease accordingly. Blood and body fluids circulate slowly, aqueous liquid cannot be metabolized and there is excessive internal yin cold. This is the chief pathogenesis of "deficient yang producing cold." In such a case, asthenic phenomena prevail, such as preference for calmness, lying with a rolled body, profuse watery urine, aqueous grainy diarrhea, etc. pallor, creeping chills and cold limbs, pale tongue, retarded pulse, etc. may also be seen. Thus "deficient yang producing cold" and "excess yin producing cold" are different in pathogenesis. The former is asthenia with cold while the latter is major cold with unclear deficiency signs.

7-2-2-2 The absolute decline of yin

This pathological state is accompanied by a relative excess of yang and hyperfunction of yin due to asthenia caused by severe consumption of *jing*, blood, body fluids, etc. and yin's failure to restrain yang. Its pathogenesis is usually characterized by a deficient heat syndrome manifested by insufficient yin fluid, lack of nourishment, restlessness and relative yang *qi* excess. It is mainly caused by the consumption of yin by the yang pathogen or injury of yin by fire produced by the five extreme emotions or depleted yin fluids due to a prolonged illness.

A deficiency of yin fluid mainly refers to deficiencies of the liver and kidney.

Kidney yin is the foundation for the formation of myriads of yin. Therefore, deficient kidney yin is important in the pathogenesis of the relative decline of yin. Since yin fluid (water) is insufficient, yang *qi* (fire) cannot be restrained and various manifestations occur, such as internal heat (fever) due to deficient yin, blazing yang due to deficient yin and excess yang caused by deficient yin, etc. For example, chest heat, hot palms and soles, "steaming of bones" and tidal fever, flushed face, emaciation, night sweat, dry throat, red tongue with little coating, minute, weak and rapid pulse, etc. are manifestations of deficient yin producing heat. Deficient yin producing heat differs from excessive yang producing heat in pathogenesis, and their clinical manifestations are also different. The former is asthenia with fever, but the latter is mainly fever with not so visible asthenic signs.

7-2-3 Interrelationship of yin and yang

On the basis of impaired yin or yang, pathological changes in one aspect influence its opposite, forming the pathogenesis of deficiencies of both yin and yang. Since the kidney stores essential *qi*, pathological processes of deficient yang affecting yin and vice versa are likely to affect the kidney.

7-2-3-1 Deficient yin affecting yang

This usually implies that declined yin fluid impairs the formation of yang *qi* or consumes yang *qi* due to lack of nourishment. Deficient yang results from an inadequate material basis from deficient yin, forming a pathological state of deficiencies of both yin and yang with deficient yin as the root cause. Take the syndrome of excessive liver yang that is commonly seen as an example. Its pathogenesis is mainly deficient yin and excess yang caused by "inadequate water to nourish wood," but, the development of the disease can further consume the essential *qi* of the kidney and affect kidney yang, resulting in the symptoms of deficient yang, such as chills, cold limbs, pallor, deep and weak pulse, etc. This eventually transforms itself into the syndrome of deficiencies of both yin and yang due to deficient yin affecting yang.

7-2-3-2 Deficient yang affecting yin

Deficient yang *qi* influences the production of yin fluid because of insufficient energy to manufacture it. Thus, deficient yin is caused by both deficient yang, forming a pathological state of deficiencies of both yin and yang with deficient yang as the major one. For example, the main pathogenesis of edema commonly seen in clinic is that yang *qi* is too deficient to promote fluids normally, and as a result water metabolism is blocked, body fluids stagnate and aqueous damp is generated internally and exuded through the skin. It develops due to a gradual consumption of yin owing to its lacking resource of yang, with symptoms of deficient yin, such as emaciation, restlessness and production of fire even *che-zong*,[1] etc. and transforms itself into the syndrome of deficiencies of both yin and yang caused by deficient yang affecting yin.

7-2-4 Disharmony of yin and yang

A special pathogenesis of the disharmony between yin and yang, which includes both deficient yang hindering yin and excessive yin hindering yang. Its pathogenesis is chiefly manifested by excessive yin stagnating internally and exuding yang. In this case both yin and yang are forced to be unconnected, resulting in complex pathological phenomena, such as true cold and false heat and true heat and false cold, etc.

7-2-4-1 Excess yin hindering yang

A pathological state where the yin pathogen stagnating internally forces yang *qi* to float outside, resulting in the disconnection and mutual exclusion of both yin *qi* and yang *qi*. Internal excess of yin cold is the root of disease, but as yang is flushed outside, false heat signs, such as flushed face, anxiety with fever, thirst, large pulse, etc. appear. It is therefore called the true-cold and false-heat syndromes.

7-2-4-2 Excess yang hindering yin

A pathological state where excessive internal pathogenic heat congeals in the deeper part of the body so that yang *qi* is blocked internally and fails to reach the limb, while yin is excluded outside. The root of the disease is excessive internal yin. But, as yin is excluded externally, false cold signs appear, such as cold clammy extremities, deep pulse, etc. in clinic. It is therefore called the true heat and false cold syndrome.

7-2-5 Depletion of yin and yang

7-2-5-1 Depletion of yang

A pathological state where yang *qi* is suddenly exhausted, resulting in a sudden severe failure of bodily functions. It is usually caused by the fact that the pathogenic factor is so violent that the anti-pathogenic one cannot conquer it, resulting in a sudden exhaustion of yang *qi*. It is also caused by deficient yang and insufficient anti-pathogenic factor, fatigue, etc. or deficient yang due to hyperhidrosis caused by severe depletion of yang *qi* and outward dispersion of deficient yang. In sudden exhaustion of yang *qi*, fatal signs such as hyperhidrosis, cold clammy skin and limbs, mental fatigue and minute faint pulse may be seen.

7-2-5-2 Depletion of yin

A pathological state with severe exhaustion of bodily functions due to a sudden depletion or loss of yin fluid within the body. In general, it is caused by the consumption of yin fluids due to excess pathogenic heat or prolonged retention of pathogenic heat. It is also caused by a severe impairment of yin fluid. In such a case, fatal signs such as asthmatic breath, thirst, anxiety, hyperhidrosis and collapse, even if the four extremities are warm may be seen.

Although depletion of yin and yang are different in pathogenesis and clinical signs, depletion of yin leads to a scattering of yang due to its lacking dependence and depletion of yang leads to exhausted yin, as yin and yang within the body are interdependent. Therefore depletion of yin can rapidly result in depletion of yang and vice versa, finally leading to the dissociation of yin and yang, causing death because of the lack of essential *qi*.

7-3 Abnormality of *qi* and blood

Abnormality of *qi* and blood refers to pathological changes, such as insufficient *qi* and blood and disorders of their physiological functions. Pathological changes of the viscera cause disharmony of *qi* and blood in the viscera. So, the pathogenesis of abnormal *qi* and blood, running parallel with the flourishing and decline of pathogenic and anti-pathogenic factors and disharmony between yin and yang, is the basis for the pathogenesis of various pathological changes of viscera and meridians, etc.

7-3-1 Abnormal *qi*

Abnormality of *qi* includes deficient *qi* due to insufficient production or excessive consumption of *qi*, and hypofunction and abnormal movement of *qi*, etc. The first two are mainly manifested in deficient *qi*, the last in pathological changes of disorders of *qi*, such as *qi* stagnation, *qi* regurgitation, *qi* blockage and *qi* exhaustion.

7-3-1-1 Deficient *qi*

A pathological state of consumed *qi*, dysfunction, visceral hypofunction and weak body resistance. It is chiefly caused by insufficient *qi* due to deficiency of congenital endowment, malnutrition or dysfunctional lung and kidney. It also results from internal injuries from fatigue and lack of physical exercise, prolonged illness, etc. For example, listlessness, general lassitude, weak limbs, vertigo, perspiration, susceptibility to colds, etc. are all manifestations of *qi* deficiency.

Being closely related with blood and body fluids, *qi* deficiency influences them leading to shortage and retarded circulation of blood and body fluids that result in various pathological processes of blood and body fluids and exhausted *qi*, etc.

7-3-1-2 Abnormal movement of *qi*

This refers to pathological processes, such as *qi* stasis, *qi* regurgitation, *qi* blockage and *qi* exhaustion, caused by abnormal *qi* movements.

Ascending, descending, entering and leaving of *qi* are the main *qi* movements as well as the basic cause of the contradictory movement of the viscera, meridians, yin-yang, *qi* and blood.

The functional activities of the viscera and meridians and the interrelation of the viscera, meridians, *qi* and blood, yin and yang all depend upon the movement of *qi* to stay balanced. For example, the harmony between body functions, such as the lung's respiration, the spleen sending the puried nutrients upward and the stomach sending the turbid matter downward, the balance between yin and yang of the heart and kidney, and the interconnection between water and fire (descending heart fire and ascending kidney water), the liver's functions are all normal manifestations of the smooth flow of *qi*. If *qi* movement is impaired, pathological changes of the five yin and six yang viscera, the superficial and deep (or external and internal) portions of the body, four limbs and nine apertures,[2] etc. may appear. In general, disorders of the *qi* mechanism can be generalized by: *qi* stasis (obstruction of *qi* flow), *qi* regurgitation (overactive *qi* in its ascending movement or inactive *qi* in its descendance), trapped *qi* (insufficient force of *qi* in its ascending movement or excess force of *qi* in its descendance), *qi* blockage (blockage of *qi* in going-out) and *qi* exhaustion (outward exhaustion of *qi* due to its failure to be retained internally).

a. *Qi* stasis is mainly caused by obstruction, such as internal depression of the emotions or phlegm, damp, retained food, congealed blood, etc. that influence the flow of *qi*, forming local blockages of *qi* that lead to the dysfunction of viscera and meridians. If *qi* stagnates at a certain location, distension, fullness and pain, even congealed blood, *tan-yin* (phlegm and excess exudates), etc. may appear. The liver is concerned with ascendance and the lung, descendance, the spleen is concerned with ascendance and the stomach descendance and both interrelationships are important in regulating *qi*. Therefore, stagnation of *qi* can be seen not only in stagnation of lung *qi*, stagnation of *qi* due to depressed liver or stagnation of the spleen and stomach, but in all dysfunctions of these viscera.

b. *Qi* regurgitation: An abnormal state of ascending and descending *qi* and the regurgitation of visceral *qi* caused by injuries from emotional factors, improper diet, obstructing phlegm and turbid matter, etc. It is most frequently seen in viscera, such as the lung, stomach and liver. If *qi* stagnates in the lung, the lung fails to perform its clearing and descending functions and the *qi* regurgitates, resulting in coughing. If *qi* stagnates in the stomach, the stomach fails to propel downward, causing nausea, vomiting, belching and hiccup. If *qi* stagnates in the liver, liver *qi* regurgitates, resulting in pain and distension of the head, flushed face, congestive eyes and irascibility. Regurgitation of blood together with *qi*, or hemoptysis, hematemesis, or fainting due to obstruction by regurgitating blood may also result if *qi* stagnates in the liver.

Generally speaking, *qi* regurgitation is mainly the excess type, although it is also occasionally of the deficiency type. If the lung cannot carry on its purifying and descending functions, because of its weakness or the kidney's failure to absorb *qi*, regurgitation of lung *qi* can result. The stomach's failure to perform its descending function due to its weakness can also lead to regurgitation of stomach *qi*.

c. Trapped *qi*: A pathological state mainly characterized by *qi*'s failure to ascend. The stability of the location of the viscera within the body depends upon the normal movement of *qi*. Therefore, when *qi*'s ascending force is weakened due to *qi* deficiency, certain visceroptosis, such as gastroptosis, prolapse of uterus, etc. may be caused. Since the body obtains *qi* from diet, *qi* is produced by the spleen which is concerned with ascendance. The spleen and stomach are the resource of *qi* and blood, thus trapped *qi* easily appears when they are weak. Therefore, trapped *qi* is often called the middle *qi* trap (a collective term for *qi* of the spleen and stomach) accompanied by distension, fullness, heaviness and dropping of the loin and abdomen, frequent desire for urination, shortened breath, general weakness, low voice, forceless pulse, etc.

d. *Qi* blockage and *qi* exhaustion: These are pathological states mainly characterized by an abnormal entering and leaving of *qi* and which occurs in severe cases, such as *jue* (fainting) syndrome[3] and *tuo* (collapse) syndrome.[4]

Qi blockage is a pathological state of *bi-jue* syndrome[5] which suddenly occurs mainly due to the external blockage of the turbid pathogen or extremely depressed *qi*, and even obstruction of outgoing *qi*. For example, the *bi-jue* syndrome caused by the filthy and the turbid (substance of odour), the *bi-jue* syndrome due to exogenous febrile disease, excess heat, fainting due to sudden mental trauma, etc., the pathogenesis of which is the obstruction of outgoing *qi*.

Qi exhaustion: A pathological state of exhaustion of the physiological functions suddenly appearing owing to the anti-pathogenic factor's failure to conquer the pathogenic one, or a persistently weakened anti-pathogenic factor so that *qi* cannot be maintained internally but is exhausted externally or *qi* exhausted together with blood due to hemorrhage, hyperhidrosis, etc. or *qi* exhaustion together with body fluids.

7-3-2 Abnormal blood

Abnormal blood includes pathological changes, such as an insufficiency of blood or excessive consumption of blood due to hemorrhage, prolonged illness, or blood deficiency due to the accelerated circulation of blood due to blood heat; blood congealment caused by retardation of blood circulation.

7-3-2-1 Blood deficiency

A pathological state of insufficient blood or the decreased nourishing function of blood. It may be caused by excessive loss of blood and delayed formation and supplement of new blood, obstruction of blood generation due to a weak spleen and stomach, malnutrition, a weak blood-forming function, shortage of the resource of blood or persisting consumption of *ying* (nutrients) and blood caused by prolonged illness, chronic consumption, etc.

As tissues and organs such as the viscera and meridians, all depend upon the nourishment of blood, symptoms of general weakness, such as systemic or local malnutrition, gradual hypofunction, etc. may occur when blood is deficient. For example, dull complexion, pale lips, tongue, and nails, vertigo, palpitation, fever, mental fatigue and general lassitude, emaciation, numbness of hands and feet, difficult flexion and extension of joints, dry and uncomfortable eyes, blurred vision, etc. are all clinical signs of blood deficiency.

7-3-2-2 Congealed blood

Obstruction of blood circulation due to *qi* stasis or retarded blood circulation, or blockage of collateral meridians by phlegm and turbid matter or stagnation of cold blood due to the entry of pathogenic cold into blood, or blood consumed by pathogenic heat which has entered blood, etc. all can form blood stagnation, even congealed blood. Therefore, congealed blood is the product of blood stagnation and can also obstruct the meridians (vessels), becoming a further cause of stagnation of blood.

As the pathogenesis of blood stagnation is chiefly the unsmooth flow of blood, any pain has a definite location and is not relieved by cold or warmth. Palpable abdominal masses may form and block certain areas, accompanied by signs of retarded blood circulation and blood stagnation, such as dull complexion, scaly skin, dark-purplish lips and tongue, ecchymosis, etc.

Blood stagnation may block *qi*, forming a malignant circulation with *qi* stasis leading to further blood stagnation and vice versa.

7-3-2-3 Blood heat

A pathological state when pathogenic heat exists in the *xue* (blood) phase[6] and blood circulation is accelerated. It is usually caused by pathogenic heat entering the blood and pernicious fire produced by the five extreme emotions.

Since blood circulates when warmed, it accelerates or even affects the meridians (vessels) and extravasates when blood is heated. Pernicious heat can also consume blood and body fluids. Therefore, its clinical picture is characterized by heat signs as well as consumed blood, hyperactive movement of blood and yin injury.

7-3-3 Dysfunction of the relationship between *qi* and blood

Qi pertains to yang while blood, to yin. They are interdependent.

Qi warms, transforms and controls blood; blood nourishes and carries *qi*. Hence abnormal *qi* movement influences blood. For example, *qi* deficiency can lead to difficult generation and inevitable deficiency of blood. Weakened *qi* leads to stagnation of blood, and lowers *qi*'s control over hemorrhage. Stagnant *qi* is followed by blockage of blood, whereas the disorder of *qi* mechanism is followed by trapped blood together with *qi*, even epistaxis, bloody stools and metrorrhagia. Similarly, *qi* is affected when blood becomes deficient and its circulation abnormal. For example, deficient blood leads to deficient *qi*, blood stagnation and *qi* stagnation; blood exhaustion may be accompanied by *qi* exhaustion. The dysfunction of *qi* and blood includes *qi* and blood stagnation, *qi*'s failure to control blood, exhaustion of *qi* associated with severe hemorrhage, deficient *qi* and blood and failure to nourish meridians, etc.

7-3-3-1 Stagnant *qi* and blood

They often exist simultaneously. They are caused by obstructed blood circulation and external injuries from sprains and strains, etc. In normal circumstances, the liver which is concerned with dispersion and discharge and stores blood plays a vital role in regulating the *qi* mechanism, so that stagnant *qi* and blood are usually closely related to a malfunction of the liver. Secondly, since the heart controls blood vessels and promotes blood circulation, a malfunction of the heart causes congealed blood, which leads to stagnant *qi*. Distension, fullness and pain, ecchymosis and abdominal masses are frequently seen in clinic when there is *qi* and blood stasis.

7-3-3-2 Inability of *qi* to control blood

A pathological state that includes hemorrhaging, like hemoptysis, hematemesis, epistaxis, ecchymosis, bloody stools, hematuria, metrorrhagia, etc. If the ability of *qi* to control blood decreases, blood may consequently extravasate. Metrorrhagia, bloody stools, hematuria, etc. are due to insufficient middle *qi* (gastrosplenic *qi*) and deficient *qi*.

7-3-3-3 Exhaustion of *qi* associated with severe hemorrhage

A pathological state when *qi* is lost together with blood and causes hemorrhage, forming deficient or exhausted *qi* and blood. It is often caused by blood loss in external injuries or metrorrhagia, postpartum hemorrhage, etc. Since blood is the carrier of *qi*, its exhaustion can lead to depletion of *qi*.

7-3-3-4 Deficient *qi* and blood

A pathological state where deficient *qi* and blood exist simultaneously. It is usually caused by chronic consumptive diseases or blood loss occurring before the exhaustion of *qi* associated with severe hemorrhage; or deficient *qi* occurring before a gradual decrease of blood, such as pale or withered yellowish complexion, lack of *qi* and disinclination to talk, listlessness and asthenia, emaciation, palpitation, insomnia, dry skin, numb limbs, etc. may be simultaneously seen.

7-3-3-5 Hypofunction of *qi* and blood in nourishing meridians

A pathological state where deficient *qi* and blood or disharmony between them causes a decline in their intersupporting functions and the meridians, tendons, muscles and skin are not well enough nourished, resulting in abnormal movement or sensation of the tendons and muscles of the trunk and limbs, dry skin, itching, and sometimes scaly skin.

7-4 Abnormal body fluid metabolism

Imbalanced metabolism of body fluids includes the abnormal distribution of body fluids and imbalance between the formation and excretion of body fluids. The result is that an insufficient formation, excessive consumption and excretion of body fluids occur, resulting in a retarded circulation of body fluids within the body, forming pathological changes, such as stagnation, retention and overflow of fluids. Normal metabolic balance can be maintained on the basis of the harmony of the viscera. The formation, distribution and excretion of body fluids cannot depart from *qi*'s movement. Only if the movement of *qi* is normal can body fluids stay balanced. Only if *qi* is functioning normally can body fluids be formed, distributed and excreted. So far as the physiological functions of the viscera are concerned, the formation of body fluids cannot be separated from the transportation and digestion of the spleen and stomach. The distribution and excretion of body fluids cannot be separated from the spleen's spreading functions, the kidney and bladder's evaporating function and the triple energizer's clearing and regulating functions. The cooperation between the physiological functions of the viscera constitute the regulating mechanism for the body's fluid metabolism, so it can maintain harmony in the formation, distribution and excretion of body fluids. If *qi* movement becomes imbalanced and its function is abnormal or the functions of the viscera such as the spleen, lung and kidney become abnormal, abnormal body fluid metabolism will result with insufficient or retained body fluids, producing aqueous damp or *tan-yin* (phlegm and excessive exudates) internally.

7-4-1 Insufficiency of body fluids

Insufficient body fluids which fail to nourish and moisten the internal organs and external openings, skin and hair is usually caused by the consumption of body fluids due to pathogenic dryness or fire produced by the five emotions or fever, but is also caused by profuse sweating, vomiting, diarrhea, blood loss, or the excessive use or misuse of pungent and dry drugs, etc.

Since *jin* (thin clear fluid) and *ye* (thick turbid fluid) have different features, locations and physiological functions, the manifestations of deficient body fluids are also different. For example hyperhidrosis and thirst due to high temperatures in midsummer, dry mouth, nose and skin frequently seen in dry weather, sunken eye, even charley horse, etc. appearing during severe vomiting, severe diarrhea, and frequent urination are all signs of the consumption of *jin*. Being thick and turbid and less movable *ye* has the main function of nourishing the viscera, enriching the bone marrow, brains, spinal cord, and lubricating the joints. It is neither easily impaired and consumed, nor rapidly supplemented whenever consumed. A bright and red tongue with no or little coating, dry lips and tongue without desire for drinking, emaciation, withered skin and feet, etc. at the late stage of febrile diseases or consumption of yin during a prolonged illness are all clinical signs of dried yin fluid and movement of endogenous wind.

In general, consumption of *jin* is not necessarily accompanied by the exhaustion of the *ye* but the exhaustion of *ye* is accompanied by injury to the *jin*.

7-4-2 Distribution, excretion and obstruction of body fluids

The distribution and excretion of body fluids are two key links of fluid metabolism. If they are dysfunctional, abnormal stagnation of body fluids within the body will result and they will become the primary cause of pathological substances, such as endogenous aqueous damp, *tan-yin*, etc.

The obstruction of fluid distribution leads to retarded circulation within the body or retention in local areas, so they are not transported. As a result, aqueous damp is internally produced and *tan-yin* is formed. The obstruction of body fluid distribution has different causes, which include the malfunction of the lung's dissipating, purifying and descending functions, or the spleen's transporting and digesting functions and distributing *jing*, or the liver's dispersing and discharging functions and whether the triple energizer aqueducts are obstructed or not. For example, phlegm stagnates in the lung when the lung fails to perform its dissipating and descending functions. If the spleen is hypofunctional in its transporting and digesting aqueous damp and distributing *jing*, body fluid circulation can be slowed down, inducing pathogenic damp and phlegm.

If the liver fails to perform its dispersing and excreting functions, the *qi* mechanism can be obstructed and *qi* becomes stagnant, leading to retention of fluid and production of phlegm and excessive liquid in the middle energizer. The obstruction of the triple energizer directly influences not only the circulation of body fluids, but also their excretion. Among all the above-mentioned mechanisms, the most important one is the obstruction of the transporting and digesting functions of the spleen. *Plain Questions* states, "Edema and swelling from pathogenic damp are due to splenic disorder."

The obstruction of the excretion of body fluids mainly refers to the hypofunction of body fluids in transforming themselves into sweat and urine and leading to retention of aqueous liquid that exudes into the subcutaneous region and results in edema. The transformation of body fluids into sweat chiefly relies on the kidney. Although the hypofunctional lung and kidney may lead to water retention and result in edema, kidney *qi* also plays a role in controlling excretion because fluid can also be transformed into urine that will be discharged from the body when the lung fails to perform its dissipating function. When the junction between the skin and muscle is blocked, the excretion of sweat is obstructed and fluid is retained. When kidney *qi* is hypofunctional and the formation and excretion of urine are obstructed, overflowing aqueous damp can occur, resulting in edema.

The organs concerned with the distribution and excretion of body fluid influence each other although they are different and the result of their malfunction is the retention of aqueous damp and *tan-yin* that cause various pathological changes.

7-4-3 Disharmony between body fluids, *qi* and blood

As was previously described, the formation, distribution and excretion of body fluids depend upon *qi* activities of the viscera and the movement of *qi* because *qi* circulates together with body fluids, carrying and spreading them over the entire body. At the same time, body fluids are needed to keep blood and vessels enriched and unobstructed. Therefore, harmony between body fluids, *qi* and blood is an important aspect to guarantee normal physiological activity. Whenever the harmony is lost, the following pathological changes may appear.

7-4-3-1 Retention of body fluids and obstruction of *qi*

This refers to a pathological state where the obstruction of fluid metabolism and retention of aqueous damp and *tan-yin* lead to a blockage of *qi*. For example, in the blockage of the lung by *shui-yin* (excessive aqueous fluid), stagnation of lung *qi* and the lung's failure to perform its dissipating and descending functions, fullness of the chest and cough, asthmatic and hasty breathing and difficulty lying flat may occur. In "aqueous *qi* affecting the heart," obstructed heart *qi* and restrained heart yang with palpitation and cardialgia may appear and retention of *shui-yin* may follow. Retention of *shui-yin* in the middle energizer and obstruction of the *qi* mechanism of the spleen and stomach may result if the purified *qi* fails to ascend and the turbid matter fails to descend, with dizziness and lassitude, distension and fullness in the epigastrium and abdomen and dyspepsia. *Shui-yin* stagnating in the four extremities may lead to the obstruction of the meridians manifested by heaviness, distension and pain of the limbs and trunk, etc.

7-4-3-2 Exhaustion of *qi* associated with body fluids

This mainly refers to a pathological state when *qi* and body fluids are exhausted due to excessively consumed body fluids by high fever, exhaustion of body fluids by hyperhidrosis, where the impairment of body fluids leads to an internal generation of fever due to deficiency or endogenous pathogenic wind due to dried blood. Body fluids are an important component of blood and share the same source with acquired *jing*. If they are injured by high fever, consumed by burns or lost through blood loss and exhausted body fluids, or consumptive fever due to yin deficiency, exhausted body fluids and dried blood may result, manifested by anxiety, dry nose and throat, or heat in the chest, palms and soles, emaciation, dry skin, or scaly skin accompanied by itching or peeling, etc.

7-4-3-3 Exhaustion of body fluids and dryness of blood

This chiefly refers to exhaustion of body fluids, leading to dryness of blood and endogenous heat of deficiency or dryness of blood and pathogenic wind. Body fluids are the component of blood, originating from the acquired essence of cereals together with blood. If they are injured by high fever or consumed by burns, impaired by blood loss or fever due to pulmonary tuberculosis, anxiety, dry nose and throat, or fever at palms and soles, muscular emaciation, dry skin, or scaly skin with itchy skin or peeling may appear.

7-4-3-4 Consumed body fluids and congealed blood

This mainly refers to a pathological state when consumed or impaired body fluids lead to stagnation and obstruction, usually caused by high fever, burns, or vomiting, diarrhea, hyperhidrosis, etc. Consumed body fluids can cause the volume of blood to decrease and blood to circulate unsmoothly, resulting in congealed blood, dark-purple tongue and petechiae, ecchymosis or maculopapule, etc. may appear because of insufficient body fluids.

7-5 "Five endogenous pathogens"

The "five endogenous pathogens" refers to a pathological phenomenon similar to that caused by pathogenic wind, cold, damp, dryness and fire (intense heat), but produced internally as pathological changes of *qi*, blood, body fluids and viscera, etc. As the diseases occur in the interior, they are termed endogenous dryness, endogenous cold, endogenous damp, endogenous fire, etc. respectively and the "five evils" are by no means pathogenic factors, but a pathogenic change caused by the physiological dysfunction of *qi*, blood, body fluids, viscera, etc.

7-5-1 Wind *qi* moving internally

As wind is closely related to the liver, it is therefore called "liver wind moving internally" or just liver wind. It is a manifestation of wind moving internally in the course of disease, causing pathological reactions such as vertigo, convulsions, tremor, etc. The root cause is excess yang, or deficient yin failing to restrain yang, so that yang increases without any restraint. Violent muscle spasms are due to wind and vertigo and tremor are due to hepatic disorder. *Plain Questions* pointed out that these manifestations are not only similar to pathogenic wind, but related to the liver.

This pathological state is caused by overactive and adverse flow of yang *qi* within the body. There are many causes of adverse flow of yang *qi* within the body. They are chiefly: transformation of liver yang into wind, wind symptoms produced by extreme heat, wind produced by deficient blood, etc.

7-5-1-1 Transformation of liver yang into wind

This is usually caused by injury from emotional factors, fatigue, consumed liver yin and kidney yin so that yin is deficient and yang is in excess, and floating yang fails to descend. If this condition lasts long, the more yang floats, the more deficient yin will become, and fail to restrain yang, since liver yang transforms itself into wind because it is not restrained. In mild cases, muscular twitching, numbness and tremor of the limb, vertigo or facial paralysis, or hemiplegia may be seen, but in severe cases, regurgitation of blood associated with *qi* and sudden fainting, or *tuo* (collapse) syndrome or *bi* (blockage) syndrome create an imbalance.

7-5-1-2 Wind symptom produced by extreme heat

This is usually seen in febrile diseases. As pathogenic heat consumes body fluids and nutritional blood and impairs the Liver Meridian, so tendons and vessels lack nourishment. Excess yang heat produces wind symptoms, resulting in *jin-ye* syndrome,[7] convulsions, flapping of the ala nasi, upward fixation of the eye, etc. accompanied by high fever, mental confusion, delirium, etc.

7-5-1-3 Wind symptom produced by deficient yin

This is usually seen in febrile diseases and caused by the impaired yin or severe consumption of yin fluid. Its main pathogenesis is that exhausted yin fluid fails to nourish tendons and vessels, producing endogenous wind symptoms. It belongs to the symptom caused by asthenia, with spasmotic tendons and muscular twitching, or tremor of the hands and feet. Its pathogenesis and clinical picture are different from those of transformation of liver yang into wind and wind symptoms produced by extreme heat.

7-5-1-4 Wind symptom produced by deficient blood

This is usually caused by insufficient blood or excessive loss of blood, or consumed nutritional blood due to a prolonged illness, deficient liver blood, malnourished tendons and vessels, or the blood's failure to nourish collateral meridians. Numb limbs and trunk, muscular twitching, even rigid hands and feet may be seen in this condition.

There is also a wind symptom produced by dried blood, which is caused by the exhaustion of blood by prolonged illness, or internal congealed blood and obstruction of the formation of new blood. Its pathogenesis is deficiencies of both body fluids and blood, so the skin is not nourished and *qi* and blood in the meridians are in disharmony. Itching, peeling, dry or scaly skin may be seen.

7-5-2 Internal cold

Internal cold is also called endogenous cold. As yang *qi* declines and its warming function decreases, cold due to asthenia is produced internally or pathogenic cold diffuses. Its pathogenesis is as follows: Deficient yang leads to excess yin, while excess yin, leads to endogenous cold, manifested as deficient yang losing its warming function and cold due to asthenia produced internally or contraction of blood vessels and slowed circulation of blood, e.g., pallor, cold trunk and limbs, or rigid tendons and vessels, arthralgia, etc. The spleen is the acquired foundation and source of *qi* and blood, and the yang can reach the muscles and four extremities. Kidney yang is the root of the body's yang *qi* and can warm the viscera and tissues. Therefore deficient spleen and kidney yang is likely to cause the spleen and kidney to become hypofunctional, with cold signs due to deficiency, particularly deficient kidney yang.

Deficient yang *qi* will lead to dysfunctions of *qi*. Yang will fail to produce yin and metabolic activities will be blocked due to lack of energy, leading to accumulation or retention of yin pathological products, such as aqueous damp and *tan-yin*. *Plain Questions* states, "Diseases with dilute and clear discharges are due to cold." Frequent urination with profuse, watery urine, dilute and clear nasal discharge, saliva and sputum or diarrhea, or edema, etc. are thus usually caused by deficient yang failing to transform body fluids into *qi*.

Internal cold due to deficient yang and excess yin and cold syndrome is caused by the affection of exogenous cold or too much unripe and cold food. Although different in nature, endogenous cold and exogenous cold are often connected with each other. The difference between them is that endogenous cold is mainly deficiency accompanied with cold, and exogenous cold is cold accompanied by some deficiency signs due to injury of yang by pathogenic cold. The invasion of pathogenic cold impairs yang *qi*, resulting in deficient yang and a body deficient in yang *qi* is likely to be affected by pathogenic cold because of its weakened resistance against the exogenous factor.

7-5-3 Internal dampness (also called endogenous damp)

The spleen's failure to transform and digest food and aqueous damp, and distribute body fluids causes the accumulation and retention of aqueous damp, phlegm and turbid matter in the middle energizer. As dampness is produced internally usually due to a weak spleen, it is also known as dampness due to a weak spleen.

The production of endogenous damp is usually caused by obesity and excess phlegm and dampness, or indulgence in unripened, cold food or rich food. The distribution of body fluids is blocked. The result is that aqueous liquid gathers forming pernicious damp and stagnates forming pathogenic phlegm, or is retained forming *yin* (excess exudates) or accumulates to form water. Hence, the spleen's failure to perform its transporting and digesting function is the focal point which causes internal damp, as was described in *Plain Questions*, "Edema and swelling from dampness is due to spleen disorder."

Since the spleen's transporting and digesting functions depend upon the warmth and functions of kidney yang, endogenous damp is not only a pathological product formed because deficient spleen yang fails to transform body fluids, but is also closely related to the kidney. Since the kidney controls aqueous liquid and kidney yang is the foundation of all kinds of yang, the kidney influences the transporting and digesting functions of the spleen. A problem of the kidney or spleen can produce internal damp and turbid matter. As pathogenic damp is yin in nature, excess damp can impair yang *qi*, resulting in internal damp stasis which affects the spleen and kidney yang, resulting in a deficient yang and excess damp syndrome.

Damp is heavy, turbid, mucoid and lingering, and usually blocks *qi*. Its clinical manifestations vary according to the area it blocks. If it stagnates in the meridian, fullness and heaviness of the head as if it were tightly bandaged, heavy limbs and trunk or difficulty in movement may be seen. *Plain Questions* states, "Spasm and stiffness of the neck are due to dampness." The affection by endogenous damp leads to chest distress and cough. The blockage of the middle energizer by endogenous damp features epigastric distension and fullness, poor appetite, creamy or sweet mouth, thick mucoid tongue coating. Stagnant endogenous damp in the lower energizer is followed by abdominal distension and loose stools, difficulty in urination, overflowing aqueous damp of the skin and the junction between the skin and muscle. Although dampness can block the upper, middle and lower energizers, it mainly blocks the middle energizer. Hence, stagnation of endogenous damp due to a weak spleen is the most common syndrome.

In addition, although exogenous damp and endogenous damp are formed differently, they often influence each other. The spleen is likely to be affected by exogenous damp and the spleen's failure to perform its transporting function leads to the production of endogenous damp. Therefore, the person with a hypofunctional spleen and excess endogenous damp is likely to be affected by exogenous damp.

7-5-4 Dryness caused by consumed body fluids

Dryness caused by consumed body fluids is also called endogenous dryness. It is a pathological state where the tissues and organs of the body are not nourished due to deficient body fluids, resulting in general dryness. It is caused by exhaustion of yin fluids due to a prolonged blood illness and *jing* which results in deficiency of yin fluid and consumption of yin by pathogenic heat or transformation of pathogenic damp in dryness in the course of certain febrile diseases. Since deficient body fluids do not moisten the viscera internally and the junction between the skin and muscle and openings externally, pernicious dryness and heat are generated internally and pathological dryness is commonly seen in clinic as a result.

In general, severely consumed yin fluid may cause endogenous dryness while consumption of body fluids by excess heat may lead to production of endogenous dryness and heat. Endogenous damp may occur in the viscera and tissues, particularly in the lung, stomach and large intestine. A yin deficiency syndrome with endogenous heat and exhausted body fluids is frequently seen, e.g., dry mouth, throat and lips, dry tongue, even bright, red and cleft tongue, dry nose and eyes, fragile nails, constipation, dark scanty urine, etc. If the lung is mainly affected, pernicious dryness may be accompanied by dry cough with no sputum even hemoptysis. If the dryness is chiefly focused on the stomach, stomach yin will be deficient, with bright red tongue with no coating as the most typical signs. If the intestine is also involved, it may be accompanied by constipation.

7-5-5 Internal fire

Fire produced internally is also called endogenous fire or endogenous heat. It is a pathological state where pernicious fire (heat) disturbs the interior due to excess yang, deficient yin, stagnant *qi* and blood or pathogenic heat.

Fire and heat have the same classification and both pertain to yang, so they have almost the same pathogenesis and clinical picture. Yet, they are divided into deficiency and excess types in their formation. Their pathogenesis is mainly as follows: Normally yang maintains *shen* (Spirit), softens the tendons and warms the viscera and tissues, so called "minor fire." But, if it occurs in excess, yin fluid will be severely consumed. The pathological excess is thus called "vigorous fire."

Fire (intense heat) produced by stagnant pathogens includes:

a. Exogenous pathogenic factors, such as wind, cold, dryness, damp, etc. can all turn into excess yang due to stagnation and transform themselves into heat or fire in the pathological process, e.g., transformation of stagnant cold into heat, transformation of stagnant damp into fire, etc.

b. Pathological metabolic products (e.g., phlegm, stagnant blood) and accumulated food, parasites, etc. can also be transformed into fire due to stagnation. Its main pathogenesis is actually caused by stagnant yang *qi* in the body that produces heat or fire and internal stagnation of excess heat due to excess. Fire (intense heat) produced by the five extreme emotions is called "emotional fire." It usually refers to the emotional irritation which can influence the balance between yin and yang, *qi* and blood and visceral physiology, resulting in *qi* stasis, and transformation of prolonged stagnant *qi* into heat, e.g., internal injury from emotional factors and mental depression often leads to a depressed liver and stagnant *qi* that produce "liver fire."

Deficient yin inducing vigorous fire belongs to fire (intense heat) due to deficiency that is usually caused by deficient *jing* and blood, severely consumed yin fluid, deficient yin and excess yang. In general, systemic heat signs due to deficiency are usually seen in internal heat induced by deficient yin. Fire (heat) signs usually concentrate on a certain area of the body, e.g., toothache, sore throat, dry mouth and tongue, "steaming of bones," malar flush, etc. due to blazing fire caused by excess yang.

7-6 Pathogenesis of meridians

The pathogenesis of meridians refers to the disorders caused by pathogenic factors upon the meridian system, which mainly include excess and deficiency of *qi* and blood in the meridians, abnormal circulation of *qi* and blood in the meridians and obstructed circulation of *qi* and blood in the meridians.

7-6-1 Relative excess and deficient *qi* and blood in the meridians

Excess *qi* and blood in the meridian may accelerate the function of the viscera, tissues and organs that are connected with the meridian, thus breaking the balance between the meridians and viscera causing disease. Inversely, deficient *qi* and blood in the meridians can impair the visceral function, tissues and organs that are connected with the meridians also causing disease. Hence, excess and deficient *qi* and blood in the meridian directly influence the viscera connected with the meridians.

7-6-2 Adverse *qi* and blood in the meridians

Adverse *qi* and blood in the meridian means that abnormally ascending and descending *qi* in the meridians influences the normal circulation of *qi* and blood resulting in diseases.

Adverse *qi* and blood in the meridians usually causes the dissociation of yin *qi* and yang *qi* within the body, e.g., *Plain Questions* states, "If *qi* in the Bladder Meridian of Foot-*taiyang* is in disorder and yin *qi* and yang *qi* are dissociated, heaviness, swelling and distension of the head, inability to walk, vertigo and sudden fainting may result. This is because the meridian originates from the inner canthus, runs upward to reach the forehead, joins the Governor Vessel Meridian at the vertex and then enters the head to connect with the brain, while its lower branch descends to the popliteal fossa and traverses the calf.

Adverse *qi* and blood in the meridians also leads to dysfunction of the viscera connected with the meridians. Adverse *qi* in the meridian of foot-*taiyin* can lead to gastrosplenic dysfunction so clear *qi* fails to ascend and causes diarrhea, and turbid *qi* fails to descend and causes vomiting, and clear and turbid *qi* mix which results in severe vomiting and diarrhea. Adverse *qi* and blood in the meridian is also one of the causes of hemorrhage. Hemoptysis, hematemesis and epistaxis caused by regurgitating *qi* are related to the adverse flow of *qi* in the meridian; hemoptysis caused by liver fire invading the lung is due to upward, adverse and disordered *qi* in the meridian induced by fire (intense heat) in the Liver Meridian. Epistaxis caused by excess heat in the Stomach Meridian is also ascribed to adverse and disordered *qi* in the Stomach Meridian.

7-6-3 Obstruction of *qi* and blood circulation in the meridians

Obstruction of *qi* and blood in the meridians not only influences the viscera connected to the meridians, but also the function of the area where the meridian traverses, e.g., the exterior syndrome with the symptoms of sore muscles throughout the whole body is caused by the exogenous pathogenic factor invading the body surface and obstructing *qi* of the meridian on the body surface; unsmoothly-flowing *qi* in the Liver Meridian of Foot-*jueyin* is often the main cause of hypochondriac pain, goiter, breast masses, etc.

In addition, unsmoothly-flowing and obstructed *qi* and blood in the meridians are the main causes of stagnant *qi* and blood in a meridian.

7-6-4 Failure of *qi* and blood in the meridians

The failure of *qi* and blood in the meridians is a critical sign showing that *qi* and blood are completely exhausted. Because of different locations of the meridians and different functions of the viscera connected with the meridians, the symptoms that appear during the exhaustion of *qi* and blood are also different. As was described in *Plain Questions*, "In the failure of *qi* in the meridian of *taiyang*, upward fixation of the eye, opisthotonos, *che-zong*, pallor, sweating from exhaustion may appear, resulting in death. In the failure of *qi* in the meridian of *shaoyang*, deafness may occur, as well as loose joints, upward fixation of the eye with fright that causes death if it lasts one and a half days, with the first sign of dark-bluish and pale complexion. In the failure of *qi* in the meridian of *yangming*, there may be twitching mouth and eyes, fear, delirium, yellow complexion, analgesia and the pulse loses its slow, moderate and rhythmic character. In the failure of the meridian of *shaoyin*, dull complexion, partially exposed tooth roots, abdominal distension and obstruction of the upper and lower portions of the body may be seen. In the failure of the meridian of *taiyin*, abdominal distension and obstruction, dyspnea, belching, vomiting, hiccup caused by vomiting, flushed face caused by hiccup, obstruction of the upper and lower portions of the body when hiccup stops, dull complexion, dry skin and hair when the obstruction of meridians appears, resulting in death. In the failure of *qi* in the meridian of *jueyin*, heat sensation in the middle energizer, belching and dryness of the upper openings of the esophagus,[8] enuresis and anxiety, rolling tongue and shrinking testes may appear, resulting in death." These are the "failure of the twelve meridians." Because of the interconnection of the *qi* in the twelve meridians, they will all be exhausted if *qi* in one meridian is exhausted. In clinic the development and prognosis of the pathological process can be ascertained by observing manifestations of the failure of meridians, *qi* and blood.

7-7 Pathogenesis of *zang-fu* (viscera)

The pathogenesis of the viscera refers to the internal pathogenesis of the disharmony of normal functions of the viscera in the course of the development of disease. Either external affection or internal injury causes dysfunction of the viscera and disharmony between the viscera, yin and yang, and *qi* and blood. Therefore, it is an important pathogenic theory and is a foundation for *bianzheng* and *lunzhi* (planning treatment according to diagnosis).

The pathogenic theory of the disharmony of the viscera was first seen in the nineteen types of pathogenesis in *Plain Questions*. The explanation of the "normal transmission" or "abnormal transmission" are changes of visceral diseases according to the interacting roles of the five-element theory. Zhang Zhongjing applied it in prevention and treatment of visceral diseases and put forward the viewpoint in *Synopsis of the Golden Bookcase*, which laid a foundation for the pathogenic theory of disharmonious viscera that "Having realized a liver trouble, one should know that it would affect the spleen and the spleen should first be strengthened beforehand."

The chief manifestations of the disharmony of the viscera are: The dysfunction of the viscera and disharmony between the yin and yang, *qi* and blood of the viscera. The former has been described in Chapter II. The latter is the main content of this section.

7-7-1 Disharmony between yin and yang, *qi* and blood of the five yin viscera

Qi pertains to yang and blood to yin. As both of them warm and stimulate the viscera, they are collectively termed "yang *qi*." As yin and blood nourish the viscera, tissues, and soothe the nerves, they are collectively termed "yin blood." Generally speaking, yin and yang of the viscera control the physiological activities of the viscera, that is, excitation or restraint, ascendence or dissipation, descendence or congealment.

The yin and yang of the kidney are regarded as the foundation for the yin and yang of the five yin viscera. Hence, prolonged disharmony between the yin and yang of the viscera affects the kidney. *Qi* and blood in the viscera are derived from nutrients in food. Deficient *qi* and blood in the viscera are intimately related to their resources, the spleen and stomach, *qi* and blood. Therefore, the disharmony between the yin and yang of the viscera and that between *qi* and blood are different to a certain extent.

The main pathogenesis of the disharmony between yin and yang, *qi* and blood of the viscera is described as follows:

7-7-1-1 Disharmony between yin and yang, *qi* and blood of the heart

Pathological problems are manifested as abnormal circulation of heart blood and mental or emotional changes, etc. that are caused by disharmony between heart yin and heart yang or heart *qi* and heart blood. Since yin and yang, *qi* and blood have different actions upon physiological functions, such as the heart's control of blood and governing the Mind, etc., different pathological manifestations may appear in different pathogenesis, such as the disharmony between the yin and yang, *qi* and blood of the heart.

a. The disharmony between heart yin and heart yang is the main manifestation of an imbalance of yang *qi* of the heart.

The excess of yang *qi* of the heart, i.e., heart fire. That caused by pathogenic heat and internal stasis of phlegm-fire is usually an excess type; that caused by excessive mental labour which causes heart yin and heart blood to be severely consumed is of a deficient type; that caused by injury from emotional factor, and fire produced by the five emotions is an excess type. Yet, the deficiency and excess of heart fire can often transform into each other. The excess may severely consume yin blood, leading to vigorous fire induced by deficient yin; deficient fire may also be mixed up with phlegm-heat and pathogenic heat. Although the pathological manifestations of deficient fire and excess fire differ, their influences upon physiological functions are similar.

The main influences of the absolute or relative excess of heart yang *qi* upon physiological functions are:

a. Disturbing the Mind: Yang *qi* is concerned with the motion and ascendence; excess heart yang would lead to disturbance of the mind, resulting in mental irritation with pathological manifestations, such as palpitations, anxiety, insomnia, dreaminess, talkativeness, even raving, confusion, etc.

b. Hot and rapid blood: Excess yang leads to heat, and fire (intense heat) is produced by excess *qi*. Excess yang *qi* would lead to hot and rapid blood, which is the main pathogenesis of the physiological function of the heart's control of blood. In such cases, palpitations, rapid extravasation of hot blood may result, with pathological manifestations of various hemorrhages, etc.

c. Blazing and downward heart fire: Fire flares up and the heart opens to the tongue. If heart fire flares up along the meridian, pathological manifestations, such as tongue rupture, and pain in the tip of tongue, dry mouth and nose, etc. may be seen. The heart and small intestine are closely related. If heart fire transfers downward to reach the small intestine along the meridian, pathological symptoms, such as dark-yellowish urine, burning hot painful sensation in urination, etc. may be seen.

d. Deficient heart yang *qi*: Deficient *qi* and heart yang are usually caused by consumptive disease. It is often seen in deficient chest *qi* and its hypofunction in passing through the Heart Meridian (vessel) and promoting *qi* and blood; deficient and declined kidney yang and aqueous *qi* affecting the heart; the weak spleen and *qi*, internal generation of phlegm and the turbid matter that block the heart vessel, and stagnant blood and *qi*, etc. can all affect the heart, resulting in a relative decline of heart yang *qi*. It may often appear at a critical stage of certain acute diseases usually caused by the anti-pathogenic factor's failure to conquer a violent pathogenic factor, and sudden exhausted yang.

It is divided into deficient heart *qi* and deficient heart yang, which due to their similarities are often jointly described. Their influences upon physiological functions of the heart's control of the mind and blood are mainly as follows:

a) The deficient heart (mind) is usually caused by the fact that the heart's control of the mind is not invigorated by yang *qi*, so that mental and emotional activities are weakened and restrained and no excitation is likely to occur. Pathological symptoms such as mental fatigue and listlessness, neurosis, retardation, somnolence, indolent disinclination to talk, low voice, etc. may appear.

b) Cold and congealed blood: Blood circulates when warmed and stagnates when cooled. Insufficient yang *qi* of the heart and the hypofunctional heart's failure to control blood can cause internal generation of cold and unsmooth blood circulation, leading to congealed blood, even to the obstruction of the Heart Meridian and forming the disease or syndrome of congealed and obstructed heart blood, with cold limbs and trunk, pallor or dull dark-purplish complexion, palpitation and chest distress, stabbing pain, perspiration, even hyperhidrosis, exhausted yang collapse, unsmooth and weak, or slowed, or frequent, or irregular or regularly intermittent pulse, etc.

In addition, deficient heart yang and pathological processes of the lung and kidney often influence each other. For example, deficient yang *qi* of the heart can be caused by deficient lung *qi*: deficient yang *qi* of the heart can also influence lung *qi* and cause abnormal respiration. Therefore, cough, regurgitation of *qi* and even breathing that can be carried on only by sitting, but not lying flat are often simultaneously seen when heart yang *qi* is deficient. This is caused by deficient chest *qi* and hypofunction or deficient heart yin. Kidney yang can also influence the heart. Deficient heart yang may result when overflowing water affects the heart due to deficient kidney yang. Deficient heart yang can also affect kidney yang, resulting in oliguria and edema, etc.

e . The disharmony between heart yin and heart blood is mainly manifested by deficient heart yin, severely consumed heart blood or congealed and obstructed heart blood.

a) Deficient heart yin is usually caused by excessive mental labour, malnutrition due to prolonged illness, severely consumed heart yin or internal injury from emotional factors, persistently consumed heart yin, or heart yin consumed by blazing fire of the heart and liver. Yin's failure to restrain yang, and excess heart yang and deficient yin and excess yang lead to internal generation of fire (intense heat) due to deficiency with pernicious heat in the chest, palms and soles. As the yin fails to restrain floating yang *qi*, the mind is influenced with mental restlessness, or insomnia due to anxiety caused by deficiency. If the function of the heart to control blood is influenced, a minute and rapid pulse and red tongue may be seen. If the nutritional yin fails to maintain itself internally and body fluids are excreted together with yang, pathological symptoms, such as night sweat may occur.

b) Impaired heart blood is usually caused by blood loss or deficient blood or internal injury from emotional factor and consumed heart blood. If heart blood is deficient, the blood vessel will be vacant and no blood is controlled by the heart at all, with a minute forceless pulse; if blood is too deficient to nourish the heart (mind), neurosis will occur, with absentmindedness and even trance seen; if blood is too deficient to hold heart yang and the yang is dissociated with the yin, the Spirit will not be well kept, resulting in insomnia and dreaminess; if blood is too deficient to nourish the heart, palpitation and anxiety will result, even fear; if blood is too deficient to make the face brilliant, pathological symptoms, such as pallor and dull tongue, etc. may be seen.

c) Congealed and obstructed heart blood is also called the obstructed heart meridian (vessel). It refers to the pathological change of unsmooth blood and obstructed heart vessel. Deficiency of yang *qi* and blockage of blood and vessels by pernicious cold can lead to congealed and obstructed heart blood. Accumulated phlegm and turbid matter and obstructed blood vessels can also lead to obstructed heart blood; fatigue and lack of physical exercise and cold affection or mental irritation can often induce or aggravate it. Deficient and impaired yang *qi* arouses the failure of yang *qi* to warmly promote blood, resulting in the unsmooth circulation of blood. As congealed blood obstructs the heart vessel, *qi* and blood in the vessel circulate unsmoothly, resulting in fullness, distension and pain in the chest, etc. If the heart vessel is obstructed by congealed blood, and *qi* and blood are blocked, there will be vigorous palpitation,[9] perspiration and *tuo* (collapse) syndrome and *jue* (fainting) syndrome, etc.

7-7-1-2 Disharmony between yin and yang, *qi* and blood of the lung

Gases from inside and outside the body exchange in the lung. Its main physiological functions are to control *qi* (air) and respiration, and it is concerned with dissipation, purification, descendence and unobstructing the aqueduct. All blood passes through the lung, in order to assist the heart to promote blood circulation. Therefore the disharmony of the yin and yang, *qi* and blood of the lung may cause pathological symptoms, such as abnormal respiration, and formation of *qi* and obstructed water metabolism, etc. and also influence the heart's control of blood, leading to abnormal blood circulation.

Yet, the lung is to a certain extent special in pathology, e.g., its elevating and dissipating actions are concluded by the dissipating function of its *qi*. As blood in all the vessels passes through the lung deficient blood in the lung is extremely rare and usually invades deficient lung yin, but not that of blood. Therefore, the disharmony between the yin and yang, *qi* and blood is mainly manifested as the disharmony of the lung's *qi* and yin.

a. Disorders of lung *qi*: As the lung controls *qi* and respiration in the entire body and is concerned with dissipation, purification and descendence, and regulates the *qi* mechanism of the body, the disorder of lung *qi* is mainly manifested in the abnormal dissipation, purification and descendence and deficiency of lung *qi*.

Abnormal dissipation, purification and descendence of lung *qi* are the two aspects of the ascending and descending of lung *qi*. Although both of them are different, they often influence each other. It is usually caused by the invasion of the body surface and the lung by an exogenous pathogenic factor or internal blockage of the lung vessel by phlegm and turbid matter, or the invasion of the lung by wild liver fire. It is also formed by insufficient lung *qi* or deficient lung yin, etc.

Lung *qi*'s failure to spread *qi* can influence respiration, resulting in an abnormal *qi* mechanism, itching throat and cough, etc. and can also lead to stagnant defensive *qi* and the junction between the skin and muscle may close. If lung *qi* is deficient and fails to spread, defensive *qi* will be weak, with spontaneous sweating and common cold. If lung yin is deficient, the yang will not be restrained and body fluids excreted together with the yang, with night sweat, etc. will be seen.

Inability of lung *qi* to purify and descend refers to that lung *qi* is hyperfunctional in descending and clearing the respiratory tract, with cough and regurgitation of *qi*, profuse sputum and asthmatic breath, etc. seen.

Deficient and impaired lung *qi* is usually formed by the prolonged inability of the lung to dissipate and purify, or deficient *qi* due to prolonged illness or severe consumption of lung *qi* by fatigue. If lung *qi* is deficient, its respiratory function will decrease, gases exchanged in the interior and exterior of the body will be deficient, resulting in short breath, etc. If it influences the distribution and metabolism of body fluids, *tan-yin* (phlegm and excess exudates) will form, even edema. Or it may cause deficient defensive yang *qi* and the loose junction between the skin and muscle, and weaken body resistance, resulting in spontaneous sweating due to a weak body surface.

b. Disorder of lung yin refers to consumed yin fluid in the lung and blazing fire (heart fire) due to deficiency. It is usually caused by pathogenic heat or injury of the lung by internally-stagnant phlegm-fire, or fire produced by the five extreme emotions and consumption of lung yin by prolonged cough. If the lung fails to be moistened, the ascending and descending movements of *qi* become abnormal, or internal heat is spontaneously produced due to deficient yin, and hemorrhage occurs because of injury to the collateral meridians of the lung by pernicious fire due to deficiency and there may be symptoms of dryness and heat due to deficiency, e.g., dry cough with no sputum, or little mucoid sputum, short breath, tidal fever and high sweat, malar flush, heat in the chest, palms and soles, even bloody sputum, etc. If deficient lung yin and consumed body fluids last a long time, the kidney may be affected, leading to deficiencies of the lung and kidney.

7-7-1-3 Disharmony between yin and yang, *qi* and blood of the spleen

The main functions of the spleen are to transport and digest food, send the purified nutrients upward and control blood. Since these functions are chiefly done by the yang *qi* of the spleen, the dysfunction of the spleen in transportation and digestion is mainly caused by the deficient yang *qi* of the spleen to send the purified nutrients upward and transport and digest food, because deficient yin blood of the spleen exerts less influence upon its functions than its yang *qi*. These are the characteristics of the disharmony between the yin and yang of the spleen. The splenic function of controlling blood is actually the manifestation of the controlling action of the yang *qi* of spleen.

a. Disharmony between spleen yang and spleen *qi*: The disorder of the yang *qi* of the spleen is usually caused when the deficient yang *qi* of the spleen fails to perform its transporting and digesting functions, *qi* and blood lack their resource, or aqueous damp internally generated affects kidney yang, resulting in deficiencies of spleen yang and kidney yang; the deficient yang *qi* of the spleen fails to send the purified material upward and the middle *qi* is trapped, resulting in collapse; or deficient *qi* fails to control blood, resulting in blood loss. Disorders of splenic yang *qi* are mainly manifested by deficient spleen *qi*, deficient spleen yang and stagnant aqueous damp.

Deficient spleen *qi* (deficient middle *qi*) is usually caused by injury from improper diet, dysfunction of the spleen, prolonged illness or fatigue and lack of physical exercise. It leads to a hypofunctional spleen, with dyspepsia, light-coloured and tasteless mouth. The weakened function of the spleen to send the purified nutrients upward influences the stomach's ability to send the turbid matter downward, leading to vertigo, distension and fullness of the epigastrium and abdomen, loose stools and diarrhea, etc. The spleen's failure to perform its normal functions and insufficient refined food lead to general deficiencies of *qi* and blood. Deficient spleen *qi* leads to the hyperfunction of the spleen's ability to control blood. Blood loss, failure of deficient spleen *qi* to send the purified nutrients upward or the obstruction of spleen *qi* leads to the obstruction of *qi* in the middle energizer, with prolonged diarrhea and prolapse of the rectum, visceroptosis, etc.

The decline of the spleen is usually due to deficient spleen *qi* or declined *mingmen* (vital portal) fire[10] and the spleen lacking warmth. Deficient spleen yang can lead to internal generation of cold with signs of deficiency, such as cold and pain in the epigastric and abdominal region, aqueous-grainy diarrhea, diarrhea before dawn, etc. Deficient spleen yang can cause the failure of the spleen to warm aqueous damp and internal retention of aqueous damp, or the formation of *tan-yin* or edema due to overflowing aqueous damp in the skin.

Obstructed aqueous damp is caused by the failure of the splenic yang *qi* to transport and digest the refined principle derived from food, or blocked fluid metabolism, abnormal movement of *qi* and retained aqueous damp. The weak spleen and stagnant damp may cause *tan-yin* or edema.

The deficiency-excess syndrome forms because deficient spleen yang fails to transport and digest aqueous damp and the body is likely to be affected by exogenous pathogenic factors, or endogenous and exogenous pathogenic factors block the middle energizer, which transforms itself into cold and damages spleen yang, resulting in excess damp and deficient yang and into heat that causes endogenous damp-heat. As endogenous damp and heat in the middle energizer, "fumigate and steam," the liver and gallbladder are affected by pathogenic heat and body fluids are excreted, and jaundice with yellowish eyes may be seen.

b. Disorder of spleen yin refers to deficiencies of both spleen *qi* and spleen yin. It is usually caused by the failure of deficient spleen *qi* to transport and digest body fluids and insufficient body fluids. Deficient spleen *qi* and the spleen's failure to perform its transporting and digesting functions may result in abdominal distension, loose stool, dyspepsia, etc. In the case of deficient body fluids dry mouth and tongue, red tongue with little coating, etc. may be seen. Deficient spleen yin leads to deficient stomach yin; the stomach's failure to perform its function of sending the turbid matter downward when the stomach is not assisted by the spleen may lead to regurgitation of *qi* with retching, hiccup, etc. seen.

7-7-1-4 Disharmony between yin and yang, *qi* and blood of the liver

The main physiological function of the liver is dispersing, discharging and storing blood. It is concerned with motion, ascendance and resolution. Liver *qi* and liver yang are often in excess; liver yin and liver blood in deficiency. This is the characteristic of the pathogenesis of the disharmony of the yin and yang, *qi* and blood of the liver.

a. Disharmony between liver *qi* and liver yang is usually seen in excess. Liver *qi* and liver yang are rarely seen in deficient *qi* and yang of the liver. Excess liver yang usually occurs when deficient liver yin cannot restrain liver yang. Hence, the pathogenesis of the disharmony between liver *qi* and liver yang is mainly manifested by stagnant liver *qi* and blazing liver fire, etc.

Stagnant liver *qi* is usually due to mental irritation, depression and loss of the dispersing and discharging functions of the liver that result in stagnant *qi*, with distention, fullness and pain in the area where *qi* stagnates, or palpable masses in local areas where phlegm and *qi* and blood are mixed. If *qi* stagnates in the liver, distension and fullness in the hypochondria or pain in the right hypochondrium may be seen. If liver *qi* is blocked or phlegm, and *qi* and blood combine in the Liver Meridian, goiter, "plum-stone" syndrome[11] in the throat, distension and pain or masses in the lower abdomen or contracting pain in the testes, and dysmenorrhea, even amenorrhea may result. In addition, if liver *qi* stagnates or invades the stomach, the stomach *qi* will ascend adversely, causing eructation and acid regurgitation, even epigastric pain if it invades the spleen, pain and diarrhea will appear alternately.

Blazing liver fire is usually caused by a depressed liver and stagnant *qi* which produce pernicious fire, or injury to the liver due to overanger and sudden overactivity of liver *qi*, or injury from emotional factors and pernicious fire produced by the five emotions, and excess heart fire that induces liver fire. As it is caused by excess ascending yang *qi*, pathological symptoms, such as distension and pain in the head, malar flush and congestive eyes, irascibility, sudden tinnitus or deafness, etc. may occur. As yang *qi* of the liver ascends in excess and depressed fire impairs yin blood internally, yin blood is easily consumed and vigorous fire (induced by deficient yin) may result. When the collateral meridians (small vessels) of the lung and stomach are damaged by liver fire, it leads to hempotysis, hematemesis and expistaxis; extreme regurgitation of *qi* fire (excess *qi*) leads to the blood flourishing in the upper part of the body, resulting in *jue* syndrome.

b. Disorder of liver yin and liver blood: The pathogenesis of the disorder of liver yin and liver blood is characterized by their deficiencies. Since deficient yin leads to excess yang, the internal movement of liver wind caused by the unrestrained ascent of yang *qi* is related to deficient yin blood of the liver.

Deficient liver blood is usually caused by hemorrhea or prolonged illness or the weak generation of *qi* and blood by the spleen and stomach. In general, deficient blood would first affect the liver as the liver is the viscus that stores blood. If deficient liver blood fails to nourish the tendons and vessels, numb limbs and joints and difficulty in moving may result. When blood fails to nourish the head and eyes, vertigo, blurred vision, dry and uncomfortable eyes may result. Deficient blood is likely to produce internal patho-genic dryness and wind, leading to the internal movement of pernicious wind due to deficiency, with pathological symptoms, such as itching skin, spasmotic tendons, muscu-lar twitching, *checong*, (An infant extends and flexes its arms and legs intermittently when suffering from convulsions) etc.

The rise of excess liver yang is usually caused by the failure of deficient liver yin to restrain liver yang so that the liver yang moves adversely, or by emotional disorders and regurgitation of *qi* fire and consumed liver yin, which develop into deficient and excess yang. Since liver yin and kidney yin come from the same source, deficient kidney yin (inadequate water) to nourish the liver (wood) often results in an excess rise of liver yang, with pathological symptoms, such as vertigo, tinnitus, malar flush, congestive eyes, blurred vision, irascibility, wiry rapid pulse, etc. At the same time, as liver yin and kidney yin are deficient, weakness in the lower portion of the body, such as lumbago, weak legs, etc. may be seen.

The internal movement of liver wind has a wide range, e.g., excess pathogenic heat induces internal wind; excessively consumed liver blood and malnourished tendons and vessels make liver wind move internally, etc. It is more frequently seen in deficiencies of the liver and kidney yin to restrain yang *qi* and an excess rise of yang *qi* of the liver, accompanied by tremors of the hands and feet, convulsions, or muscular twitching, even sudden fainting, unconsciousness, convulsions and spasmotic *jue* syndrome, etc.

7-7-1-5 Disharmony between yin and yang, *qi* and blood of the kidney

The essential *qi* of the kidney that injures yin and yang is called the congenital foundation. The main physiological function of the kidney is to store *jing* and control aqueous liquids. Disharmony of yin and yang, *qi* and blood of the kidney (refined principle) can influence the kidney's storage of *jing* so that the kidney is not enriched, which results in the unfavourable growth and development of genital functions. If the renal function of controlling water is influenced, general water metabolism may be obstructed, with oliguria, or edema, polydipsia, profuse watery urine, etc. seen.

Disharmony of the yin and yang, *qi* and blood of the kidney has its own features, because essential *qi* in the kidney is the foundation of renal yin and yang, while renal yin and yang are the yin and yang of the entire body. There is often deficiency of kidney *qi* and blood.

a. Deficient essential *qi* of the kidney: Kidney *jing* pertains to yin and kidney *qi* to yang. Deficient essential *qi* of the kidney includes deficient kidney *jing* and weak kidney *qi.*

Deficient kidney *jing* is usually seen in deficient *jing* in senility or congenital deficiency, or caused by prolonged illness and malnutrition. It can influence growth and development during infancy, the production of *tiankui* during youth, and hinders the development and maturity of the sexual gland. In middle age, it can lead to presenility, sexual hypofunction, with spermatorrhea, prospermia, impotence, etc. When it causes insufficiency of cerebrospinal fluid, lowered intelligence, retarded movement, atrophy and weakness of the leg, etc. may be seen.

Weak kidney *qi* is caused by insufficient essential *qi* during childhood or declined kidney *jing* and *qi* in old age, or impairment of kidney *qi* by excess sexual activity, or prolonged illness. The influence of weak kidney *qi* upon the function of kidney is mainly the kidney's failure to control micturition and defecation and to retain essential *qi* that is likely to be lost, with nocturnal emission, prospermia, etc. seen; if it influences the renal function of absorbing *qi*, floating *qi*, hasty breath immediately after exertion, etc. may be seen. If it fails to control micturition and bowel movements, runny stools, profuse watery urine, or enuresis, dribbling of urine, or incontinence of stools and urine, etc. may result.

b. Disharmony between kidney yin and kidney yang: Kidney yin and kidney yang are the foundation of the body's yin and yang. Kidney yin is also called primordial yin, or *mingmen* (vital portal) water. Kidney yang is also called primordial yang, or *mingmen* fire. They represent the opposing states of cold and heat, calmness and motion, descending and ascending, going-out and coming-in movements of the functions of the kidney. Only by restraining each other and keeping a harmonious balance can the normal functions of the kidney be maintained. Disharmony between the yin and yang of the kidney is mainly manifested by deficient renal yin and yang.

Deficient kidney yin is usually caused by injury to yin by a prolonged illness. The fire of the five yin viscera, the fire produced by the five emotions and the fire produced by long retention of pathogenic heat can severely consume not only the yin of other yin viscera but also kidney yin, leading to deficient kidney yin if the condition lasts a long time. Deficient kidney yin leads to unrestrained kidney yang (*mingmen* fire) and an excess of king fire,[12] even internal heat induced by deficient yin and vigorous fire induced by deficient yin. It may also be caused by blood loss and consumed body fluids or taking too many warm, dry drugs for tonifying yang or excess sexual activity that injures the primary fire and consumes kidney yin, leading to vigorous fire induced by deficient yin, emaciation, heat in the chest, palms and soles, "steaming of bones" and tidal fever, malar flush, night sweat and red tongue with little coating, weak, minute and rapid pulse.

Deficient kidney yin is actually declined *mingmen* fire. But they are different in severity in clinical identification of syndrome. Deficiency in kidney yang is usually caused by deficiencies of heart and spleen yang and consumed kidney yang, or excess sexual activities. Deficient yin can lead to an internal generation of yin cold, with remarkable cold signs.

The influence of deficient kidney yang upon the physiological functions of the kidney is mainly manifested by genital hypofunction, or hypofunction of water metabolism, with pathological signs such as impotence, infertility, or edema, etc. Deficient yang and declined fire fails to warm spleen yang and deficiencies of spleen and kidney yang lead to the failure of the spleen and stomach to carry on their transporting and digesting functions, with thin and grainy stools, diarrhea before dawn, etc.

7-7-2 Disorder of the six yang viscera

7-7-2-1 Disorder of the gallbladder

The main physiological function of the gallbladder is to store and excrete bile so as to assist the transporting and digesting functions of the spleen and stomach. Since the bile is formed by liver *qi* and its secretion and excretion are controlled and regulated by the dispersing and discharging functions of the liver, the obstruction of bile is closely related to the dispersing and discharging functions of the liver.

The obstruction of bile can be caused by injury from emotional factors disturbing the liver's function to carry on its dispersing and discharging functions, and can also be caused by the obstruction of "fumigating and steaming" damp-heat in the middle energizer which further aggravates the depression of the liver causing more *qi* stasis and blocking the transporting and discharging functions of the spleen and stomach, leading to exudation of bile through the skin and causing jaundice.

In addition, the upward disturbance of stagnant heat mixed with phlegm in the Gallbladder Meridian can influence the mind, resulting in anxiety and insomnia, etc.

7-7-2-2 Disorder of the stomach

The stomach, the "sea of water and food," receives and digests food and sends the turbid matter downward. A common disorder is the obstruction of food and failure to propel downward which results in distension, fullness and pain in the epigastric region and regurgitation of stomach *qi*, resulting in belching, hiccup, etc.

Dysfunctions of the stomach are mainly caused by deficient stomach *qi*, deficient stomach yin, stomach cold and stomach heat (fire).

a. Deficient stomach *qi* is usually caused by injury of stomach *qi* from prolonged improper diet, congenital weakness or severe impairment of primordial *qi* due to prolonged illness, etc. It may cause distension, fullness and faint pain in the epigastrium, hiccup, etc.

b. Deficient stomach yin mainly refers to the dysfunction of the stomach caused by exhausted yin fluid in the stomach that is usually due to prolonged retention of pathogenic heat at a late stage of febrile disease or exhaustion of yin fluid by prolonged illness. When stomach yin is deficient, its function of receiving and digesting food declines, with poor appetite, bright, red and dry tongue, even mirror-like tongue surface, etc. the failure of the stomach to propel downward may cause pathological symptoms of regurgitation of stomach *qi*, such as distension and fullness of the epigastrium, frequent nausea, retching, even declining stomach *qi*, resulting in erosive mouth ulcers and sores, etc.

c. Stomach cold is usually caused by overeating unripened or cold food, taking too many cold drugs all which injure stomach yang *qi*, or the body is attacked by exogenous cold. This makes the stomach remarkably hypofunctional in digesting food, with pathological symptoms of frequent dyspepsia, and results in *qi* stasis due to the disorder of *qi* mechanism, congealed blood, slowed blood circulation, contraction of collateral meridians and excruciating pain in the epigastric region, which is relieved by heat, etc.

d. Stomach heat (fire): Pathogenic heat and fire have the same classification. It is called "stomach fire" when excess heat in the stomach transforms itself into fire (intense heat) and flares up. Stomach heat and fire are caused by the invasion of the stomach by pathogenic heat or too much alcohol, pungent and rich food that promote pernicious fire and heat or stagnant *qi*, conduction of pernicious fire and heat, congealed blood, phlegm, endogenous damp and retaining food which transforms into pernicious heat and fire. It can also be caused by the invasion of the stomach by overactive gallbladder fire. Both gastric heat and fire can result in the hyperfunction of the stomach, with pathological symptoms, such as *caoza* (epigastric upset), insatiable hunger, etc. Excess heat and fire consume body fluids, leading to the internal stagnation of pathogenic dryness and heat, the stomach's failure to propel downward, with pathological symptoms, such as bitter taste in the mouth, thirst and indulgence in drinking, constipation, etc. and deficient stomach yin in severe cases. Blazing stomach fire may lead to regurgitation of stomach *qi*, with pathological signs such as nausea, vomiting up sour, bitter and yellowish liquid, etc. toothache and painful gums, or epistaxis. If pernicious fire and heat affect the collateral meridian of the stomach, hematemesis due to ascending blood may result.

7-7-2-3 Disorder of the small intestine

The small intestine is a very important viscus in the digestive system. Its main functions are to receive and digest food and differentiate purified nutrients from the turbid matter. Therefore, if it is dysfunctional, it will fail to receive food, with abdominal pain immediately after eating, diarrhea or vomiting, etc. and it will fail to digest food with abdominal distension, dyspepsia, etc. and to differentiate the purified from the turbid, with abdominal pain and borborygmi, vomiting and diarrhea, etc. According to the theory of visceral symptoms, the functions of the small intestine are classified into pathological changes of the spleen and stomach because of their close relationship.

In addition, pathological symptoms, such as dribbling urine, stabbing pain, etc. are due to descending pathogenic damp-heat or downward transfer of excessive heart fire to the small intestine along the meridian, called small intestine fire in the theory of viscera symptoms.

7-7-2-4 Disorder of the large intestine

The chief function of the large intestine is to transport and further digest waste products. Its dysfunction results in abnormal bowel movements. It may be caused by the failure of stomach *qi* to descend, losing its clearing and descending functions, resulting in internal stasis, or pernicious dryness and heat, exhausted *qi*, etc., with dry stools, constipation, etc. If the stagnant combines with *qi* and blood of the large intestine, red-white dysentery, tenesmus, etc. may be seen. If the middle *qi* (gastrosplenic *qi*) is obstructed and the kidney is weak, prolonged diarrhea, uteroptosis, prolapse of the rectum and incontinence of stools, etc. may be seen.

7-7-2-5 Disorder of the urinary bladder

The function of the bladder is to store and discharge urine. When it malfunctions abnormal urination, such as frequent urination, hasty micturition, dysuria, cloudy urine, dribbling urine, anuria, or enuresis, or incontinence of urine, etc. may occur.

The bladder's storage and discharge of urine depends upon bladder *qi*, and dysfunction of the bladder is caused by abnormal *qi* movement. For example, a substantial pathogenic factor or deficient kidney yang *qi* can lead to *qi* disorders, with obstruction of urination, anuria, etc. If the kidney fails to perform its controlling and storing functions and *qi* is not vigorous, the flow of *qi* will be abnormal, with enuresis, incontinence of urine, etc. appearing.

7-7-2-6 Hypofunction of the triple energizer *qi*

The triple energizer is one of the six yang viscera as well as a collective term for the upper, middle and lower energizers. As it is a passage through which body fluids ascend, descend, go out and come in, the *qi* functions of the entire body are affected by the *qi* of the triple energizer.

Dysfunctions of the *qi* of the triple energizer include: The disorder of the *qi* mechanism of the heart, lung, spleen, stomach, intestine, liver, gallbladder, kidney and bladder and abnormal *qi* movement that leads to the abnormal function of the viscera concerned. For example, the heart's control of blood circulation, the lung's respiration function, the digestion function of spleen, stomach, intestines, liver, gallbladder, kidney and bladder all depend upon the harmony of the movement of *qi*, which can be summed up as the functions of the triple energizer *qi*.

As well *qi* in the triple energizer regulates fluid metabolism of the five yin viscera, because the triple energizer is a passage through which *qi* and body fluids pass as well as one whose *qi* has an important function. Hence, loss of the regulating function of the lung is ascribed to dysfunctional *qi* in the upper energizer. Failure of the stomach to transport and digest aqueous liquid, distribute *jing* (vital principle), and to send the clear upward and the turbid downward is ascribed to dysfunctional *qi* in the middle energizer. Failure of the kidney and bladder *qi* to discharge the turbid and problems with the intestines are ascribed to dysfunctional *qi* in the lower energizer. Therefore, dysfunctional *qi* in the triple energizer obstructs the body's water metabolism.

7-7-3 Dysfunction of the unusual organs

7-7-3-1 Dysfunction of the brain

Thoughts and emotions, sight, hearing, smell, taste and movement are all physiological functions of the brain. Hence, pathological changes may immediately cause obstruction or disharmony of the above functions. As the brain is formed by the marrow, deficient essential *qi* of the kidney, inability of *jing* (vital principle) to produce the marrow, insufficient cerebrospinal fluid may result. Dysfunction of the brain will result in pathological symptoms, such as lowered intelligence, difficulty seeing, hearing and speaking, difficult movement and atrophic and weak limbs. Since the brain is situated at the highest position of the body and fully depends upon ascending yang *qi*, the inability of yang *qi* to ascend may result in pathological symptoms, such as vertigo, hypofunction of the ears and eyes, etc.

7-7-3-2 Dysfunction of marrow and bone

Marrow is located in bones, including the bone marrow, spinal cord and brain. The bones are a framework for the body. Marrow is derived from *jing* (vital principle), enriching and nourishing bones. Dysfunctions of the marrow and bones are mainly manifested by delayed growth and development, soft, weak and fragile bones. The dysfunctions can be caused by congenital weakness, acquired malnutrition, or yin fluid consumed by long-standing pathogenic factor, or cold in the lower energizer due to asthenia and insufficient *jing* (vital principle) and blood and lead to pathological processes, such as insufficient bone marrow and weak fragile bones.

7-7-3-3 Dysfunction of blood vessels

The vessel is the passage through which *qi* and blood circulate. They are regarded as normal when unobstructed. Malnourishment of the vessel due to dried body fluids, obstructed *qi* mechanism due to internal blockage of phlegm and turbid matter, and stasis and obstruction of endogenous cold, etc. may cause an unsmooth flow in the vessels, resulting in *qi* and blood stagnation. Conversely, stagnant *qi* and blood can also influence the blood vessels. The vessels can also make *qi* and blood circulate normally within them. This function is actually the function of *qi* in controlling blood. Thus, pathological symptoms of various hemorrhages can be seen when spleen *qi* is too weak to control blood.

7-7-3-4 Dysfunction of the uterus

Dysfunction of the uterus is mainly manifested by abnormal menstruation, vaginal discharge, fetus and delivery, the causes of which are chiefly as follows:

a. Disharmony between *qi* and blood, pregnancy, delivery and breast-feeding all depend upon blood. Blood relies on *qi*. Only if *qi* and blood are in harmony can blood perform its function effectively. Otherwise, there will be problems with the uterus.

Blood heat, inability of the liver to store blood or to carry on its dispersing and discharging function and inability of the spleen to control blood or that of *qi* to govern blood can all result in metrorrhagia, with early menstruation, profuse menstrual flow, delayed menstruation, etc. If blood regurgitates together with pernicious fire, cyclical hematemesis and epistaxis may occur during or after the menstrual period.

If the uterus is weak and cold due to *qi* stasis, stagnant blood or deficient *qi* and blood or deficient yang *qi*, deficient and cold primordial *qi* in the lower portion of the body, unsmooth circulation and stagnation of blood in the uterus may result, with delayed menstruation, oligomenorrhea, or dysmenorrhea, or amenorrhea or abdominal masses seen.

The dysfunction of the uterus caused by a downward transfer of pathogenic cold-damp or damp-heat is actually due to the disharmony between *qi* and blood.

b. Dysfunctions of the heart, liver, spleen and kidney and dysfunction of the uterus: Dysfunctions of the heart, liver, spleen and kidney can cause not only disharmony between *qi* and blood but also dysfunction of the uterus. Uterus problems are also often caused by emotional factors, fatigue and lack of physical exercise, excess sexual activity, etc. For example, injury of the heart from meditation and prolonged consumption of heart blood, injury of the spleen from meditation and difficulty in producing *qi* and blood, injury of the liver from anger and loss of the dispersing and discharging functions of the liver, injury of the kidney from excess sexual activity, impaired kidney *jing*, deficient *tiankui*, etc. can all lead to the dysfunction of the uterus, with pathological symptoms, such as abnormal menstruation, pregnancy and delivery, etc.

c. Deficient *qi* and blood in the Strategic Vessel Meridian and Conception Vessel Meridian and dysfunctional uterus: Both the Strategic Vessel Meridian and the Conception Vessel Meridian originate from the uterus. The former is the sea of blood and the latter controls the uterus and fetus. Enriched *qi* and blood in these meridians are the material basis for the function of the uterus. The factors influencing the enrichment of *qi* and blood in the Strategic Vessel Meridian and Conception Vessel Meridian come from the kidney. But, as the two vessel meridians pertain to the liver and kidney, the physiological dysfunction of the liver and kidney can cause deficient *qi* and blood in the meridians, resulting in the dysfunction of the uterus. As the Strategic Vessel Meridian pertains to the *Yangming* Meridian, the dysfunctions of the spleen and stomach and deficient *qi* and blood in the *Yangming* Meridian fail to enrich *qi* and blood in Strategic Vessel Meridian and Conception Vessel Meridian which results in abnormal function of the uterus.

To sum up, the function of the uterus is a component of the physiological functions of the whole body, and its dysfunctions are closely related to the state of physiological functions of the whole body.

Notes

[1.] Clonic convulsion. An infant extends and flexes its arms and legs intermittently when suffering from convulsion.

[2.] Eyes, nose, ear, mouth, anus and urethral meatus.

[3.] Sudden fainting with cold clammy limbs, and gradually regaining consciousness.

[4.] The pathological manifestations of the terminal state of a disease due to extreme loss of yin, yang, *qi* and blood, such as profuse sweating, cold and clammy limbs, mouth open and eyes closed, incontinence of stool and urine, barely palpable pulse, etc.

[5.] *Bi* (block) syndrome and *jue* syndrome.

[6.] The last stage of an acute febrile disease.

[7.] Convulsive disease (opisthotonos and lockjaw in febrile disease) and *jue* (fainting) syndrome.

[8.] The orifices of the head.

[9.] The sensation of the heart throbbing vigorously, frequently seen in organic heart disease.

[10.] Also called kidney yang or primordial yang or true yang or true fire or kidney fire or vital fire. The functions of the kidney are the source of body heat. Pathological cold manifestations are caused by deficient kidney yang, and heat manifestations are caused by "excess of kidney yang," or "excess of kidney fire."

[11.] A condition where the patient feels a foreign body like the stone of a plum obstructing the throat, with dysphagia. There is neither redness nor swelling of the throat.

[12.] Referring to heart fire because the ancients compared the heart to a king.

8. FOUR TECHNIQUES OF DIAGNOSIS

The four techniques of diagnosis include inspection, auscultation-olfaction, inquiry and palpation.

Inspection means that the physician observes any changes which might affect the patient's general appearance, including his or her mental state and *shen* (Spirit), complexion and physical form. Auscultation-olfaction means that the physician observes any changes which might affect the patient's voice and smell. Inquiry means that the physician asks the patient or the people who brought the patient in to understand the development of the disease and its symptoms. Palpation means that the physician feels the patient's pulse and touches his or her abdomen, hands and feet and other parts of the body.

Since the body is an organic integral, local pathological processes can influence the whole body and pathological processes of the viscera can be reflected by the sense organs, four extremities, body surface, etc. The cause, feature and internal connection of disease can therefore be understood through diagnosing various symptoms of a disease by inspecting the patient's complexion, hearing, voice and feeling the pulse to collect data for *bianzheng* and *lunzhi* (planning treatment according to diagnosis).

The inspection, auscultation-olfaction, inquiry and palpation are different techniques for investigating a disease, and thus, they must be combined in clinical application. Only in this way can a disease be systematically understood and a correct diagnosis made.

8-1 Inspection

Inspection is to observe abnormal changes of the patient's *shen* (Spirit), complexion, body, tongue and secretions and excreta in order to predict pathological changes of the viscera. In TCM theory the exterior of the body, particularly the face, tongue and its coating, are closely related to the viscera. If changes occur in the viscera, *qi*, blood, yin and yang, they are reflected on the body surface. Therefore certain internal pathological processes can be understood through inspection.

8-1-1 Examination of the body

8-1-1-1 Inspection of *shen* (Spirit)

Shen (Spirit) is a manifestation of the life force including mental and emotional states. Its basis is essential *qi* and it is visible in the physical form, movement, complexion, Spleen, etc. *Plain Questions* states, "Patients with Spirit are easily to be cured, but those with no Spirit are incurable." Bodily inspection of Spirit is important to determine the flourishing and decline of anti-pathogenic factors, the severity of disease and its prognosis.

The inspection of Spirit is to observe whether the patient's mental state is normal, whether the consciousness is clear, the movements harmonious and whether the reaction is timid in order to determine the flourishing or decline of the viscera, yin, yang and *qi* and blood and the prognosis of disease. As the eye is where the essential *qi* of the five yin and six yang viscera is shown and the "ocular connection" is the messenger of the heart, eye inspection is also important to detect spiritual changes.

Attention should be paid to the following conditions when inspecting Spirit:

a. Having Spirit: Since Spirit is based on essential *qi*, sufficient essential *qi* is the basis for vitality. If the patient has alert and bright eyes, clear consciousness, quick responses and a resonant voice, it is called "having Spirit," which shows that the patient's anti-pathogenic factor has not yet been injured, that the visceral function has not yet declined. This indicates a favourable prognosis even if the disease is severe.

b. Loss of Spirit: If the patient is apathetic with dull eyes, slow responses, has difficulty breathing, mental confusion, carphologia, gasps air or faints with the eyes closed and the mouth opened, outstretched hands, enuresis, etc., it is called "less Spirit" or "no Spirit," which indicates that the anti-pathogenic factor has been injured and the disease is severe, indicating an unfavourable prognosis.

c. False vitality is usually seen in patients who suffer from a prolonged and severe disease with extremely weak essential *qi*, e.g., those who do not like to speak, with low and weak voice or who speak discontinuously, and then suddenly begin to speak persistently; those who are extremely low in spirit and their consciousness unclear but suddenly take a turn for the better; those who have a full complexion and suddenly suffer from malar flush. These are false symptoms where the yin fails to restrain yang, and the yang is separating from the yin, to which great attention should be paid.

Mental disorders can often be seen in patients with epilepsy and mania, e.g., listlessness, little talking, low spirits, trance, abnormal crying and laughter are *dian* (epilepsy) usually due to stagnation and blockage of the mind by phlegmatic *qi*. Anxiety, restlessness after taking off their clothes, crying and cursing with rage, beating someone and destroying objects, etc. are usually mania due to disturbance of the heart by phlegm-fire. Sudden fainting, unconsciousness are usually the *xian* (epilepsy) disease due to "phlegm misting the mind" and "liver wind moving internally."

8-1-1-2 Inspection of complexion

This is the inspection of facial colour and texture. As the 12 meridians and their 365 collateral meridians ascend to the face and run through the sense organs, the complexion is the external manifestation of the viscera, *qi* and blood.

The colour and texture of a complexion vary with different constitutions, geographical environments, seasons, weather and professions.

Abnormal changes of facial colour and brilliance are manifestations of different pathological reactions of the body. Different colours reflect different diseases or syndromes, while the texture reflects the flourishing and decline of essential *qi* in the body. An examination of the degree of brilliance and moisture of the face is thus important for diagnosing the severity of the disease and predicting its development. In general, the patient with a bright and moist complexion indicates that the disease is mild and superficial, that *qi* and blood have not yet declined and the disease is curable with a favourable prognosis. A dull and withered complexion indicates that the disease is severe and deep, the essential *qi* has already been injured, with an unfavourable prognosis. Dark-bluish, yellow, red, white and black colours not only represent different pathological changes of the viscera, but also different pathogenic factors, e.g., in the disease or syndromes due to a weak spleen and extreme damp, the patient's complexion is yellowish and dull. In a patient with weak kidneys due to a prolonged illness, his or her complexion is usually dull.

The five colours reflecting various diseases are respectively described as follows:

a. A white complexion indicates deficient-cold and blood-loss syndromes and is a sign of declining *qi* and blood. It may be caused by declined yang *qi* and slowly circulating *qi* and blood or insufficient *qi* and blood due to *qi* consumption and blood loss. If it is pale and accompanied by asthenic puffiness, it is ascribed to deficient yang *qi*; if whitish with emaciation, it is ascribed to severely-consumed nutritional blood. If pallor suddenly occurs in an acute disease, it often belongs to the symptom of sudden exhaustion of yang *qi*. When an excruciating pain in the abdomen appears in an interior-cold syndrome or shivering due to cold caused by deficiency, pallor may be seen, which is caused by stagnant yin cold and rigid meridians (vessels).

b. A yellow complexion indicates a deficiency and damp syndrome. A yellow colour is a sign of a weak spleen and stagnant pathogenic damp. Therefore, a yellow complexion is frequently seen in patients whose spleen *qi* and blood are insufficient or where aqueous damp has not been eliminated. If the complexion is bright-yellow, withered and dull, it is due to a weak spleen and stomach and inability of nutritional blood to upwardly nourish the body. A yellow complexion accompanied with puffiness is due to asthenia, which is ascribed to declined spleen *qi* and internally-blocking pathogenic damp, e.g., yellow face, eyes and body surface suggest jaundice and are due to pathogenic damp-heat; a fresh yellow skin colour which is "yang yellow," is ascribed to pathogenic damp-heat; a dull yellow colour to "yin yellow," is ascribed to pathogenic cold-damp.

c. A red complexion indicates a heat syndrome. Red is the colour of blood. A flushed face results from enriched blood in the collateral meridians due to extreme heat. Thus, a red complexion suggests a heat syndrome. The burning red complexion is ascribed to fever caused by an exogenous pathogenic factor or an excess heat syndrome; malar flush is caused by the deficiency-heat syndrome due to deficient yin and excess yang; pallor with occasional redness suggests a *taiyang* syndrome.[1]

d. A dark-bluish complexion indicates a cold syndrome, pain syndrome, stagnant blood syndrome and infantile convulsion. A dark-bluish colour signifies congealed cold and *qi* and a blocked meridian. As cold is concerned with contraction, extreme cold retained in the meridian leads to a rigid meridian and congealed blood that may cause a dark-bluish complexion. If yin cold is internally excessive with cardialgia and abdominal pain, pallor and a dark-bluish complexion may occur. If heart *qi* is too weak to promote blood circulation, dark-grayish and dark-purplish mouth and lips may result, which is usually caused by deficient *qi* and stagnant blood. Infantile fever and dark-bluish complexion, particularly seen on the bridge of the nose and the area between the eyelids and surrounding lips, is usually the sign of an infantile convulsion syndrome.

e. A dull complexion indicates a weak kidney, *shuiyin* (excess watery fluid) and stagnant blood syndrome. A black colour suggests yin cold and excess fluids. The reason why cold fluid and yin pathogen are in excess is chiefly due to declined kidney yang. The kidney is the viscus of water and fire and the root of yang *qi* as well. Deficient fire due to deficient yang can lead to internal excess of water cold, loss of warm nourishment of blood, with a dull complexion. Black colour in the surrounding orbital region is seen in *shui-yin* diseases[2] or syndrome of overflowing water due to weak kidney or vaginal discharge syndrome[3] due to descending pathogenic cold-damp. A full and dry complexion is ascribed to the prolonged consumption of kidney *jing*.

8-1-1-3 Examination of the body stature

Whether the body stature is robust or not indicates whether functions of the five yin viscera flourish or decline. Generally speaking, if the interior body flourishes, the exterior will be strong; if the interior body declines, the exterior will be weak.

Obese patients with white and lusterless skin and low spirits have "excess in body stature but deficiency in *qi*," which is a deficient yang syndrome. Emaciation, yellow complexion, narrow chest, and dry skin are often seen in an insufficient yin blood syndrome. Atrophic muscles are frequently seen in patients with exhausted essential *qi*. Malformations, such as a "pigeon chest," "tortoise back," etc. are ascribed to insufficient congenital endowment and mainly denote exhausted lung *qi*, weak spleen and stomach, and impaired kidney *jing* diseases.

8-1-1-4 Inspection of body stature and movement

This is the observation of the patient's stature and movement, which reflect pathological changes. Different diseases are manifested by different body statures and positions. "Yang is concerned with motion, while yin with quiescence." Patients who like to move suffer from a yang syndrome, while those who dislike movement from a yin, e.g., the patient in a lying position who can turn around easily suffers from yang, heat and excess syndromes. The patient who can hardly turn around due to body weight and appears listless, suffers from yin, cold and deficiency syndromes. The patient lying in a supine position with extended feet and who often uncovers the blanket, and dislikes heat, suffers from a heat syndrome. The patient lying in bed with a curled body and with a preference for warmth suffers from a cold syndrome. When a patient sits with the head up it is ascribed to excess lung syndrome due to excessive phlegm and saliva. When the patient sits with the head bent down with shortness of breath, and disinclination to talk, it is due to a weak lung syndrome or inability of the kidney to absorb *qi*. When a patient cannot lie down and has *qi* regurgitation when lying down, it is due to insufficient heart yang and aqueous *qi* affecting the heart. When the patient coughs and needs to rest in winter it is due to internal affection of yin (excess fluid).

It is helpful for the diagnosis to observe patients who act abnormally, e.g., occasional tremor of the eyelids, mouth or finger of convulsive disease; if seen in general weakness due to a prolonged illness, it is due to insufficient *qi* and blood and malnourished meridians. Convulsions of the four extremities are commonly seen in *xian* (epilepsy) syndrome,[4] tetanus, acute/chronic infantile convulsions, etc. Rigid hands and feet are ascribed to the rigidity of liver trouble or stagnant pathogenic cold in tendons and vessels or consumed blood and malnourished fascia. Weak and inflexible feet or hands are *wei* (atrophy) syndrome.[5] Inability of movement or numb hands and feet on either side of the body is paraplegia due to apoplexy; a pain and muscular atrophy of the hand and foot on either side of the body is due to the exhaustion of blood by pathological wind and deficient anti-pathogenic factor and retaining the pathogenic factor. Stiff neck and back, opisthotonos, convulsions of the four extremities are due to *jin* (convulsive) disease.[6]

8-1-2 Inspection of the local body

8-1-2-1 Evaluation of the head and hair

This is the observation of the head and hair colour changes. All yang meridians merge at the head. The marrow is controlled by the kidney. As hair is connected with the flourishing kidney and brilliance of blood, the condition of the kidney, *qi* and blood can be known by examining the head and hair.

a. Observation of the head notes the shape of the head.

An extremely large or small head of the infant accompanied by maldeveloped intelligence is ascribed to consumed kidney *jing* ; a sunken fontanel, deficiency syndrome; a protruding fontanel, a heat syndrome; the delayed fontanel with the vertex, deficient kidney *qi* and maldevelopment; involuntary shaking head in adults and infants is a wind syndrome.

b. Observation of the hair notes changes in the quality and colour of hair, e.g., sparse hair which falls out easily, or dry and withered hair indicates the syndrome of deficient *jing* and blood; suddenly occurring localized hair loss is ascribed to deficient *qi* and blood caused by wind affection; alopecia in youth to a weak kidney or heat in blood. Premature greying without other signs of an ailment is not a pathological state.

8-1-2-2 Inspection of the eye

The eye is the window of the liver, and the essential *qi* of the viscera ascends to the eyes. Therefore, abnormal eye changes not only relate to the liver but also reflect the visceral problem.

Besides observation of the spirit from the eye, attention should be paid to the change of their external shape and colour, etc. Congestion and swelling of the eye denote pathogenic wind-heat in the Liver Meridian; a sunken orbit, consumed body fluids; red and erosive canthi, pathogenic damp-heat; the open eyes of infant in sleep, deficient essential *qi*. Icteric sclera is often seen in jaundice; slightly white canthi, deficient *qi* and blood; excess heat in meridians, the congestive eye. It is a yang syndrome if one likes to see someone upon waking; it is a yin one if one closes the eyes and does not like to see anyone; upward fixation of the eye, or squint, or looking straight forward is seen in liver wind and is the sign of moving endogenous pathogenic wind.

8-1-2-3 Inspection of the ear

The ear is the window of the kidney, pertains to the yang meridians and the place where the big meridian gathers. In observing the ear, attention should be paid to its colour and interior, e.g., a dry and black helix is ascribed to severely consumed kidney *jing* and can be fatal; a red ear denotes suppuration and *tin* ear[7] and results from pathogenic damp-heat in the liver and gallbladder.

8-1-2-4 Inspection of the nose

The nose is the window of the lung, where the Stomach Meridian passes and air exchanges as well. In observing the nose its secretions and appearance are noted.

Clear nasal discharge indicates exogenous pathogenic wind-cold; turbid mucus is caused by exogenous pathogenic wind-heat; turbid nasal discharge for a long period of time with offensive smell, rhinorrhea caused by an external affection or endogenous pathogenic heat stagnating in the Gallbladder Meridian. Congestion in the tip of the nose or its surrounding area or red papules such as rosacea that is due to endogenous pathogenic heat in the lung and stomach, and the erosive and sunken nose bridge is commonly seen in leprosy or syphilis; flapping of the ala nasi is frequently seen in endogenous pathogenic heat in the lung or asthmatic breath caused by exhausted essential *qi* in the lung and kidney.

8-1-2-5 Inspection of the lips, teeth and throat

a. Lips: The spleen reflects itself on the lips. In observing the lips, their colour and degree of moisture and change of their shape should be noted. Slightly white lips indicate deficient *qi* and blood; dark-purplish ones are often due to stagnant pathogenic cold and blood; dark-red lips are due to pathogenic heat in the *ying* (nutrition) and *xue* (blood) phases. Dry, cleft lips may be seen in exogenous pathogenic dryness and body fluids consumed by extreme heat; salivation (during sleep) is ascribed to a weak spleen and extreme pathogenic damp or heat in the stomach and also parasite retention. Cracked lips are due to upward spreading of accumulating heat in the spleen and stomach; deviated mouth, apoplexy; umbilical convulsion, internally-moving liver wind or endogenous pathogenic wind produced by a weak spleen. The persistently opened mouth is commonly seen in *tuo* (collapse) syndrome.

b. Teeth and gums are closely related to the bones and are controlled by the kidney and the Stomach Meridian which connects with the gums and the eyes. The teeth are closely related to the kidney, while the gums are related to the stomach.

When observing the teeth, their colour, degree of moisture and shape should be noted, e.g., dry teeth are due to severe consumption of body fluids by extreme heat in the stomach; extremely dry teeth are due to exhausted kidney *jing* and inability of kidney water to ascend; loose and sparse teeth with exposed roots are due to a weak kidney or blazing fire due to deficiency, grinding one's teeth during sleep is commonly seen in patients affected by pathogenic heat in the stomach or parasite retention.

Attention should be paid to the change of their colour during observation of the gums. Slightly white gums denote deficient blood; congestive and swelling gums, blazing stomach fire; bleeding gums with redness and swelling, the collateral meridian injured by stomach fire (intense heat) due to deficiency.

c. Throat: As the throat is a pathway of the lung and stomach, other meridians, such as the Heart Meridian, Kidney Meridian, Liver Meridian, Spleen Meridian, Stomach Meridian, etc. all connect with it, so a number of pathological processes can be reflected by the throat.

While observing the throat, attention should be paid to abnormal changes of its colour and shape. A congestive, swollen and painful throat is ascribed to pathogenic heat accumulating in the lung and stomach; a congestive, swollen throat with yellowish-white spots is ascribed to extreme pathogenic heat in the lung and stomach; a fresh-red and delicate throat with mild pain, blazing fire is due to deficient yin; a chronic slightly red throat without swelling is due to floating fire due to deficiency; a throat with a grayish-white pseudomembrane that cannot be removed but which bleeds and reproduces immediately after being rubbed is caused by diphtheria and pertains to the syndrome of lung heat and consumed yin.

8-1-2-6 Inspection of the skin

The skin corresponds internally with the lung, and is a protective screen for the body with defensive *qi* flowing in it.

Attention should be paid to the change of skin colour and texture. Yellow skin of the face and eye indicates jaundice; puffy skin indicates overflowing aqueous damp that causes disease; dry and withered skin is caused by consumed body fluids, etc. In addition, great attention must be paid to pathological changes, such as *ban-zhen*,[8] white blisters,[9] carbuncle, cellulitis, T-shaped furuncle,[10] etc.

a. *Ban-zhen* is a sign of skin disease. There are also certain diseases that are associated with them, for instance, *feng-zhen* (wind skin rash), *ma-zhen* (measles), *yin-zhen* (urticaria), etc. They are often seen in exogenous febrile diseases and subcutaneous hemorrhages and can form reddish or purplish patches. Those which cannot be felt with the fingers are *ban*, often seen in acute fever, and are signs of pathogenic heat invading the *ying* (nutrition) and *xue* (blood) phases. Those with reddish or purplish miliary elevation on the skin which can be felt with fingers are *zhen* (papule). Those commonly seen in exogenous febrile disease are caused when pathogenic heat stagnating in the lung and stomach cannot be expelled outside the body, but inwardly invade *ying* (nutrition) and *xue* (blood). Those which exude through muscles are *ban*, while others which exude through the skin and blood vessel are *zhen*. Observation of *ban-zhen* is chiefly to note changes of their colour and shape.

The ruddy and shining ones are benign. If they are dark-red, they are caused by extreme toxic heat; if purplish, extreme toxic heat and severely consumed yin fluid; if slightly red or purplish, insufficient *qi* and blood or exhausted yang *qi*.

Those that are evenly distributed are benign. If they are few and scattered, they are caused by mild and superficial pathogens; if they are dense and their colour cannot be changed by pressure, they are due to deep and severe toxic heat; those with unevenly distributed spots, sink immediately after they appear, and are due to deficient antipathogenic factor and the inward trapping of the pathogen.

Those seen in miscellaneous disease and caused by internal injury are ascribed to heat affecting blood; if they are dark-purplish in colour, and large in shape, they are signs of deficient *qi*'s failure to control blood and are associated with stagnant blood.

b. White blisters   Small glistening and transparent vesicles appearing on the skin and protruding, containing yellowish serous fluid. They are frequently seen on the chest and neck, or occasionally on the limbs, caused by stagnant pathogenic damp in the skin and incomplete sweating.

Whitish glistening blisters indicates a favourable prognosis called *jin-pei* and are signs that pathogenic damp-heat reaches the body surface outwardly. Dry white blisters called *ku-pei* are unfavourable, a reflection of exhausted body fluids. Since pathogenic damp is stingy and stagnant and does not easily expose transparently, it is likely to relapse.

c. Carbuncle, cellulitis, T-shaped sore and furuncle all belong to surgical boils whose shapes and symptoms can be seen on the body surface. Those wide in local invasion, red, swollen, hot, painful and rooted are carbuncle, pertaining to a yang syndrome; those swollen, deeply located with unchanging colour are cellulitis, pertaining to a yin syndrome; those having a narrow range, miliary and firmly rooted or numb or itching, white in their heads and painful are T-shaped sores; those originating from the body surface, round, red, swollen, hot, painful and soft immediately after suppuration are furuncles.

8-1-3 Inspection of the tongue

Observation of the tongue, also known as "tongue diagnosis," is an important component of diagnosis of disease. Tongue diagnosis has a long history. It was recorded as early as in the *Internal Classics*. It has been developing for thousands of years, and has now been established as a systematic theory.

8-1-3-1 Relation between the tongue and viscera

The tongue is the window of the heart, and the spleen also reflects itself on the tongue. As the tongue is connected with a number of viscera via the meridians, such as the branch of Heart Meridian of Hand-*shaoyin*, Spleen Meridian of Foot-*taiyin*, Kidney Meridian of Foot-*jueyin*, etc., the essential *qi* of the viscera can ascend to nourish the tongue and pathological processes are also reflected on it, therefore observing the tongue can help diagnose pathological changes of the viscera.

The connection between a portion of the tongue and a certain viscus was discovered and thus the tongue is divided into four sections; the tip, centre, root and edge which respectively correspond to the heart and lung, spleen and stomach, kidney, liver and gallbladder. The technique of diagnosing pathological changes of the viscera through different portions of the tongue is valuable for clinical reference. (Fig. 42)

8-1-3-2 Tongue diagnosis

Observation of the tongue notes changes of the tongue proper and its coating. The tongue proper is composed of muscles, vessels and tissues, while its coating is a layer of mossy substance on its surface produced by stomach *qi*. The normal tongue is soft, flexible and light-red and is coated with a layer of thin, moderately-moistened coating with evenly distributed granules on it. It is often described as a light red tongue with a thin whitish coating.

Different pathological conditions and their coating are respectively introduced as follows:

Observation of tongue proper

a. Observation of tongue colour

a) Pale tongue: A tongue less red than normal indicates a deficiency and cold syndrome, is a sign of weak yang *qi* and deficient *qi* and blood, caused by insufficient blood due to deficient yang and deficient *qi* and blood. It is commonly seen in a disease of deficient yang and blood.

b) Red tongue: A tongue redder than normal indicates a heat syndrome caused by invading pathogenic heat that results in extreme *qi* and blood and possibly seen in a heat syndrome due to internal excess as well as endogenous pathogenic heat due to deficient yin.

c) Dark-red tongue: indicates the depth and severity of pathogenic heat invading the body. In a febrile disease caused by an exogenous factor, it denotes that pathogenic heat has invaded deep into *ying* (nutrition) and *xue* (blood) and is frequently seen at the late stage of the febrile disease. In miscellaneous diseases of internal injury, it is often seen in patients with a prolonged and severe illness and is ascribed to flaring fire (intense heat) caused by deficient yin.

d) Purplish tongue: indicates heat and cold syndromes. The dark-purplish tongue with less fluid indicates that pathogenic heat is preponderant, yin fluids consumed and blood stagnant. A slightly purplish or dark purplish and moistened tongue is ascribed to extreme internal yin cold and congealed blood. The tongue with purplish spots is due to the congealed blood syndrome.

b. Observation of tongue shape notes the state of the tongue proper and its abnormal changes.

The examiner should note whether the tongue proper is flourishing or withered, old or delicate. The bright and moist tongue indicates that body fluids are sufficient; the dry and thin tongue is withered, indicating consumed body fluids. The tongue with rough veins and withered shape and colour is cold, denoting excess and heat syndromes. The tongue with veinules and fat and withered shape indicates a deficient and cold syndrome. At the same time, it should be noted whether the tongue is fat, large, cracked, thorny and indented.

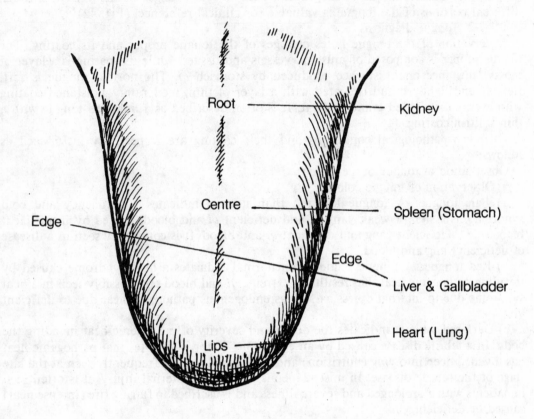

Fig. 42. The correspondence of the viscera to different portions of the tongue

a) Enlarged or flabby tongue: The tongue is larger than normal. It is divided into the flabby, delicate tongue and the swelling, distending tongue. The flabby delicate tongue with light colour is ascribed to a deficient spleen and kidney, stagnant body fluids and blocking *shui-yin* (excess watery fluid) and phlegm-damp. The swollen distended tongue with a dark colour is due to extreme pernicious heat in the heart and spleen. An enlarged tongue with dark-purplish colour is ascribed to poisoning.

b) Thin tongue: The thin and small tongue is a sign of deficient yin blood. The thin tongue with light colour is due to deficient *qi* and blood, while the thin dry tongue with dark-red colour is caused by blazing fire due to deficient yin and consumed body fluids.

c) Cracked or fissured tongue: The tongue surface has marked cracks or fissures caused by consumed body fluids which fail to moisten the tongue surface. If it is dark-red with fissures, it is due to the consumption of body fluids by extreme pernicious heat and impaired yin *jing* (vital principle); the pale tongue with fissures is often a reflection of deficient blood. A cracked tongue in a healthy person is of no significance in clinical diagnosis.

d) Indented tongue: It has indentations along its edge and is pressed by the edges of the teeth. Indented and enlarged tongues are often caused by a weak spleen. A pale, moist tongue indicates a weak spleen and extreme pathogenic damp.

e) Thorny tongue: The papillary buds over the tongue increase and swell and feel thorny when touched. A thorny dry tongue is caused by extreme pathogenic heat, and the more extreme the heat, the more thorny the tongue. The viscus in which pathogenic heat is situated can be known according to the location of the thorn, for example, the thorn at the edge of the tongue, means extreme liver and gallbladder fire; the thorn at the centre of the tongue means extreme stomach and intestinal heat.

c. Observation of tongue stature mainly notes the change of the movement of the tongue proper.

a) Stiff tongue: The tongue is stiff and inflexible or fails to roll, causing stuttering. If it is seen in febrile diseases due to external affection, it is caused by pathogenic heat invading the pericardium and internally blocking phlegm and turbid matter; or it is caused by body fluids consumed by high fever and extreme pathogenic heat. If seen in a miscellaneous disease, it is often a sign of apoplexy.

b) Atrophic and soft tongue: The tongue is soft and cannot extend, roll and turn around. It is mainly due to deficient *qi* and blood, consumed yin fluids and malnourished tendons and vessels. If a tongue is light-coloured and atrophic in a prolonged illness, it is due to deficient *qi* and blood; if dark-red and atrophic, exhausted yin. If it is dry, red and atrophic in a newly-encountered disease, it is due to the consumption of yin by burning heat.

c) Tremulous tongue: cannot be controlled. If it is seen in a prolonged illness, it is due to deficient *qi* and blood or weak *qi*. In febrile diseases it is due to external affection and is mainly a sign of endogenous pathogenic wind produced by extreme heat or internally moving wind due to deficiency.

d) Wagging tongue: The patient sticks his or her tongue out and moves it up and down, left and right. It is due to the affection of the heart and spleen by pernicious heat and can be seen in the toxic pestilential factor attacking the heart or weakened antipathogenic factor. It is often a sign of endogenous pathogenic wind or maldeveloped infantile intelligence.

e) Deviated tongue: is usually due to apoplexy, or is a sign of apoplexy.

f) Curving tongue: contracts and cannot extend. It is a sign of a fatal case. The light-coloured or dark-bluish and moist tongue is due to stagnant pathogenic cold in tendons and vessels; a tongue fat in shape is due to internally-blocked phlegm and turbid matter; a dark-red tongue is due to consumed body fluids in febrile disease.

d. Observation of tongue coating: The tongue coating is produced due to an upward steaming of stomach *qi*. A healthy person has a thin layer of whitish coating on the tongue, which is moderately moist and not slippery indicating normal stomach *qi*. The affected tongue coating is formed due to an upward steaming of stomach *qi* with a pathogenic factor. Observation of normal changes of tongue coating aids in diagnosing disease.

e. Observation of the tongue coating's colour: Tongue coatings can be white, yellow, grey and black. Since the colour is related to the pathogenic factor, the tongue's colour can show the features of a disease.

a) A white tongue coating is generally seen in exterior-cold syndromes. A thin, whitish coating is the normal tongue coating. When affected by a pathogenic factor that is still in the superficial part of the body, it does not change remarkably. The thin, whitish coating of a tongue can thus be the evidence that the pathogenic factor has not yet been transmitted into the deep part of the body. A light-coloured white-coated tongue is often seen in the interior-cold syndrome. If a white tongue coating is distributed over the tongue surface as white powder piles on it, it is called a powder-piling tongue coating. It is caused by an exogenous pathogenic factor and extreme internal toxic heat and is often seen in pestilence and internal carbuncle.

b) A yellow tongue coating indicates heat and interior syndromes. Since a yellow tongue coating is caused by pathogenic heat, it indicates a heat syndrome. In general, the yellower the tongue coating, the more severe the pathogenic heat. A slight yellow tongue coating indicates mild heat, while a deep-yellow coating indicates stagnant pathogenic heat. A yellow tongue coating also denotes an interior syndrome, while the tongue coating changing into yellow denotes an exogenous syndrome, or superficial pathogenic factor transmitting into the deep portion of the body and transforming itself into heat. Since a yellow tongue coating indicates pathogenic heat in the interior of the body, it is commonly seen in association with a dark-red coating. If the tongue is light-coloured, enlarged and delicate with a yellow, slippery and moist coating seen, the disorder of stagnant aqueous damp due to deficient yang should be considered.

c) A grey tongue coating indicates an interior syndrome and can be seen in interior-heat and cold-damp syndromes as well. As it may develop into a black coating, grey and black coatings are often seen simultaneously. The former can be derived from the white one and also seen simultaneously together with the yellow one. If it is grey and moist, it is due to stasis of endogenous pathogenic cold-damp or internal retention of *tan-yin* (phlegm and excess exudates); if grey and dry, it is due to consumed body fluids by pernicious heat or blazing fire due to deficient yin.

d) A black tongue coating indicates an interior syndrome, extreme pernicious heat and cold. It is frequently derived from the grey or red-yellow one, and seen at the severe stage of disease. The black, dry and cracked coating, even the thorny black one is mainly due to body fluids exhausted by burning heat; the black and moist one, is due to deficient yang and extreme cold. Thus, it is significant to distinguish pathogenic cold from pathogenic heat through the grey black coating of the tongue and to observe the degree of moisture of the tongue coating.

f. Observation of the quality of the tongue proper is chiefly to observe changes of thickness, moisture, viscosity, peeling and the root of the tongue coating.

a) Thickness: Whether a tongue coating is thick or thin is judged by whether the tongue can be seen, i.e., it is a thin coating through which the tongue surface can vaguely be seen. Otherwise, it is a thick one.

Observation of the thickness of the tongue coating can help determine the severity and development of the disease. In general, a tongue coating is thin when the pathogenic factor is situated in the body surface and the disease is mild and superficial. The tongue coating is thick when the pathogenic factor goes into the deep portion of the body and the disease becomes more severe or food, yin (excess fluid), phlegm and damp stagnate internally. The tongue coating becomes thinner when the pathogenic factor is subdued internally and expelled externally and the disease takes a turn for the better.

b) Moisture: A normal tongue coating is moist which is a sign of ascending body fluids. The moisture of the tongue coating mainly indicates changes of body fluids.

A dry coating is a dry tongue surface when touched, and it is called a rough coating when it feels rough, both of which are due to the failure of body fluids to ascend and is often seen in a disease where body fluids are consumed by extreme pernicious heat. It is termed a slippery coating when there is excess liquid on the tongue and the surface feels slippery and moist. It is a sign of internal retention of aqueous damp.

When a dry tongue coating becomes moist, it is a sign that pathogenic heat is gradually disappearing or that body fluids are gradually increasing which indicates that the patient's condition is improving. When a moist tongue becomes dry, this indicates that body fluids have been consumed, and the pathogenic factor has become a heat one.

c) Viscosity: The tongue surface is covered by a layer of turbid and sticky substances that are fine, dense, and hard to be scraped. It is frequently seen in pathological processes of yang *qi* restrained by a yin pathogen, such as damp and turbid matter, *tan-yin*, food retention, etc.

Crusty tongue coating: The coating on the tongue appears like a soft, loose, and thick crust of residue which can be easily scraped. It is formed by ascending turbid matter in the stomach, which is steamed by extreme yang *qi*.

d) Peeling: The tongue coating is lost, so that the tongue surface looks like a mirror. It is also called a mirror tongue. It is a sign of exhausted stomach yin and severely impaired stomach *qi*. If the coating is not completely lost and the tongue coating peels at places, it is termed a partial loss of tongue coating and is also a sign of injury to both stomach *qi* and stomach yin. The partially turbid matter has not been eliminated, and the anti-pathogenic factor has been affected. The disease condition is comparatively complex.

e) Rooted or rootless tongue: A rooted coating is when the coating is firm, substantial and closely sticks to the tongue surface, and can hardly be scraped. A rootless coating is when the tongue coating is not substantial, seems to be painted on the tongue surface, is easily scraped and does not seem to grow from the tongue. The tongue coating is important for differentiating anti-pathogenic and pathogenic factors, deficiency and excess, and the presence or absence of stomach *qi*. Generally speaking, a rooted tongue coating is seen in cases of excess and heat syndromes and indicates the existence of stomach *qi*. A rootless coating is seen in deficiency and cold syndromes, indicating declining stomach *qi*.

8-1-3-3 Relation between the tongue proper and its coating

A disease is a complex process and the change of the tongue proper and its coating are the reflection of the intricate complex pathological changes on the tongue. Therefore, attention should be paid to the relation between the tongue proper and its coating and any changes of the two should be analysed jointly to determine their indications.

Under normal circumstances, the changes of the tongue proper and its coating are unified in their indications, e.g., a yellowish coating and a red dry tongue are often seen in endogenous pathogenic heat due to excess, while a white coating and a light-coloured, and moist tongue are often seen in endogenous pathogenic cold due to deficiency. However, in the course of disease, the change of the tongue proper and its coating do not always accord with each other, for instance, a dark-red tongue is originally due to a heat syndrome and a white coating is often seen in a cold syndrome, but the dark-red tongue and its white coating can also be seen simultaneously. In acute febrile disease due to an exogenous pathogenic factor, a dark-red tongue with a white and glossy coating are due to pernicious heat at *ying* (nutrition) phase and pernicious damp at *qi* (vital energy) phase; in miscellaneous diseases due to internal injury, they are frequently seen in the disease or syndrome of phlegm and turbid matter, and food retention caused by pernicious blazing fire (intense heat) due to deficient yin. If a dark-red tongue with a white coating is seen, it is a sign of body fluid consumption by pathogenic dry-heat. The dark-red tongue is due to pathogenic damp obstruction and congealed pathogenic heat; the white coating is caused when pathogenic dryness rapidly transforms itself into pathogenic fire and the disease develops rapidly. Pathogenic dry-heat has entered the *ying* (nutrition) phase and body fluids have been severely consumed when the tongue coating does not change to yellow. Therefore, they differ from common febrile diseases with yellow tongue coating.

Since a tongue and its coating reflect a condition from different angles, their conditions should be taken into consideration and synthetically analysed, so as to aid clinical identification of syndromes.

8-1-3-4 Clinical significance of tongue diagnosis

Clinical practice has found that tongue changes reflect the flourishing and decline of *qi* and blood, pathogenic factors, the location and development of disease as well as determine the transformation and prognosis of disease. In certain cases the tongue can even be regarded as evidence for identification of syndromes.

In general, observing the tongue proper is mainly for differentiating the deficiency and excess states of the viscera. Observing the tongue coating is mainly for differentiating the depth of the pathogenic factor and the existence of stomach *qi*.

The clinical significance of tongue diagnosis is as follows:

a. Judging the flourishing or decline of anti-pathogenic factor; whether the viscera, *qi* and blood are flourishing or not is reflected by the tongue surface. E.g., a ruddy tongue indicates flourishing *qi* and blood; a light-coloured tongue, declining *qi* and blood; a thin, white and moist coating, flourishing stomach *qi*; a mirror-like tongue with no coating, declining stomach *qi* or severely-consumed stomach yin.

b. Differentiating the depth of disease: In exogenous disease, a thick tongue coating often reflects the depth of disease, e.g., a thin tongue coating indicates the initial stage and superficial location of disease. The thick coating indicates the pathogenic factor gradually entering the deep portion of the body and the deeper location of disease. A dark-red tongue indicates that pathogenic heat has entered *ying* (nutrition) and *xue* (blood) phases, the deeper location of a severe disease.

c. Distinguishing the feature of pathogenic factors: Different changes of tongue indications can reflect different pathogenic factors, e.g., a yellow tongue coating is caused by pathogenic heat; a white one, pathogenic cold; a curdy and glossy coating is caused by disease due to retention of food, phlegm and turbid matter. Ecchymosis and petechia occurring on the tongue are signs of stagnant blood.

d. Predicting the tendency of disease: Since changes in the tongue coating reflect the anti-pathogenic and pathogenic factors and the depth of disease, observing the coating can show the developmental tendency of a disease. This is significant, particularly in acute febrile disease, e.g., a transformation of the white tongue coating into a yellow or black one is due to the pathogenic factor invading the body from a superficial to deep level, from a mild to severe form and from cold to hot. Transformation of a moist coating into a dry one means that body fluids are gradually being consumed by excess pernicious heat. Transformation of a dry or thick coating into a moist or thin one signifies resumption of fluid production and a gradually declining pathogenic factor.

It should also be pointed out that patients who are seriously ill with a small change of tongue indication or healthy persons with abnormal tongue indications are sometimes seen in clinic. Hence, only by analysing the past history and other symptoms and signs can an accurate diagnosis be made when inspecting the tongue.

8-1-3-5 Notes on tongue diagnosis

While observing a tongue, attention should be paid to light, the extension of the tongue and the colour of the coating.

a. Light: When observing the tongue, sufficient light is needed and let the light shine directly into the patient's mouth. If a tongue is observed at night, observation should be repeated in the daytime if necessary.

b. Extension of the tongue: A patient is required to extend his or her tongue outward and expose it slightly downward, and the surface should be flat and not rolling. Care should be taken not to have it extending outward by force lest its colour should be influenced.

c. Coating colour: The tongue coating can be coloured by certain food or drugs, which is termed the "coloured tongue coating," e.g., olives, plum or mulberries can make it yellow; smoking can make it grey, etc. Whenever the tongue coating does not accord with the disease condition, ask the patient about diet and medication so as to avoid any misunderstandings.

In addition, a tongue coating may become thick or thin due to food or scraping; it may also become red when taking hot or irritating food; its surface may often become dry when the patient has a stuffy nose or breathes through the mouth.

8-1-4 Observation of excreta

Excreta comprises sputum, saliva, vomiting, stools, urine, tears, nasal discharge, vaginal discharge, etc. The colour, quality, volume and other changes are necessary reference data for identifying the syndrome.

In general, clear and thin excreta suggests a cold syndrome. Yellow, turbid (or cloudy), mucoid and stringy excreta suggest a heat syndrome. This is because stagnant blood leads to stagnant yang *qi*, and stagnant aqueous damp, so that aqueous liquid is clear, thin and cold and the excreta, clear and thin and body fluids are condensed by pernicious fumigating and burning heat, so that the excreta is yellow, turbid and sticky.

8-1-4-1 Sputum and saliva

White, clear and thin sputum indicates a cold syndrome, and yellow white and mucoid saliva indicates a heat syndrome. Scanty saliva that can hardly be excreted or discharged signifies dry phlegm. White profuse sputum that is easily expectorated is damp phlegm. Thick purulent blood is caused by toxic heat in the lung, the lung carbuncle syndrome.[11] Bloody sputum or fresh blood coughed up is caused by injury of lung collateral meridians by pathogenic heat.

8-1-4-2 Vomit

Clear and thin sputum and saliva are due to cold *yin* (excess watery exudates). Clear and thin vomit mixed with food without sour taste and foul odour is due to deficient stomach *qi* due to cold. Yellow and bitter vomit is due to heat affection to the liver and gallbladder and the stomach's failure to propel downward. Sour and smelly vomitus is due to heat affection to the stomach or food retention. Bloody sputum or fresh blood coughed up is due to the injury of lung collateral meridians by pathogenic heat.

8-1-4-3 Stools

Loose, dark-yellow and mucoid stools are due to pathogenic damp-heat in the intestine. Watery stools mixed with undigested food is due to pathogenic cold-damp. Jelly-like stools mixed with purulent blood is caused by dysentery in which white stools indicate that the disease is located at the *qi* phase, and dark-red stools indicate the *xue* (blood) phase. Red-white stools indicate disordered *qi* and blood. It is called "distal blood" when defecation is followed by passing black blood; it is called "proximal blood" when bright red blood is passed before defecation.

8-1-4-4 Urine

Clear, profuse urine indicates a deficient-cold syndrome; dark-concentrated urine, a heat syndrome; cloudy urine, descending damp and turbid, weak spleen and kidney *qi*; hematuria, the vessel injured by pathogenic heat; urine containing gravel is stone *lin*[12] while milky urine is called milky *lin*.[13]

8-1-5 Observation of the veinules of the infant's index finger

Small superficial veinules of the infant's finger are the collateral meridians that expose the anterior border of the palmar side of the index finger. They are also branches of the Lung Meridian of Hand-*taiyin*. Hence, examination of the veinules and diagnosis of pulse at the *cun* section are of similar significance in clinic. As the infant's pulse is rather small, and an infant always cries and moves at random during diagnosis, the true pulse indication is influenced and its skin is thin and delicate and its small superficial veinules are comparatively obvious. Pulse diagnosis is performed by observing the small superficial veinules of the index finger of infants under three years old.

The small superficial veinules of the index finger are divided into three sections: the wind strategic pass, the *qi* strategic pass and the life strategic pass. The small superficial veinules of the proximal phalanx of the infant's index finger is called the wind strategic pass, those of the middle phalanx are called the *qi* strategic pass, and those of the distal phalanx, the life strategic pass. (Fig. 43)

8-1-5-1 Techniques for observing the finger's veinules

Hold the end of the infant's index finger with the index finger and thumb of the left hand, gently rub the palmar side of the infant's index finger from its root with the thumb of the right hand several times so as to make the small superficial veinules more visible for observation.

8-1-5-2 Observing the small superficial veinules of the finger

a. The colour of the small superficial veinules of the index finger are slightly red and seen in the wind strategic pass. After illness, they become bright-red, which is due to an exterior syndrome or external affection of pathogenic wind-cold; the purplish-red one, a heat syndrome; the dark-purplish one, obstructed blood vessels that indicate a serious case; the light-coloured one, a deficiency syndrome; the black one, an excess syndrome; the dark-bluish one is seen in convulsions and varieties of pain syndromes as well.

b. Length: In general, the small superficial veinules seen at the wind strategic pass indicate a superficially located pathogenic factor and in mild cases; those seen at the *qi* strategic pass, indicate a deeply invading pathogenic factor; those seen at the life strategic pass indicate severe cases; if they extend to reach the fingernail, the disease is extremely serious.

c. Floating or sinking: Small superficial veinules of the finger indicate an exterior disease; those not seen indicate an interior disease.

Since abnormal changes of colour, location, length of small superficial veinules of the index finger may reflect the pathogenic factor, the flourishing or decline of the anti-pathogenic factor and the depth and severity of disease, examining them can aid in determining the disease condition and its prognosis. However an accurate diagnosis must be made in association with the data acquired by other diagnostic techniques. (Fig. 43)

8-2 Auscultation-olfaction

Auscultation is chiefly to listen to the patients' speech, respiration and cough, etc. so as to distinguish a cold disease from a heat disease and a deficiency disease from an excess disease.

Olfaction is mainly to smell the patients' respiratory gases, secretions and excreta in order to determine the disease.

8-2-1 Auscultation

8-2-1-1 Speech

a. Strength of speech: The patient's speech reflects the flourishing and decline of anti-pathogenic and pathogenic factors. In general, speaking continuously in a high tone with restlessness indicates excess and heat syndromes; speaking feebly and little with calmness indicates deficiency and cold syndromes. If no sound can be produced, it is called aphonia, which is divided into deficiency and excess types. Aphonia seen in the external affection of pathogenic factor, or obstructed *qi* duct at the late stage or pregnancy belongs to an excess syndrome; aphonia seen in internal injury, deficient lung and kidney yin, failure of body fluids to ascend, is a chronic or recurrent deficiency syndrome. A deep and harsh voice is often seen in an exogenous disease and obstructed pathogenic damp and the turbid matter due to lung *qi*'s failure to spread and is also due to an obstructed *qi* (gases) duct. Groaning, crying out in alarm, etc. often relate to general ache and distension.

b. Delirium results from the pathological changes of the heart (Mind).

Mental confusion with incoherence and high voice is delirium, which is often seen in the excess syndrome of the Mind blurred by pathogenic heat; semi-consciousness, discontinuously uttering and subdued grumbling and muttering by a semi-conscious patient pertain to the deficiency syndrome due to severely injured heart *qi* and mental disorder. Speaking wildly due to loss of reason is madness which is commonly seen in *kuang* (mania) syndrome[14] and caused by the disturbance of the heart by pathogenic phlegm-fire. The patient mutters to himself and stares when seeing someone. This is often seen in *dian* (epilepsy) syndrome[15] and is a sign of deficient heart *qi* and the failure of *jing* (vital principle) to nourish the mind. Stuttering suggests the pathological change of upwardly-disturbing pathogenic wind-phlegm.

8-2-1-2 Respiration

a. Feeble and coarse breath: Feeble breath indicates deficient lung and kidney *qi* and pertains to the impairment and deficiency caused by internal injuries; forceful and coarse breath in a high voice indicates extreme internal pathogenic heat and an obstructed *qi* (gases) duct and pertains to an excess-heat syndrome.

b. *Xiao* and *chuan* (wheezing dyspnea): Dyspnea and short hasty breath sometimes accompanied by flapping of the ala nasi or an open mouth and elevated shoulder and inability to lie flat is called *chuan*; dyspnea characterized by a wheezing sound in the throat, *xiao*.

Chuan is divided into deficiency and excess patterns. An asthmatic and coarse breath and a high voice is that of the excess pattern and results from substantial pathogen in the lung and an unsmooth *qi* mechanism. Short, asthmatic breath and low voice with a long exhalation and a short inhalation discontinuously is *chuan* of the deficiency pattern, resulting from deficient lung and kidney *qi*.

c. Lack of *qi* and sighing: Feeble breath and lack of *qi* in respiration results from deficient *qi*. A deep breath with a prolonged expiration due to a depressed chest like sighing, results from mental depression and the liver's failure to perform its dispersing and discharging functions.

8-2-1-3 Cough

Cough is a reflection of the lung's failure to carry on its dissipating and clearing functions and *qi* regurgitates. During auscultation attention should be paid to the phlegmatic sound. Cough in a low and harsh voice and deficient *qi* indicates an excess syndrome; cough in a low voice indicates deficiency. A prolonged hasty, continuous cough is called whooping cough (pertussion). If the cough resembles a dog bark, care should be taken for diphtheria. A dry cough with no or little mucoid sputum results from the invasion of the lung by pathogenic dryness or is caused by dry lung due to deficient yin. If the cough is accompanied with sputum, the colour, volume and quality of sputum should be distinguished in order to diagnose the disease.

8-2-1-4 Hiccup and eructation

Both hiccup and belching are caused by regurgitating stomach *qi*, but their clinical signs and the disease they indicate are different.

Hiccup in a high, short and loud voice indicates a substantial heat affection; hiccup in a low, long and weak voice indicates a cold affection due to asthenia. Common hiccup, moderate in sound, with no discomfort, is due to an occasional affection of pathogenic wind-cold after meals or hastily swallowing food, which does not pertain to an ill state. If hiccup in a low and weak voice occurs due to declining stomach *qi* in a prolonged illness, it suggests a fatal case.

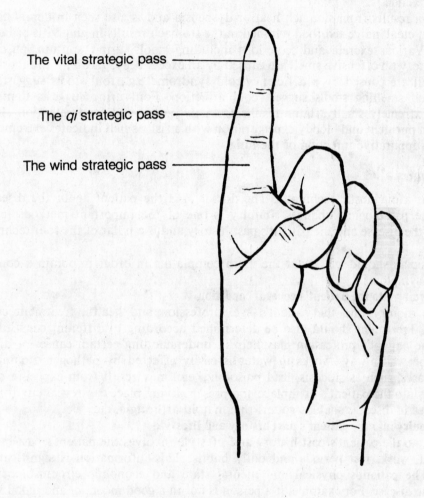

The vital strategic pass ——————

The qi strategic pass ——————

The wind strategic pass ——————

Fig. 43.   The three strategic passes of the superficial veinules of an infant

Belching is frequent after overeating. It can be caused by dyspepsia, disharmony between the liver and stomach, a weak stomach and regurgitating *qi*, etc. Belching with a sour odour is due to food retention or dyspepsia. Belching without a sour odour is due to disharmony between the liver and stomach or a weak stomach and regurgitating *qi*.

8-2-2 Olfaction

Ozostomia results from stomach heat or dyspepsia and is also seen in dental carries, dirty mouth, etc. Undigested food retained in the stomach results in gingivitis or internal carbuncle. Various excreta and secretions including stools, urine, sputum, pus, nasal discharge, etc. with offensive smell are caused by an excess-heat syndrome and those with a fishy smell are caused by a deficiency-cold syndrome e.g., foul stools suggests heat affection and smelling stools suggest cold affection. Foul urine suggests damp-heat affection. Extremely smelly flatus results from dyspepsia and food retention. Turbid sputum with purulent and bloody expectoration with a fishy smell indicates extreme toxic heat and a suppurative infection of the lung.

8-3 Inquiry

Inquiry is a diagnostic technique. The doctor asks the patient about the disease to ascertain the pathological changes. Inquiry is one of the important methods used to understand the disease and the patient's past history and is a pillar of the four techniques of diagnosis.

The physician should ask about the main complaints in order to obtain a complete view of the symptoms.

8-3-1 Inquiry into the patient's general condition

After an inquiry into the patient's age, profession and health, treatment can be determined. Treatment should also be determined according to different constitutions. Knowing the patient's profession may help in understanding certain causes of disease, e.g., someone who always works in water is easily affected by pathogenic damp and certain diseases, such as silicosis, lead poisoning, etc. may result from exposure on the job. Inquiry into the patient's birthplace and present living place can reveal environmental influences in diseases such as goiter, rheumatoid arthralgia, etc.

8-3-2 Inquiry into the patient's past history and lifestyle

Inquiry into the patient's past history and lifestyle involves the patient's past medical history, diet, work, rest periods and daily habits. This information is significant for diagnosis. The patient's physical and mental state and economic circumstances also influence the disease. For example, if a person is not in a good mood, *qi* and blood would be depressed, causing the problem of depressed liver and stagnant *qi*, etc. In diet, preference for one of the "five tastes" often leads to a relative flourishing or decline of visceral *qi*. Preference for warmth to coolness is usually due to relative excess yin *qi*; preference for coolness to warmth, is due to relative excess yang *qi*. If a person leads a hard life and is fatigued or lacks physical exercise, the disease or syndrome caused by too much strain may be seen. An extremely easy and comfortable life can impede the spleen's transporting function. This usually results in a phlegm-damp problem. An irregular life often leads to disease.

8-3-3 Inquiry into the patient's family and medical history

The patient's family medical history can aid in diagnosing certain infections and hereditary diseases, such as pulmonary tuberculosis, mania, etc.

The patient's past health condition and major illnesses can be used as a references for diagnosing present problems. For instance, one who usually suffers from overactive liver yang is likely to suffer from windstroke (apoplexy).[16] Mania often relapses in the patient who is mentally overstimulated. Hence it is helpful to inquire about the patient's past history for diagnosing the present disease.

8-3-4 Inquiry into the disease process

Inquiry into the disease process is to inquire the whole course of the disease (occurrence, development and treatment, etc.), which is important for diagnosis. The nature of disease can be understood by inquiring the cause of disease, for example, a disease caused by exogenous pathogenic wind-cold in winter is usually an exterior-cold syndrome; a disease caused by depression is trouble with stagnant liver *qi*, etc. Whether the disease is a deficiency or excess type can be understood by inquiring into the course of disease, e.g., sudden deafness is usually ascribed to the excess syndrome due to deficient kidney yin. To inquire the treatment and effect can be regarded as references for application of drugs according to identification of syndromes. For example, it may not be a heat syndrome if no therapeutic effect is achieved after the patient has taken drugs of a cold nature; it may be a cold syndrome if the symptoms have improved after the patient has taken drugs of a hot nature. If the chief symptoms of distension and fullness are aggravated after taking drugs for promoting *qi* flow and subduing distension, the trouble will be a deficiency syndrome caused by a weak spleen and stomach which fail to digest food. It is thus seen that only by inquiring into the whole course of disease can a correct diagnosis be made.

8-3-5 Inquiry into present symptoms

TCM also pays special attention to the present symptoms. Summing up the diagnostic techniques of medical experts in earlier generations, Zhang Jingyue, a medical expert of the Ming Dynasty (1368-1644) formulated the Ten Rhythmic Questions. Medical experts in later generations revised and supplemented them as: "The first: chills and fever; the second: sweating; the third: head and body; the fourth, bowel movements; the fifth, diet; the sixth, chest; the seventh, hearing; the eighth, thirst; the ninth, past history; the tenth, the cause, drugs and response to them, menstrual changes and a little pediatritics about variola and massages."

8-3-5-1 Chills and fever

Chills and fever, i.e., creeping chills and fever are common symptoms. It is called creeping chills when the patient still feels cold even when wearing more clothes and standing near a source of heat. It is called aversion to cold when the sensation of cold is relieved when the patient wears more clothes and warms himself near a source of heat. Fever not only refers to a higher temperature than normal, but also to the patient's sensation of general or local fever, e.g., fevers in the chest, palms and soles.

Chills and fever chiefly occur when there is a strong pathogenic factor and are linked to the flourishing and decline of the yin and yang of the body. In general, when a pathogenic factor causes disease, pathogenic cold causes chills and pathogenic heat, aversion to heat; when yin and yang are in disharmony, excess yang leads to fever and declining yang and excess yin leads to chills. Chill is a yin sign, while fever is a yang sign. If there are chills and fever, whether they appear simultaneously or alone, their onset, characteristics and accompanying symptoms, etc. must be cleared up.

Commonly-seen chills and fever:

a. Chills and fever seen at the initial stage of the exterior syndrome caused by exogenous pathogenic factor are the signs that the exogenous pathogenic factor is stagnating in the body surface and that defensive yang *qi* is struggling against the pathogenic factor. As exogenous factors vary with wind-cold and wind-heat, there are severe chills with low-grade fever and mild chills with high fever.

Severe chills with low-grade fever is characteristic of exogenous pathogenic wind-cold. As pathogenic cold attacks the body surface and impairs the yang, the disease manifests as severe chills; as cold is contracting and stagnant and depresses defensive yang *qi*, fever results with pain in the body and head, no sweat, superficial and tight pulse, etc.

Exogenous pathogenic wind-heat manifests as high fever with mild chills. As pathogenic wind-heat is the yang pathogen that causes excess yang, fever is high. As defensive *qi* is not so strong and the pores open when the pathogen attacks the body surface, slight aversion to wind-cold occurs, often accompanied by thirst, perspiration and superficial rapid pulse.

b. Chills with no fever pertain to the deficiency-cold syndrome when the patient fears cold but has no fever. Since weak internal yang *qi* leads to cold and fails to warm the body surface, manifestations of a deficiency-cold syndrome, such as pallor, cold limbs, lying with a curved body, preference for more clothes and blankets, etc. are seen simultaneously. Fear of cold or cold and pain in the affected area can also be seen because of a direct attack of the viscera by exogenous pathogenic cold and impaired yang *qi*, which is so-called "extreme yin causing cold."

c. Fever with no chills:

a) Strong fever: It is called strong fever when the patient has a persistent high fever and no aversion to cold, which is mainly seen in the interior-excess syndrome when exogenous pathogenic wind-cold invades the deep portion of the body and transforms itself into pernicious heat or exogenous pathogenic wind-heat transmits inward. As the anti-pathogenic factor is dominant but the pathogenic factor is also substantial, the internal heat is in excess and spreads outward, which is "extreme yang causing heat." It is often associated with profuse sweating, polydipsia, etc.

b) Tidal fever: Tidal fever is when the body temperature rises at regular intervals or is even higher (usually in the afternoon) just like the tide. There are the following patterns:

Tidal fever due to deficient yin is fever occurring in the afternoon or evening. It pertains to deficient yin producing internal pernicious heat, and is characterized by fever in the chest, palms and soles, sometimes with a sensation that the heat spreads from the inside of the bone to the outside of the skin. It is thus called "tidal fever due to steaming of bones," often accompanied by night sweats, malar flush, dry mouth and throat and red tongue with little fluid.

Tidal fever due to pathogenic damp and warmth (mild heat) is characterized by a high fever in the afternoon, and a latent fever characterized by the patient's skin, which is not hot at the very beginning, but hot after being felt for a longer time. The disease lies in the spleen and stomach because pathogenic damp is obstructed by pernicious heat. It is often accompanied by chest distress and vomiting, a sensation of heaviness in the body and head and loose stools.

Yangming tidal fever is caused by an internal combination of pathogenic heat and dryness in the stomach and intestine. It is also more serious in the afternoon. It is often accompanied by an abnormal illness and pain aggravated by pressure, constipation, perspiring hands and feet and yellow and dry or thorny tongue coating.

c) Prolonged low-grade fever: occurs for a long time with the body temperature somewhat higher than normal (within 38°C), or the patient feels hot but the body temperature is not elevated.

Prolonged low-grade fever has a complex pathogenesis. For instance, tidal fever due to yin deficiency or fever in summer mentioned above, i.e., "chronic summer fever," etc. manifest as persisting low-grade fever due to deficient qi.

In fever due to deficient qi, pallor, poor appetite and general weakness, shortness of breath and disinclination to talk, pale tongue and weak pulse can also be seen. It is mainly caused by a weak and impaired spleen qi, middle qi (gastrosplenic qi) and the failure of purified yang to ascend.

d) Alternate chills and fever: Alternate chills and fever is when creeping chills and fever attack alternately. They are characteristic of the semi-exterior-interior syndrome[17] and a sign that the anti-pathogenic factor is vying with the pathogenic one.

In malaria chills and strong fever occur alternately at regular intervals (one to three times a day). The malaria pathogen causes chills when it vies with the yin and causes fever when it vies with the yang or alternate chills and fever at regular intervals, characterized by excruciating headache, repeated and prolonged fever subsiding after perspiration.

8-3-5-2 Sweating

Sweat is fluid formed by body fluids steamed by yang qi. Pathological changes of sweating can be seen in the syndromes of external affection and of internal injury. Ask the patient about the time, location, quality and accompanying symptoms of sweating.

Commonly-seen sweat symptoms:

a. Differentiation of sweat in an exterior syndrome: Since an exterior syndrome is located on the body surface, the nature of the exogenous pathogenic factor and flourishing or decline of the anti-pathogenic factor can be distinguished by understanding whether sweating occurs or not as an exterior syndrome. The exterior syndrome with no sweat is caused by exogenous pathogenic cold, such as the exterior-excess syndrome of febrile disease;[18] an interior syndrome with sweat, exogenous pathogenic wind, such as taiyang windstroke,[19] the external affection of exogenous pathogenic wind-heat and the exterior syndrome of the repeated affection of the exogenous pathogenic factor are due to weak defensive yang qi.

b. Spontaneous sweating: Sweating aggravated after exertion is termed spontaneous sweating, which is caused by deficient qi and hyperfunctional defensive qi. It is often accompanied by the symptoms of deficient yang qi, such as mental fatigue, general weakness, shortness of breath and fear of cold.

c. Night sweat: Sweating during sleep which ceases after awakening is mainly caused by deficient yin and internal pernicious heat, and is often accompanied by fever in the chest, palms and soles, insomnia, malar flush, dry mouth and throat.

d. Profuse sweating: Continuous sweating associated with high fever, polydipsia and desire for cold drinks. A full large pulse indicates an excess heat syndrome caused by internal yang heat which causes profuse sweating.

Hyperhidrosis accompanied by rapid breathing, mental fatigue and weakness, cold clammy extremities and faint pulse is a critical sign that yang *qi* and primordial *qi* are nearly exhausted. It is thus called "sweating from exhaustion."

e. Sweating with rigour: Sweating following rigour, which is the manifestation of the struggle between anti-pathogenic and pathogenic factors and the turning point of the development of disease. Fever subsiding after sweating, normal pulse and cool body fluids are the signs that the disease has taken a turn for the better; restlessness and rapid pulse following sweating are signs that the anti-pathogenic factor has failed to conquer the pathogenic factor.

f. Forehead sweating: Sweating limited to the forehead is frequently seen with polydipsia, yellow tongue coating and floating rapid pulse. If it is seen after a severe disease or in the aged with asthmatic breath, it indicates a deficiency syndrome. If it suddenly occurs at the late stage of a severe disease, it is a critical sign that deficient yang fluid is exhausted together with *qi*.

g. Sweating on either side of the body: Sweating seen on either side of the body or the upper (or lower) portion of the body is caused by the obstruction of the meridian by pathogenic wind-phlegm or wind-damp or the unsmooth flow of *qi* and blood in the affected side.

h. Sweating from palms and soles: Profuse sweating from palms and soles accompanied by a dry mouth and throat, constipation and yellow urine, and minute pulse is due to stagnant pathogenic heat in the yin meridian because the palm and sole are where the meridian of *hand-jueyin* and the meridian of *foot-shaoyin* traverse. Profuse sweating on the chest is caused by worry and injury of the heart and spleen by overexertion.

Attention should also be paid to differentiate cold and hot sweating besides various sweat symptoms in clinic. Cold sweating is chiefly due to deficient yang and weak defensive *qi*; hot sweating is due to external pathogenic wind-heat and weak defensive *qi* or internal pernicious heat.

8-3-5-3 Inquiry into pain

Pain can be caused by excess, e.g., external affection or stagnant *qi* and blood or congealed phlegm and turbid matter, or parasites, food retention, etc. block the meridian and impede the smooth flow of *qi* and blood. "Where there is a blockage, there is a pain." Pain is also caused by deficiency, e.g., deficient *qi* and blood or impaired yin *jing* and malnourished viscera and meridians.

a. Location of pain: As each part of the body is connected with a certain viscus and meridian, it is significant to know in which viscus and meridian a pathological change occurs to ascertain the source of the pain.

a) Headache: All the yang meridians gather in the head. Most of the twelve meridians and the eight extra meridians are linked with the head, especially the three yang meridians which directly traverse the head.

Headache caused by certain exogenous pathogenic factors, such as wind, cold, summer-heat, damp, fire (intense heat) and obstructed or ascending phlegm and turbid matter disturbing the clear yang, is mainly an excess syndrome.

Headache caused by the failure of impaired *qi*, blood and *jing* and body fluids to upwardly nourish the head pertains to a deficiency syndrome. The location of headache in the meridian can be determined according to the distribution of the meridian, e.g., pain in the neck pertains to the meridian of *taiyang*; pain in the forehead the meridian of *yangming*; migraines, the meridian of *shaoyang*; and vertical pain, the meridian of *jueyin.*

b) Chest pain: Since the chest is where the heart and lung are located, pathological changes of the heart and lung, such as deficient yang *qi*, a surprise attack of exogenous pathogenic cold, stagnant blood blockage, obstructing phlegm and turbid matter, collateral meridian injured by pernicious fire (intense heat) may lead to an obstructed *qi* mechanism and pain.

Chest distress with fullness and pain is caused by *tan-yin*. Distension and referring pain relieved by belching is caused by stagnant *qi*. Chest pain with expectoration of pungent blood is caused by lung carbuncle. Chest pain and asthmatic breath accompanied by fever, expectoration or rusty sputum is caused by affection of the lung by heat. Chest pain referring to the chest and the chest *bi* (blockage) syndrome[20] are due to disturbed heart yang and stagnant phlegm and turbid matter. If a paroxysmal pain in the precordia is accompanied by a feeling of chest distress, colical pain, even greyish complexion, profuse cold sweat, it is "real cardiac pain."

c) Hypochondriac pain: The hypochondria are where the Liver Meridian and Gallbladder Meridian are distributed. Pain there may be caused by an unsmooth flow of liver *qi*, stagnant liver fire, affection of the liver and gallbladder by pathogenic damp-heat, stagnant *qi* and blood and *xuan-yin*.[21]

d) Epigastric pain is seen in such diseases as the invasion of the stomach by pathogenic cold, food retention in the epigastric region and the invasion of the stomach by regurgitating liver *qi*.

e) Abdominal pain: The abdominal region is divided into the upper, lower and lateral abdomen. The abdominal region above the umbilicus pertains to the spleen and stomach; that below the umbilicus, the kidney, bladder, large and small intestines and uterus, that on either side of the lower abdomen is where the Liver Meridian traverses. The different viscera the meridian pertains to can be determined according to their location.

Abdominal pain, classified into excess and deficiency, stagnant cold, accumulated heat, stagnant *qi*, congealed blood, food retention and parasites, etc., is mainly an excess syndrome; deficient *qi*, congealed blood and cold due to deficiency is a deficiency syndrome.

f) Lumbago: As the loin is the residence of the kidney, lumbago is mainly seen in pathological processes of the kidney. Lumbago caused by the obstruction of the meridian by pathogenic wind, cold and damp or obstruction of the collateral meridians by congealed blood is an excess syndrome; lumbago caused by deficient *jing* and *qi* or inability of the impaired yin and yang to warm and nourish the body is a deficiency syndrome.

g) Pain in the four extremities: Pain in the four extremities or their joints, or muscles or meridians is chiefly due to the blockage of *qi* and blood by invading exogenous wind and cold. It can also be caused by the spleen and stomach's failure to transport essential *qi* derived from food to the limbs. Pain in the heel or the lumbar vertebra is mainly due to a weak kidney.

b. Features of pain: Owing to different causes and pathogenesis of pain, it varies with characteristics. Asking about its characteristics can aid in differentiating its cause and pathogenesis.

a) Distending pain may appear in many portions of the body, most frequently seen in the epigastrium and abdomen. Distension and pain are mainly due to stagnant *qi*.

Distension in the epigastric region results from stagnant cold and *qi* in the middle energizer; pain in the chest and hypochondria is due to the depressed liver and stagnant *qi*. Distending pain in the head is mainly seen in the disease or syndrome of an excess rise of liver yang or blazing liver fire.

b) Pain with a heavy sensation is mainly seen in the head, limbs and loin. Since damp is heavy, turbid and sticky, damp stasis in the meridian makes one feel heavy. If pain with a heavy sensation is felt in the head, and pain and heavy limbs and loin are felt, it is a damp syndrome.

c) Stabbing pain: One of the characteristics of pain due to stagnant blood is more frequently seen in the chest and hypochondria, on either side of the lower abdomen or lower abdomen and epigastric region.

d) Colical pain: is usually formed due to the obstruction of *qi* mechanism by substantial pathogen, e.g., a "real cardiac pain" caused by stagnant and obstructed cardiac blood, epigastric and abdominal pain caused by roundworms; pain in the lower abdomen caused by stone *lin*.

e) Burning pain: Pain with a burning sensation and preference for coolness. It is frequently seen in the hypochondriac or epigastric region and caused by the affection of collateral meridians by pathogenic fire or extreme yang caused by deficient yin.

f) Cold pain: Pain with a cold sensation and reference for heat. It is often seen in the head, loin and epigastric and abdominal regions and caused by the obstruction of collateral meridians by pathogenic cold or the failure of the viscera and meridians to be warmed and nourished due to deficient yang *qi*.

g) Faint pain: Pain not so excruciating but tolerant and persistent. It is mainly caused by deficient and obstructed *qi* and blood and frequently seen in the pain in the head, epigastric abdomen and loin due to deficiency.

h) Contracting pain: Convulsive or contracting pain is usually caused by malnourished tendons and vessels. As the liver is concerned with tendons, it is related to liver trouble.

Besides the location characteristics and duration of pain, it should be noted whether it is relieved by pressure or not. In general, pain that occurs in a newly-encountered disease which is persistent and aggravated by pressure is caused by an excess syndrome; that which occurs in a prolonged illness at intervals or is relieved by pressure is caused by a deficiency syndrome.

8-3-5-4 Sleep

As *Miraculous Pivot* states, "Exhausted yang *qi* and excess yin *qi* lead to insomnia and exhausted yin *qi* and excess yang *qi*, somnolence." Asking about the normal changes of sleep may often indicate the flourishing or decline of yin and yang. Normal changes of sleep are chiefly as follows:

a. Insomnia is characterized by difficulty in falling asleep, waking easily, and inability to fall asleep after waking, or disturbed sleep. It is a pathological symptom where the yang does not correspond to the yin and *shen* (Spirit) is not well kept. It is caused by deficient yin blood and excess yang heat, resulting in disturbed mind and difficulty in falling asleep. For example, insomnia with anxiety can occur due to yin deficiencies of heart and kidney and excess heart fire. Continuous palpitations due to a weak heart and spleen and disturbing pathogenic factors, such as phlegm-fire and food retention can also cause insomnia. A depressed gallbladder and stomach trouble caused by food retention are also causes of insomnia.

b. Somnolence is frequently seen in the disease or syndrome of deficient yang and excess yin and obstructing and stagnating pathogenic phlegm-damp. For instance, somnolence with dizziness is usually caused by the obstructed pathogenic phlegm-damp and the clear yang's failure to ascend; desire for sleep due to mental fatigue and awakening immediately after being called, mimic sleep and mimic waking are the signs of deficient yang of the Heart Meridian and Kidney Meridian. When seen in an acute febrile disease, insomnia is mainly the sign of the pathogenic factor entering the pericardium and mental confusion is due to extreme pernicious heat.

8-3-5-5 Diet and appetite

Patients should be asked about their drinking and eating habits, their appetite, whether they prefer cold or hot food and the taste and odour in their mouth.

a. Thirst: Whether thirst appears or not reflects the flourishing or decline and distribution of body fluids. In the pathological process, no thirst signifies that body fluids have not yet been consumed and there is no pathogenic heat. Thirst chiefly suggests consumed body fluids or their failure to ascend due to stagnation. They should be differentiated in accordance with the characteristics of thirst and their accompanying symptoms.

Generally speaking, thirst with frequent drinking of water is commonly seen in a heat syndrome. Severe thirst with preference for cold drinks is caused by consumption of body fluids by excess pernicious heat. Thirst with preference for drinking a small amount of hot water or thirst where the water is vomited immediately after being drunk and difficulty in urination are due to internal retention of *tan-yin* and aqueous liquid's failure to ascend. Thirst with frequent drinking of small amounts is commonly seen in acute febrile diseases and mainly pertains to pathogenic heat entering the *ying* (nutrition) and *xue* (blood) phases. A dry mouth with the desire to rinse it, but without desire for swallowing water may be seen in congealed blood. Drinking caused by severe thirst and profuse urine indicates a "wasting and thirst" disease.

b. Appetite: Appetite is significant for judging the patient's gastrosplenic function and for determining a prognosis.

Poor or no appetite and dyspepsia are often manifestations of gastrosplenic dysfunction. Taking little food in a prolonged illness and seen with withered-yellow complexion, emaciation and general lassitude is due to a weak spleen and stomach. Taking little food accompanied by chest distress, abdominal pain, heavy trunk and limbs, and a thick and glossy tongue coating is mainly caused by the spleen's failure to transport pathogenic damp.

Anorexia or aversion to erosive smelly food is frequently seen in food injury. Anorexia possibly occurring in pregnant women is due to *qi* regurgitating in the Strategic Vessel Meridian and the stomach's failure to propel downward. Aversion to rich food is frequently seen in the disease or syndrome of the affection of the liver, gallbladder, spleen and stomach by pathogenic damp-heat.

Ravenous appetite and hunger after eating is insatiable hunger. When accompanied by emaciation, it is due to extreme stomach fire and a weak stomach.

Hunger with little appetite is caused by deficient stomach yin and upward disturbing fire due to yin deficiency. Polyphagia and frequent hunger with loose stools and dyspepsia are due to a weak spleen.

Preference for eating unripened rice, mud, etc. is particularly seen in children, which is a common sign of parasite retention. Preference for certain foods in pregnant women is not generally a pathological state.

In a disease process, increased appetite indicates a gradual recovery of the stomach and decreased appetite indicates a weak spleen and stomach. It is a sign of the immediate failure of gastrosplenic *qi* when the patient who originally could not eat suddenly becomes ravenous. This is called *chuzhong*. It is a manifestation of a "momentary recovery of consciousness just before death."

c. Taste: Ask a patient about abnormal tastes and ordours in the mouth. A bitter mouth is frequently seen in a heat syndrome, particularly in the pathological change of the affection of the liver and gallbladder by substantial heat. A sweet and greasy mouth is the affection of the spleen and stomach by pathogenic damp-heat. Acid regurgitation is pathogenic heat accumulating in the liver and stomach. A sour odour in the mouth is the internal retention of food. A tasteless mouth indicates a weak spleen.

8-3-5-6 Stools and urine

Attention should be paid to the shape, colour, time, volume, frequency and accompanying symptoms.

a. Stools: Abnormal stools can be divided into dry and loose. It is termed constipation when dry and firm stools are difficult to excrete at long intervals and decreased frequency of defecation, which is mainly caused by pathogenic heat being retained in the intestine, or consumed body fluids or impaired *qi* and body fluids so that the large intestine is too dry to transmit waste products. Diarrhea is when stools are thin, soft, even watery with increased frequency and at short intervals, which is often seen in the disease or syndrome when the spleen fails to perform its transporting function. The small intestine can not differentiate the purified (nutrients) from the turbid (scum) and aqueous liquid directly descends to the large intestine. Stools that are first dry and then loose are mainly due to a weak spleen and stomach. Stools that are sometimes dry but sometimes loose are chiefly due to a depressed liver and weak spleen and disharmony between the two. Stools mixed with water, or aqueous-grainy diarrhea or diarrhea before dawn are due to a weak spleen and stomach and extreme endogenous pathogenic cold and damp. Diarrhea with yellow chyme is due to the affection of the large intestine by pathogenic damp-heat. Foul stools with undigested food is caused by injury from stagnant food. Difficult defecation with normal stools seen in the aged is due to deficient *qi*.

A burning sensation occurring in the anus during defecation is mainly due to heat affection of the rectum. Incontinence or even prolapse of the rectum is chiefly seen in prolonged diarrhea due to a weak spleen. Tenesmus is commonly seen in dysentery. Loose stools with unsmooth defecation are often symptoms of the liver's failure to carry on its dispersing and discharging functions. Asphalt-coloured stools with easy defecation are due to congealed blood. Diarrhea with an abnormal pain relieved after defecation is due to food injury; diarrhea with an abnormal pain not relieved after defecation is due to a depressed liver and weak spleen.

b. Urine: Since urine is derived from body fluids, whether body fluids are sufficient and whether the viscera concerned are normal can be ascertained through the change of urine.

Polydipsia (excessive or abnormal thirst) indicating kidney trouble is often caused by pernicious cold due to deficiency and is also frequently seen in loss of body fluids due to extreme pernicious heat or severe diaphoresis, emetics and purgation. It is also commonly seen in the disease or syndrome of the dysfunctional lung, spleen and kidney with abnormal *qi* and stagnant internal aqueous damp. Dribbling of urine is called *long* (anuria) or *bi*, which is due to descending pathogenic damp-heat, or obstructed and congealed blood and calculus pertaining to an excess syndrome, whereas dribbling caused by deficient kidney yang's failure to carry *qi* or consumed kidney yin and internally-deficient body fluids, is a deficiency syndrome.

Frequent urination with dark scanty and hasty urine is mainly caused by pathogenic damp-heat affecting the lower energizer. Profuse clear urine is caused by cold due to deficiency in the lower energizer, weak kidney *qi* and a weak bladder. Frequent urination with scanty urine is often due to internal pernicious heat caused by deficient yin.

Frequent urination with hard stools is due to spleen trouble. Decreased urine is often seen in the disease or syndrome of abnormal functioning of *qi* and internal retention of aqueous damp.

Dysuria frequently accompanied by a hasty, uneasy and burning sensation is mainly the *lin* syndrome[22] of downwardly-attacking pathogenic damp-heat; a feeling of vacancy and pain after micturation is mainly due to the decline of kidney *qi*; dribbling of urine after micturation is due to weak kidney *qi*. Incontinence of urine is also caused by weak kidney *qi* and would be a critical sign if associated with coma. Enuresis is usually the deficiency syndrome of deficient kidney *qi*.

8-3-5-7 Menstrual flow and vaginal discharge

a. Menstrual flow: Attention should be paid to the patient's menstrual flow and accompanying symptoms, the beginning of the menstrual flow and menopause.

a) Menstrual cycle: Menstruation is ahead of schedule when it begins at least a week earlier than the expected time, and sometimes even occurs twice a month, which is mainly caused by extravasation of blood by pathogenic heat or failure of weak *qi* to control blood, also by a depressed liver or congealed blood. It is late menstruation when menstruation begins at least one week later than the expected time, mainly caused by stagnant pathogenic cold and *qi* and unsmoothly-circulating blood or insufficient blood in the Governor Vessel Meridian, and often seen in obstructed phlegm or stagnant *qi* and blood. An irregular menstrual cycle is when menstruation does not occur at normal intervals and is caused by stagnant liver *qi*. An absence of menstruation or occurrence of lower backache with no menstrual flow in a few healthy and fertile women is abnormal.

b) Menstrual amount: Menstrual flow varies with an individual's constitution and age. Menstruation with excessive blood loss or prolonged duration is called menorrhagia, and is caused by pernicious heat in blood, and impaired Strategic Vessel Meridian and Governor Vessel Meridian, or failure of weak *qi* to control blood. A reduction of menstrual flow, or of the duration as well as the amount of blood are termed oliguria, and caused by deficient blood or stagnant pathogenic cold and blood or blocked pathogenic phlegm and damp. Amenorrhea is when menstruation ceases for more than three months, accompanied by illness, excluding pregnancy and breast feeding, and is caused by deficient *qi* and blood and cold. Menopause caused by a change in living environment does not belong to an ill state if no obvious symptoms occur.

c) Colour and quality: Normal menstrual flow is red in colour, neither thin nor thick in quality and without blood clots. Blood slightly red in colour and clear in quality is mainly caused by deficient blood and pertains to a deficiency syndrome; a dark-red colour and thick in quality, is due to internal blood excess and heat, an excess syndrome. Dark-purplish menstrual flow with blood clots is caused by stagnant cold and blood; a dark-red flow with blood clots is due to stagnant blood.

d) Dysmenorrhea: A common disease with abdominal and lumbar pain prior to, during or after the menstrual period. When pain occurs prior to or during the menstrual period, it is mainly due to stagnant *qi* and blood. Cold pain in the lower abdomen, which is relieved by warmth, is due to stagnant pathogenic cold. When faint pain occurs during or after menstrual period in the lower abdomen and soreness and pain is felt in the lumbar region, it is due to consumed and deficient *qi* and blood and malnourished uterus and meridians.

b. Vaginal discharge: Normally a small amount of white, odourless secretion within the vagina nourishes and moistens the vaginal wall. Vaginal discharge is when it is secreted excessively or persistently. White, profuse discharge is termed leukorrhea. Red and mucoid discharge with mimic blood is called red leukorrhea and yellowish, mucoid and smelly discharge is called yellow leukorrhea. Leukorrhea and yellow leukorrhea are more commonly seen in clinic.

When asking a patient about her vaginal discharge, attention should be paid to its volume, colour and odour. Profuse, white thin and watery discharge is ascribed to pathogenic damp caused by weak sleep; yellow mucoid and smelly discharge sometimes accompanied by itch and pain in the external genitalia is due to pathogenic damp-heat pouring downward; dark-red persistent and slightly foul discharge is due to pathogenic heat accumulating in the Liver Meridian; dark-greyish, thin, clear and profuse discharge with soreness and coldness in the loin and abdomen, is due to a weak kidney. White thin and clear discharge are mainly due to deficiency and cold syndromes; yellow or dark-red mucoid and smelly discharges are due to excess and heat syndromes.

8-3-5-8 Children

It is difficult to ask children about their diseases because some of them cannot answer the physician's questions clearly and others do not complain. Therefore the parents must also be questioned.

Besides the normal questions, the condition before and after birth, measles, chicken pox, fevers, convulsions, vaccination, infectious disease, infant diet, walking, learning to speak, hereditary diseases, and the health of the family should be asked about.

8-4 Palpation

Feeling the patient's pulse and palpating certain areas are diagnostic and examination techniques for identifying syndromes.

8-4-1 Taking the patient's pulse

In ancient times, taking the pulse meant to feel the pulse at "three sections".[23] The *cun* section is the main palpation, and pulse indications are classified into 28 types according to the location, frequency, shape and volume of pulse so as to perceive pathological changes of the body. Since pulse diagnosis fully depends upon the doctor's experience, the location and indication of the pulse should be accurately distinguished by repeated practice.

8-4-1-1 The principle of the formation of pulse indications and clinical significance of taking pulse

a. The principle of the formation of pulse indications: The heart controls blood and vessels. Heartbeat and blood circulation are promoted by *zhong qi* (chest *qi*). Blood circulates in the vessel due to the action of the heart and smooth functioning of various viscera. Only through the distribution of lung *qi* can blood spread to the entire body. *Qi* and blood are derived from the spleen and stomach. The circulation of blood is controlled by spleen *qi*; the liver stores blood, and regulates the volume of circulating blood; the kidney stores *jing*. *Qi* derived from *jing* is the foundation of yang *qi*, the motive force for the functioning of organs and tissues. Thus, the pulse is closely related to the viscera, *qi* and blood.

b. Clinical significance of pulse: Since the viscera, *qi* and blood are closely related, blood and vessels are influenced and pulse varies when the viscera, *qi* and blood malfunction. Therefore, the location of disease can be determined and a prognosis made by taking the pulse.

a) Determining the location and characteristics of a disease and the flourishing and decline of the pathogenic factor. However complex the symptoms of disease are, a disease is situated superficially or deep and the superficial or deep pulse often reflects the superficial or deep location of disease. A superficial pulse usually indicates that the disease is superficial; the deep pulse indicates a deep disease. A disease may be divided into cold and hot. The frequency of pulse may reflect the disease e.g., a slow pulse usually indicates a cold disease or syndrome, but a rapid pulse indicates a hot one. The ebb and flow of anti-pathogenic and pathogenic factors arouse pathological changes of deficiency and excess. Whether a pulse is forceful or not can reflect a deficiency or excess syndrome or disease. A weak pulse indicates a deficiency syndrome due to deficient anti-pathogenic factors; a substantial and forceful pulse indicates an excess syndrome due to a violent pathogenic factor.

b) Predicting the prognosis of disease: The pulse is useful for making a prognosis of the disease. For example, a moderate pulse seen in a prolonged illness indicates that stomach *qi* is gradually recovering and the disease will take a turn for the better; a full pulse seen in deficient *qi* due to a prolonged illness indicates a deficiency syndrome, or blood loss. Prolonged diarrhea is usually a critical sign that the pathogenic factor prevails over the anti-pathogenic one. A moderate pulse appearing in an exogenous febrile disease and gradually disappearing pernicious heat is a sign that the disease is nearly cured. If a hasty and rapid pulse with restlessness occurs, the disease will progress. Again, sweating with rigour, a normal pulse after sweating and a cool body after a fever disappears indicates that the disease will take a turn for the better. A hasty and rapid pulse with restlessness is a critical sign that the disease will progress.

It must be pointed out that the relation between the pulse and disease is complex. Generally they correspond to each other, since there is sometimes the exception that they do not correspond to each other, there are the formulations, "diagnosis according to symptoms and signs rather than pulse"[24] and "diagnosis according to pulse rather than symptoms and signs."[25] In clinical application, a correct diagnosis can be made by using the four diagnostic techniques.

8-4-1-2 Location of palpation and pulse

Pulse diagnosis through palpation and taking the pulse is done at the *cun* section on both wrists, medial to the radius.

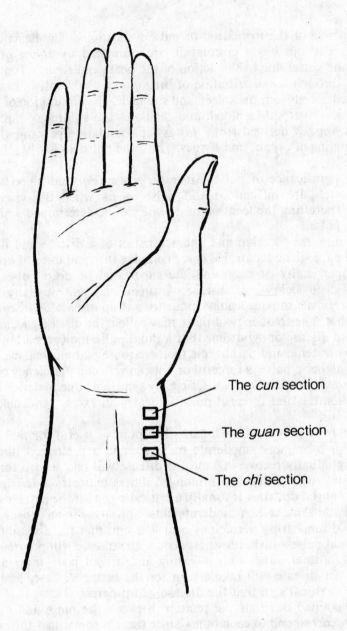

The *cun* section

The *guan* section

The *chi* section

Fig. 44.   The three sections for feeling the pulse

The *cun* section is divided into three sections, namely, *cun*, *guan* and *chi*. The section at the medial styloid process is called *guan*, with *cun* distal to and *chi* just proximal to it. They are located on either hand, six in total. The classification commonly used today is: The right *cun* section corresponds to the lung; the right *guan* section, to the spleen and stomach; the right *chi* section, to the kidney (the vital portal); the left *cun* section, to the kidney. As a whole, "the upper (*cun* section) indicates the upper (portion of the body) and the lower (*chi* section), the lower (portion of the body)." The reason why the pulse at the *cun* section can reflect the pathological change of the viscera is that the *cun* section is where the Lung Meridian of Hand-*taiyin* traverses and the meridians, *qi* and blood in the viscera meet at the lung and the Spleen Meridian of Foot-*taiyin* communicates with the Lung Meridian of Hand-*taiyin*, which originates from the spleen and stomach and are the resources of all the viscera, *qi* and blood. Therefore, the viscera, meridians, *qi* and blood of the entire body are reflected on the pulse at the *cun* section. (Fig. 44)

8-4-1-3 Ways of taking pulse

The patient should take a sitting or supine position, with the arm and heart nearly at the same level, and the wrist straight and palm upward, so that the blood circulates smoothly when feeling the pulse.

Locate the patient's pulse with three fingers, i.e., first palpate the processus styloid radii with the middle finger to locate the *guan* section, then the area just proximal to it or locate the *cun* section with the index finger, and the area just distal to the *guan* section to locate the *chi* section with the ring finger. Palpate with the three fingertips at the same level. The distribution of the pulse sections should accord with the patient's body length. Since a child's body is smaller, "locate the *guan* section with one finger (thumb)."

The techniques of pulse diagnosis of varying the distal pressure and certain manoeuvers are often used during taking the pulse. It is called "lift" to touch gently to ascertain a superficial sensation; it is called "press" to press harder to obtain a deeper sensation; it is called "search" to vary the pressure of the location of the finger to get a better feeling of pulse. There are three modes—light, medium and heavy in each of the three sections —*cun*, *guan*, and *chi*, collectively termed "three sections and nine modes."

It is called "total palpation" to feel the pulse with the index, middle and ring fingers simultaneously at the *cun*, *guan* and *chi* sections. This is a common technique of diagnosis. In order to understand pulse indications in a certain region, the pulse is felt with one finger at one location which is called an "individual palpation." In clinic these techniques are often applied in coordination.

During taking the pulse, the patient should be quiet and rest if they have just exerted themselves. The person taking the pulse must breathe evenly and smoothly concentrating on their finger sensation. The pulse should be more than 50 beats a minute.

Taking the pulse is mainly to assess changes in the patient's radial pulse. The pulse indication includes frequency, rhythm, fullness, location, degree of obstruction, etc. The location, disease characteristics and flourishing and decline of anti-pathogenic and pathogenic factors are differentiated through assessing the change of pulse. (Fig. 45)

8-4-1-4 Normal pulse indications

A normal pulse is felt four times per breath, and is moderate, forceful and rhythmic. It normally changes with changes of activity and environment. In the pulse science of TCM, the pulse is said to have "spirit," if the pulse is strong; "stomach *qi*," if the pulse

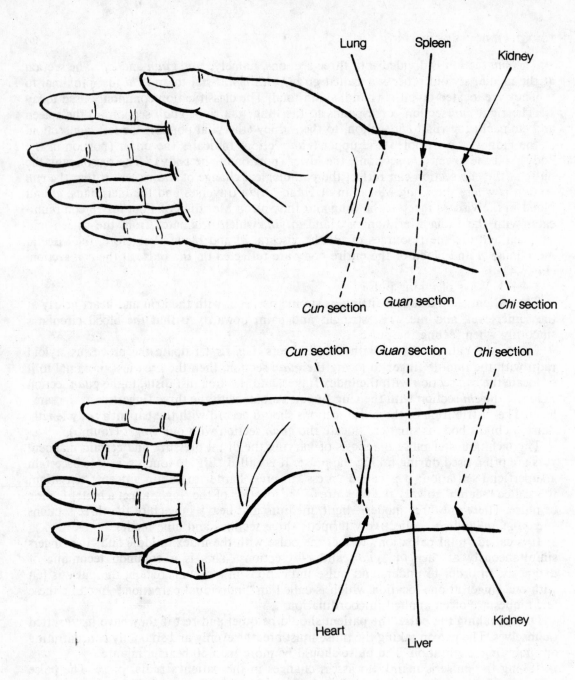

Fig. 45.   The correspondence of the three sections to the five yin viscera

is moderate and unhurried; and "root," if the pulse can be taken on deep palpation.

The pulse is related to the internal and external environments of the body. It varies along with physiological changes such as age, sex, constitution and mental state, e.g., the younger the person, the quicker the pulse. The infant's pulse is hasty and frequent, young and middle-aged people have strong pulses and the aged have weak pulses. The adult woman's pulse is softer, weaker and quicker than the adult man's. A tall person's pulse is longer than a short person's. A thin person's pulse is somewhat superficial and the obese person's pulse is deep. People who do hard physical labour or exercise, who drink alcohol, take much food, or are excited, have rapid and strong pulses. The pulse becomes weaker with hunger. Weather changes influence pulse indications, for instance, the pulse is somewhat stringy in spring and somewhat stony in winter. These changes should be distinguished from those of abnormal pulse.

It is called a "slantedly-located" pulse when a person's pulse cannot be felt at the *cun* section but runs outwardly and slantedly from the *chi* section to the dorsal hand; it is called a "dorsally-located pulse" if the pulse is felt on the dorsal wrist. Both of them are an anatomical anomaly of the radial artery and pertain to a special pulse location.

8-4-1-5 Abnormal pulse and its indications

An abnormal pulse reflects changes of a disease. In general, all pulses are abnormal ones except the pulses within the range of normal physiological changes. In recent times, pulse indications are mainly explained from the twenty-eight types which are classified according to their location, frequency, shape, rhythm, momentum and degree of obstruction. Pulses are classified as follows:

a. A superficial pulse can be easily felt with a gentle touch, but easily obliterated by a heavy press. It indicates an exterior syndrome. The superficial and strong pulse indicates an exterior-excess syndrome, and the superficial and weak pulse indicates an exterior-deficient syndrome. It often appears at the initial stage of exogenous disease, i.e., the exterior syndrome as well as in patients who suffer from a prolonged illness and are generally weak in constitution.

Similar pulses:

a) A scattered pulse is scattered and disordered to a gentle touch and disappears when heavily pressed. It is chiefly seen in a critical case of *qi* collapse and exhaustion of essential *qi* in the viscera.

b) A hollow pulse is superficial, large and hollow. It is seen after hemorrhea or hyperhidrosis.

b. A deep pulse cannot be detected with a light pressure but by heavy pressure. It indicates an interior syndrome. The forceful pulse indicates an interior-excess syndrome, and the weak pulse, an interior-deficient syndrome.

Similar pulses:

a) A hidden pulse is deeply situated and can be felt by pressing the bone. It is often seen in the *jue* (fainting) syndrome and excruciating pain.

b) A firm pulse can only be felt by a deep palpation and is firm, forceful, large, taut and long. It is frequently seen in the condition due to accumulating yin cold, such as *zhenxia*,[26] hernia, etc.

c. A slow pulse has a rate below 60 beats per minute. It indicates a cold syndrome. The forceful pulse denotes accumulating cold and the weak pulse indicates deficient yang.

Similar pulses:

a) The moderate, forceful and even pulse with a rate of 60 beats per minute, seen in a healthy person.

b) The loose and retarded pulse indicates the affection of pathogenic damp and a weak spleen and stomach.

d. A rapid pulse has a rate of over 90 beats per minute. It indicates a heat syndrome. The forceful type denotes an excess-heat syndrome and the weak pulse indicates a deficiency-heat syndrome.

Similar pulse:

A very rapid pulse of over 120 beats per minute may be seen at the late stage of febrile disease and in the exhausted yin and excessive yang in pulmonary tuberculosis.

e. Weak pulse: A general term for varieties of weak pulses; the rough, weak and empty pulses indicating deficient *qi* and blood and most frequently seen in deficient *qi*.

f. Substantial pulse: A general term for varieties of forceful pulses; the large forceful and substantive ones indicate an excess syndrome.

g. A slippery pulse feels even and smooth like pearls rolling on a dish. It indicates *tan-yin* (phlegm and excess exudates) and food retention and excess-heat syndrome and pregnancy.

Similar pulse:

A throbbing pulse is slippery, rapid and forceful. It indicates fright and pain.

h. An irregular pulse is irregular in rhythm, faint and slow and mimics scraping lightly with a knife. It indicates stagnant *qi*, congealed blood, consumed *jing* (vital principle) and deficient blood with impaired yin.

i. A small pulse is as small, soft and forceless as a thread, but can be obviously felt. It indicates deficient *qi* and blood and damp disease.

Similar pulses:

a) A soft pulse is small, soft and superficial. It can be felt by a gentle touch, but becomes indistinct on heavy pressure. It is often seen in deficiency and damp syndromes.

b) A faint pulse is extremely faint and weak and barely palpable. It is caused by declining yang seen in patients with exhausted kidney yang and sudden collapse.

c) A weak pulse is soft, deep and small. It indicates various syndromes due to deficient *qi* and blood.

j. A full pulse comes on forcefully and fades. It is due to extreme pathogenic heat.

A large pulse fills the fingertip. A large and forceful pulse indicates the excess syndrome caused by pathogenic heat; a large and forceless pulse indicates deficient and impaired yin, yang, *qi* and blood in the viscera.

k. A stringy pulse is taut and long, and feels like a violin string. It indicates gallbladder trouble, a pain syndrome and *tan-yin* (phlegm and excess exudates).

Similar pulses:

a) A taut pulse feels tense, forceful and tight like a rope to the finger. It indicates cold and pain syndromes and dyspepsia.

b) A tympanic pulse is extremely taut but hollow, and feels like the head of a drum. It is often seen in a post-hemorrhagic state or after spermatorrhea, or delivery ahead of schedule and metrorrhagia.

l. A regular intermittent pulse is a rather slow and weak pulse, with missed beats at regular intervals. It is often seen in declining visceral *qi* and heart trouble, etc.

Similar pulses:

a) An abrupt pulse is rapid and irregular. It indicates extreme yang heat, stagnant *qi* and congealed blood, phlegm and food retention, etc.

b) An irregular intermittent pulse is slow and misses beats at irregular intervals. It indicates extreme yin, cold phlegm and stagnant blood, stagnant *qi* and obstructed *qi* in the meridian.

8-4-1-6 Compound pulse and its indications

In a disease process the anti-pathogenic factor varies and more than two kinds of pathogenic factors can occur and the location and characteristics of a disease change constantly. Sometimes two or more pulses occur simultaneously, for example, the superficial slow pulse and deep-tense pulse. It is termed the compound pulse when two or more pulses appear concurrently. Some pulses are formed by several simple pulses among the twenty-eight pulses, e.g., a soft pulse is formed by small and superficial pulses; a weak one, deep and small pulses.

In general, the disease that a compound pulse indicates usually equals the total of the diseases that various simple pulses indicate. For example, a superficial pulse indicates an exterior syndrome and rapid pulse indicates a heat syndrome. Thus the disease is an exterior-heat disease. The superficial-tense pulse thus indicates an exterior-cold syndrome. The deep slow pulse indicates an interior-cold syndrome.

The compound pulses commonly seen in clinic and their indications are exemplified as follows:

A superficial-tense pulse indicates an exterior-cold syndrome caused by exogenous pathogenic cold or pain due to the wind *bi* (blockage) syndrome.[27]

A superficial-slow pulse indicates the exterior-deficiency syndrome due to impaired defensive *qi* by exogenous pathogenic wind, disharmony of *ying* (nutrition), *wei* (defence), *qi* (vital energy) and *xue* (blood) phases and the *taiyang* meridian affected by pathogenic wind.

A superficial-rapid pulse indicates an exterior-heat syndrome due to the invasion of the body surface by exogenous pathogenic wind-heat.

A superficial-slippery pulse indicates pathogenic wind-phlegm or an exterior syndrome associated with phlegm. It is frequently seen in the exogenous pathogenic factor in patients with excessive phlegm.

A deep-slow pulse indicates an interior-cold syndrome and is often seen in the disease or syndrome of deficient yin of the spleen and stomach and stagnant yin cold.

A stringy-tense pulse indicates cold and pain syndromes and is frequently seen in the disease or syndrome of pathogenic cold stagnating in the Liver Meridian or depressed liver and stagnation of *qi*, and hypochondriac pain, etc.

A stringy-rapid pulse is often seen in the diseases or syndromes, such as endogenous pathogenic fire (intense heat) produced by a depressed liver or the affection of the liver and gallbladder by pathogenic damp-heat, etc.

A slippery-rapid pulse indicates phlegm-heat, phlegm-fire or internal pernicious heat and food retention.

A full-rapid pulse indicates excess pernicious heat at *qi*, commonly seen in an exogenous febrile disease.

A deep-stringy pulse indicates a depressed liver and stagnant *qi* or internal retention of *shui-yin* (excess watery fluid).

A deep-irregular pulse indicates congealed blood, most commonly seen in stagnant cold and blood due to deficient yang.

A stringy-small pulse indicates deficient liver and kidney yin or deficient blood and a depressed liver or a depressed liver and a weak spleen.

A deep-slow pulse indicates syndromes, such as deficient spleen and kidney yang and retention of aqueous damp.

A deep-small-rapid pulse indicates deficient yin or fever due to deficient blood.

A stringy-slippery-rapid pulse is seen in the syndromes, such as liver fire associated with phlegm or the upwardly disturbing wind yang and internally accumulating phlegm-fire, etc.

8-4-1-7 Diagnosis in accordance with pulse and symptoms. Normally a pulse accords with symptoms but not always. For example, in an excess syndrome, a full, rapid and substantive pulse is seen, which accords with the symptoms and indicates that the body's anti-pathogenic factor is strong enough to combat the substantive pathogenic factor; if a deep, small, faint and weak pulse is seen, the pulse would be contrary to the symptoms, showing that the pathogenic factor prevails over the anti-pathogenic factor, resulting in a deeper invasion of the pathogenic factor. In acute cases, a deep, full, rapid and substantive pulse indicates that the anti-pathogenic factor is strong enough to resist the pathogen; in a chronic disease, a deep, faint, small and weak pulse indicates the possibility that the pathogenic factor is declining and the anti-pathogenic factor will recover. If a deep, small, faint and weak pulse is seen in a newly-encountered disease, it indicates that the anti-pathogenic factor has declined; a superficial, full, frequent and substantive pulse in a chronic illness indicates that the anti-pathogenic factor has declined and the pathogenic one has not yet been eliminated, and both new and old diseases develop abnormally.

Since it may occur that a pulse does not accord to symptoms, whether the pulse and symptoms are true or not must be cleared up and a diagnosis made according to the pulse rather than according to the symptoms.

As the pulse is only one of the manifestations of a disease, it cannot be used as the sole basis for diagnosis. Only by applying the four diagnostic techniques can an accurate diagnosis be made.

8-4-2 Palpation of certain areas of the body

8-4-2-1 Method and significance

Palpation to identify the syndrome was recorded in the *Internal Classic, Treatise on Febrile Diseases, Synopsis of the Golden Bookcase*, etc. It is a diagnostic technique to understand normal bodily changes by touching or pressing certain portions of the patient's body in order to find the location, characteristics and severity of the disease.

Palpation can be divided into touching, stroking and pressing techniques. Touching refers to touching local areas of the patient's body gently with the finger or palm, such as the forehead, four extremities, etc. to understand the (cool or hot, moist or dry) state of the skin. Feeling is stroking local areas of the patient's body, such as swollen and distended areas, etc. to ascertain the patient's local feeling and the shape and size of a mass, etc. Pressing is to press the local part of the patient's body, such as the chest, abdomen and the area where a mass grows to understand whether there is tenderness, a mass, the degree of swelling and distension, etc. These three techniques are applied in combination, the first two and then the third, first gently then a stronger pressure is applied in order to understand the pathological change.

When palpating, a doctor should manipulate lightly, avoiding sudden force. In winter the doctor's hands should be warmed before examining the patient. The doctor should advise the patient to cooperate and tell the doctor the feeling. The patient's facial expression should be observed during examination so as to find where the pain is.

8-4-2-2 Contents

a. Palpation of the skin surface: is to find out whether the skin is cold or hot, moist or dry and swollen or distended.

Not only whether the body is affected by pathogenic cold or heat can be discovered, but also the exterior/interior, deficiency/excess of the heat affection can be differentiated from the intensity and depth of pernicious heat through palpation of the skin surface. In general, when pathogenic heat is extreme, the body is usually hot; when yang *qi* declines, the body is usually cold. In a hot body when the pernicious heat is intense at the initial press, but becomes mild after prolonged pressure, it is superficial; if it becomes intense after prolonged pressure and spreads outward, it is deep; if the skin is widely hot with no steaming sensation, it is due to fever caused by general debility.

Touching the skin surface lightly can aid in detecting whether the skin is moist or not and in understanding yin and yang diseases and whether body fluids are consumed, e.g., moist and bright skin indicates that body fluids have not yet been consumed; dry or scaly skin indicates that body fluids are consumed or blood is stagnant and deficient. Detection of swelling and distension by heavy pressure can distinguish edema from gaseous distension.

In surgery, the yin and yang disease or syndrome and whether suppuration appears can be distinguished by palpating the affected area. For example, boils which are firm and not hot, with diffuse flat swelling belong to a yin syndrome and those which burn and are deeply rooted, belong to a yang syndrome. Those that are fixed, firm, hot and moderately hot, have not yet suppurated; those that are firm at their edge but soft at their centre and intensely hot have suppurated. Those that cause pain when lightly pressed indicate that the pus is superficial; those that cause pain by heavy pressure indicate that the pus is deep. Those that cannot rise when pressed down have not yet suppurated, while those with a waving sensation when pressed have suppurated.

In addition, it is helpful for diagnosis of acute febrile diseases to palpate the *chi* skin.[28] It indicates an acute febrile disease when the *chi* skin is intensely hot which is seen in exogenous diseases.

b. Palpation of hands and feet: Palpation of hands and feet is mainly for detecting coldness or hotness of the body. Whether yang *qi* flourishes or declines can be ascertained by examining the warmth or coolness of the hands and feet. Cold hands and feet are due to the deficient yin and extreme pathogenic cold; hot hands and feet are due to extreme yang heat. Whether the disease is caused by an external affection or internal injury can be examined by palpating the (warm or cool) palm and dorsum of the hand. Intensely hot palms indicate an endogenous injury; an intensely hot dorsum indicates an exogenous disease.

c. Palpation of the epigastric and abdominal regions is mainly to detect whether the skin is dry or moist by gently touching its surface, to understand whether there is a painful sensation by palpating a local area, to detect its softness or firmness in order to differentiate excess and deficiency of the viscera, features of pathogenic factors and the degree of their accumulation.

a) Palpation of the epigastric region: Whether the epigastrium is soft and tender or not can distinguish the distension and fullness[29] from the knotted-chest.[30]

b) Palpation of the abdomen: It indicates deficiency if the abdominal pain is relieved by pressure, and excess if the abdominal pain is aggravated by pressure.

It is gaseous distension when the abdomen is distending and full like a drum, with normal urination; it is ascites when liquid accumulates in the abdominal cavity, which resembles a sac containing much water with difficulty in urination. It is *zhen* and *ji*[31] if there is a palpable and immovable mass in the abdomen with pain at a definite site. In this case, the yin viscera are affected at the *xue* (blood) phase. It is *jia* and *ju*[32] when there is an intermittent feeling of an indefinite mass in the abdomen, with pain at a definite site. In this case, the yang viscera are affected at the *qi* (vital energy) phase. If the abdominal pain occurs in the surrounding umbilicus, with the mass felt in the lower left abdomen by palpation, stagnant dry stool should be taken into consideration. It is due to accumulated intestinal parasites when something indefinite accumulates in the abdomen and is firm when pressed.

It indicates intestinal carbuncle when a pain occurs in the lower right abdomen, which is aggravated by heavy pressure immediately after the pressing hand is withdrawn.

d. Palpation of acupoints: Acupoints are the foci on the body surface where *qi* and blood in the meridians gather and traverse, as well as the place through which *qi* in the viscera is transported. They can reflect physiopathological changes of the viscera through their meridian connections. Hence, understanding changes and reactions of the acupoints by palpation can also be regarded as one method for detecting and diagnosing visceral diseases. Marked tenderness or a hypersensitive reaction or nodules found in the area where *qi* in the meridians gather is an indication of disease. For example, a nodule can be palpated at *Feishu* (B. 13) or tenderness at *Zhongfu* (L. 1) in lung trouble; tenderness at *Ganshu* (B. 18) and *Qimen* (Liv. 14) in liver trouble; tenderness at *Weishu* (B. 21) and *Zusanli* (S 36) in stomach trouble; tenderness at *Shangjuxu* (*Lanwei*) (S 37) of the Stomach Meridian of Foot-*yangming* in intestinal carbuncle. These palpations can help diagnose visceral diseases.

Notes

[1] A symptom complex or real cold in the lower part of the body and false heat in the upper body. It is caused by weakness and cold in the lower energizer with floating yang. The chief manifestations are shortness of breath, tachypnea, fatigue, dizziness, palpitations, cold clammy limbs, flushed face, copious pale urine, loose stools, etc.

[2] The various diseases caused by water retention. Its meaning is the same as *tan-yin* (phlegm and excess exudates) in a broad sense, or in an implied sense.

[3] A collective term for gynecological diseases.

[4] A kind of mental abnormal disorder characterized by sudden loss of consciousness, followed by convulsions of the limbs, frothy salivation, upward turning of the eyeball, crying. The patient is normal after regaining consciousness.

[5] Wasting syndromes (atrophic debility): The diseases and syndrome complexes of atrophy and debility of the limbs and body.

[6] Opisthotonos and lockjaw in febrile diseases.

[7] A suppurative infection of the ear characterized by redness, swelling, pain, and heat and perforation of the eardrum with yellowish purulent discharge.

[8] Subcutaneous hemorrhages coalesce to form reddish or purplish patches. Those which cannot be felt are *ban* often seen in acute fevers, and are signs of pathogenic heat invading the *ying*

(nutrition) and *xue* (blood) phases. Those with reddish or purplish miliary elevations on the skin which can usually be felt are *zhen* (papule), often caused by stagnation of pernicious wind-heat with invasion of blood vessels, and which extrude from the skin.

⁹· Small whitish vesicles of the skin of the neck, chest and abdomen which appear during the course of certain damp febrile diseases, containing yellowish fluid. The whitish glistening blisters indicate a favourable prognosis while the dry ones, unfavourable.

¹⁰· An acute, suppurative inflammatory lesion of the body surface, which progresses rapidly and is fumigating and dangerous. It is small, but deep-rooted like a nail, thus its name.

¹¹· Suppurative infections of the lung: suppuration of the lung with purulent and bloody expectoration, i.e., lung abscess and gangrene of the lung.

¹²· One of the *lin* symptom complexes. Urine contains gravel, due to calculus in the urinary system. The chief manifestations are pain of one side of the lower back or intermittent colicky pain, radiating to the hypogastrium and genitalia, difficulty of urination, and occasional fine sandy gravel in the urine.

¹³· One of the *lin* symptom complexes. The chief symptoms are cloudy urine like rice water or emulsified fat, and difficulty of urination.

¹⁴· A general term for manic-depressive psychosis.

¹⁵· Same as 4.

¹⁶· Referring to the disease or syndrome characterized by sudden fainting and falling down, unconsciousness, or sudden facial paralysis, hemiplegia and incoherent speech.

¹⁷· The pathological changes are neither located in the exterior, nor in the interior but in between. The main manifestations are oscillations between chills and fever, chest distress, hypochondriac discomfort, retching, anorexia, bitter taste, dry throat, vertigo, stringy pulse, etc.

¹⁸· A type of exterior syndrome characterized by chills, no sweating, superficial and taut pulse, besides the symptoms and signs of the exterior syndrome.

¹⁹· The *taiyang* meridian affected by pathogenic wind: One of the *taiyang* diseases among the six meridians diseases due to external affections. Its main manifestations are headache, chilly sensation, fever, perspiration, superficial and slow pulse, etc.

²⁰· The symptom complex due to interference with the flow of yang *qi* and stagnation of phlegm and damp pathogens in the chest chiefly manifested as upper back pain, a feeling of suffocation in the chest, shortness of breath, cough with copious phlegm, etc.

²¹· A disease of water retention in the chest. The chief manifestations are distending discomfort in the hypochondria with occasional mild swelling, hypochondriac pain with cough, etc. It is similar to pleurisy with effusion.

²²· Abnormalities of micturation are mainly manifested by frequency of urination, urgency of urination, painful micturition or incontinence of urine. They may be classified into five types, such as stone *lin* (dysuria caused by calculus), *qi lin* (dysuria due to dysfunction of the bladder), milky *lin* (chyuria), consumptive *lin* (chronic dysuria), and blood *lin* (hematuria with pain), and includes such diseases as infection, calculus and tuberculosis of the urinary system, chyuria and prostatitis, etc.

²³· The section of the radial artery for pulse diagnosis is divided into three parts. The part at the radial styloid process is called *guan*, with *cun* distal to it and *chi* just proximal to it.

²⁴· In clinical examination, when the pulse does not accord with the symptoms and signs, when the symptoms actually reflect the condition of the illness, then the diagnosis is made according to the symptoms rather than to the pulse.

²⁵· In clinical examination, when the pulse does not accord with the symptoms, when the pulse reflects the actual condition of the illness, the diagnosis should be made according to the pulse rather than the symptoms.

²⁶· The symptom complex with a mass or swelling in the abdomen, *zhen* and *ji* are clinically characterized by a palpable and immovable mass of a definite shape in the abdomen, with pain at a definite site. In this case, the yin viscera are affected at the *xue* (blood) phase. *Jia* and *ju* are characterized by the intermittent feeling of an indefinite mass in the abdomen, with pain at no definite site. The yang viscera are affected at the *qi* (vital energy) phase.

²⁷· A *bi* (blockage) syndrome caused by a relative excess of pathogenic wind with chief manifestations of migratory pain in the limbs.

[28.] Examination of *chi* skin: The *chi* region is the forearm, and examination of *chi* is a diagnostic technique to determine the moisture, texture and temperature of the skin by manual palpation.

[29.] Subjective feeling of fullness and distressing discomfort due to obstruction of the *qi* mechanism between the chest and abdomen.

[30.] Varieties of symptoms due to an accumulation of pathogenic heat (or cold) with fluids (either phlegm or blood) in the chest and abdomen.

[31.] [32.] See 26.

9. EIGHT GUIDING PRINCIPLES

The eight guiding principles, viz., yin, yang, exterior, interior, cold, heat, deficiency and excess is one of the theoretical bases for *bianzheng* and *lunzhi* (planning treatment according to diagnosis). The information obtained by the four diagnostic techniques is analysed and summed up as the eight kinds of syndromes according to the depth of disease, its characteristics and flourishing and decline of the pathogenic and anti-pathogenic factors, etc. called identification of syndromes according to the eight guiding principles. The eight guiding principles also belong to the category of *bianzheng* (identification of syndrome) in TCM.

The contents of the eight guiding principles were mentioned as early as the *Internal Classic,* while Zhang Zhongjing applied them in diagnosis and treatment of febrile and miscellaneous diseases. "Yin Yang Pian," a chapter in *Complete Book of Jingyue* (*Jingyue Quan Shu*) further expounded them. Cheng Zhongling advocated them, thus, they have become an important component of TCM.

Diseases can be basically generalized according to the eight principal syndromes even if their manifestations are complex. They are classified into two main classifications, yin and yang syndromes. The location of a disease is classified as either superficial or deep. Diseases are also classified as either hot or cold. The disease caused by a preponderant pathogenic factor is called an excess syndrome, but that caused by a weaker anti-pathogenic factor, is called a deficiency syndrome. Identification of syndromes according to the eight guiding principles, therefore classifies diseases according to exterior-interior syndromes, cold-heat syndromes, excess-deficiency syndromes in order to guide treatment. Yin-yang syndromes are a further classification, i.e., exterior, heat and excess syndromes pertaining to yang; interior, cold and deficient syndromes pertaining to yin. Hence, the yin-yang principle is the general principle of the eight guiding principles.

The eight guiding principles sometimes show various contradictions in a pathological change, but they are interconnected, e.g., identification of exterior and interior syndromes must connect with cold or heat, deficiency or excess syndromes and those of deficiency and excess syndromes must be connected with the exterior or interior, cold or hot ones. The change of disease is not always a simple but rather is a complex condition when the exterior and interior, cold and heat, and deficiency and excess syndromes constantly intermingle. At the same time, under certain conditions, the characteristics of a syndrome may also change to a certain extent, e.g., an exterior syndrome may transform into an interior one and vice versa; a cold syndrome may change into a hot one and vice versa; an excess syndrome may change into a deficient one and vice versa. Some manifestations that are contrary to the features of disease may also appear. For instance, the true heat and false cold, the true cold and false heat, the true deficiency and false excess, the true excess and false deficiency, etc. Therefore, not only the syndromes must be skillfully grasped, but special attention must also be paid to their interconnection when identifying syndromes according to the eight guiding principles. Only in this way can a disease be correctly recognized and diagnosed.

9-1 Exterior and interior

Exterior and interior are the two guiding principles for identification of the location and depth of disease. The form of the body is exterior while the viscera are interior. The five yin viscera are interior and the six yang viscera are exterior. The meridian is exterior and the viscera are interior. The three yang meridians are exterior and the three yin meridians are interior, etc. As far as the depth of disease is concerned, because a pathogenic factor invades the deep body, an exogenous disease gets deeper; when a pathogenic factor is eliminated, the disease becomes milder. This concept is important for identification of febrile disease with the names of six meridians and acute febrile diseases according to *wei* (defence), *qi* (vital energy), *ying* (nutrition) and *xue* (blood).[1] The skin and hair, muscles and meridians are exterior while the viscera and bone marrow are interior. The disease occurring in the superficial part of the body pertains to the exterior, while that in the deep part to the interior.

The identification of exterior and interior suits exogenous diseases and is significant in ascertaining the severity and depth of disease and tendency of a pathological change, i.e., an exterior syndrome is superficial and mild, but an interior one is deep and severe. A disease progresses when a superficial pathogenic factor invades the deep body, but regresses when a deep pathogenic factor goes outward. The changes of a disease can be grasped and the disease can be treated properly when understanding the severity and progress of the disease. Diaphoretic and purgative therapies are adopted accordingly.

9-1-1 Exterior syndromes

An exterior syndrome refers to the syndrome that is situated superficially in the skin. It generally refers to the initial stage of an exogenous disease caused by the invasion of the "six excesses" into the skin, mouth and nose. Therefore, it is characterized by a rapid onset and short duration.

Clinical picture: Mainly thin white tongue coating, superficial pulse, often accompanied by pain in the head and body, stuffy nose, cough, etc.

Analysis of symptoms: The invasion of the "six excesses" into the body. As these factors stay on the body surface and hinder the normal dissipation of defensive *qi*, and the skin is not warmed as normally by the *qi*, aversion to wind and cold appears. As the lung is concerned with the skin, and the nose opens to the lung, the skin and hair affected by a pathogenic factor may influence the lung, causing the lung *qi* to fail in performing its dispersing and descending functions, resulting in stuffy nose, cough, even asthmatic breath. A pathogenic factor stagnating in the meridian makes *qi* and blood circulate unsmoothly, leading to pain in the head and body. Owing to the pathogenic factor lying in the skin and hair where the anti-pathogenic factor vies with the pathogenic one, a superficial pulse may be seen. Since the pathogenic factor has not deeply invaded, the tongue does not obviously change, and only a thin white coating appears. It is treated by diaphoresis with pungent drugs to disperse the pathogenic factors.

9-1-2 Interior syndromes

An interior syndrome is inside the body (the viscera, *qi* and blood, marrow, etc.). It is opposite to an exterior syndrome. All syndromes that are not exterior pertain to the interior syndrome. Its clinical picture varies greatly and is explained in the 9-2, 9-3, and 10-3 sections.

Analysis of symptoms:

a. An exterior syndrome further develops and the superficial pathogenic factor invades deeply.

b. The exogenous factor attacks the viscera directly.

c. Internal injuries caused by emotional factors, diet, fatigue and lack of physical exercise, etc. directly influence and cause visceral dysfunction. Since the exogenous factor is wide in range and its treatment varies, it should be determined according to the condition.

9-1-3 Identification of exterior and interior syndromes

Identification of exterior and interior syndromes is significant for identifying exterior and interior syndromes for inquiring the past history, detecting chills and fever and changes of tongue coating and pulse, etc. In general, a newly-encountered disease with a short duration pertains to an exterior syndrome and a prolonged disease pertains to an interior syndrome. The disease with fever and creeping chills is an exterior syndrome; the disease with fever, but no aversion to cold or chills and that with no fever is an interior syndrome. As to the exterior syndrome in which the tongue coating does not change frequently or a dark-red tip and edge of the tongue are only seen without other abnormal manifestations of tongue coating, an interior syndrome should be considered. A superficial pulse indicates that the disease is located superficially; while a deep pulse indicates a disease that is located deeply.

9-1-4 Relation between exterior and interior syndromes

a. The transformation of an exterior syndrome into an interior one. In a disease process, under certain circumstances, the exterior syndrome that has not improved transmits internally, with an interior syndrome appearing, called "from the exterior to the interior." In certain interior syndromes a pathogenic factor in the deeper part of the body is brought to the skin and muscles, called "from the interior to the exterior." The occurrence of this transformation chiefly depends upon the condition of the struggle between the anti-pathogenic and pathogenic factors. The transformation of an exterior syndrome into an interior one is caused by weakened body resistance against the pathogenic factor or a preponderance of the pathogenic factor or improper nursing or mistreatment, etc. The transformation of an interior syndrome into an exterior one results from proper nursing and treatment and strengthened body resistance. Generally speaking, the former denotes the trend of aggravation of a disease while the latter, devotes improvement of a disease. Therefore, it is important for predicting the tendency of the development of disease to grasp the change from the interior syndromes into the exterior syndromes. The following are examples.

The exterior syndrome transmitting inward: When creeping chills disappear, but aversion to heat is accompanied by polydipsia and desire for drinking, red tongue with yellow coating, dark-red urine, in the interior syndrome that originally had fever and creeping chills indicates that the disease is developing inwardly, and the pathogenic factor is going from the superficial part of the body to the deep part and becoming an interior-heat syndrome.

The interior syndrome transmitting outward: Fever and restlessness, cough and chest distress, then fever and perspiration, relieved restlessness or exposed rashes in the deeper part of the body are brought to the skin and muscles. For example, in patients with measles, the rashes disappear after occurrence, high fever, asthmatic breath, restlessness, etc. due to weak constitution, or wind-cold affection or early medication of drugs of a cool nature blocked defensive *qi*, which reflects that toxic rashes transmit inward and the disease transmits from the superficial part of the body to the deep body. The pathogenic factor can also transmit from the deep to the superficial part of the body if the treatment is not right. The infant's body resistance can be strengthened, and therapies, such as heat-clearing and exposing exanthema, are used to expel the pathogenic factor and promote the development of the exanthema, to clear up pernicious heat and relieve asthmatic breath and expose the exanthema.

b. Exterior and interior syndromes can appear in the same period of time. When there is an exterior syndrome complicated with an interior one, or the primary disease associated with the secondary one, such as internal injury complicated with external affection or the external affection followed by injury from improper diet, then exterior and interior syndromes are present simultaneously.

Since exterior and interior syndromes are related to cold/heat and deficiency/excess, they have different patterns. The commonly seen ones are the exterior-cold and interior-excess and interior-deficiency, etc. They are described in the section of Identification of Syndromes according to Cold/Heat and Deficiency/Excess.

9-2 Cold and heat

Cold and heat are the two guiding principles for identifying the characteristics of disease. The cold and heat syndromes reflect the relative flourishing and decline of the yin and yang in the body. The manifestation of excess yin or deficient yang is a cold syndrome; excess yang and deficient yin is indicative of a heat syndrome.

Identification of cold and heat cannot be judged according to an isolated symptom, but through all the symptoms reflecting the disease and by using the four diagnostic techniques. A heat syndrome refers to a group of hot symptoms and a cold syndrome refers to cold symptoms, e.g., an exterior-cold syndrome includes a group of cold signs, such as fever, severe aversion to cold, with little taste, no thirst, thin, white and moist tongue coating, and superficial taut pulse. It is thus diagnosed as an exterior-cold syndrome; an exterior-heat syndrome includes hot signs, such as creeping chills, high fever, slight thirst, dark-red tip of the tongue and edge of the tongue and superficial, rapid pulse. It is therefore diagnosed as an exterior-heat syndrome. Attention must be paid to that creeping chills and fever are different from those in cold and heat syndromes.

Identification of cold and heat is important in treatment. *Plain Questions* states, "Heating the cold" and "cooling the heat," i.e., drugs of a hot nature should be used for a cold syndrome and those of a cold nature, for a heat one. The therapies for the two cases are entirely different.

9-2-1 Cold syndromes

A cold syndrome includes symptoms manifesting the cold affection or deficient yang and excess yin.

Clinical picture: Creeping chills and preference for warmth, tasteless mouth and no thirst, pallor, cold limbs and rolling body in bed, clear profuse urine, loose stools, light-coloured tongue with white, moistened and slippery coating, and slow or taut pulse are frequently seen.

Analysis of symptoms: A cold syndrome is caused by external affection of yin cold or prolonged illness due to internal injury, consumed yang *qi* and excess internal yin pathogen. Yang *qi* fails to warm the body due to general weakness of affection of exogenous pathogenic cold, resulting in creeping chills and preference for warmth, cold limbs and rolling body in bed; as internal yin cold is excessive tasteless mouth with no thirst occur; since deficient yang fails to warm and transform aqueous liquid, clear cold excreta, such as sputum, nasal discharge, saliva, etc. result. If the spleen is affected by pathogenic cold or the spleen yang is weak for long, the spleen's transporting and digesting functions may become abnormal, with loose stools, a light-coloured tongue and white, moist and slippery coating. As yang *qi* is too weak to promote blood circulation, a slow pulse may be seen.

9-2-2 Heat syndromes

A heat syndrome includes symptoms of hyperfunction of the body due to heat affection or excess yang and deficient yin.

Clinical picture: Fever and preference for coolness, thirst and indulgence in cold drinking, flushed face and congestive eyes, restlessness, dark-red scanty urine, constipation, red tongue with yellow dry coating, rapid pulse, etc.

Analysis of symptoms: The external affection of pathogenic fire (intense heat) or "seven emotions" that produce pernicious fire; or pathogenic heat due to prolonged improper diet or excess sexual activity and fatigue and lack of physical exercise that result in deprived yin *jing* (vital principle), deficient yin and excess yang.

As yang heat is excessive, bodily fever and preference for coolness may result. As pernicious fire (intense heat) injures, yin and body fluids are consumed, dark-red scanty urine appears. Consumed body fluids result in thirst and preference for cold drinks. Since the fire is blazing, flushed face and congestive eyes occur. As endogenous pathogenic heat disturbs the mind, restlessness may result. Heat affection to the intestine and consumption of body fluids cause dry stools. A red tongue with yellow coating is a hot sign, while a dry tongue coating is a sign of injury of yin. Since blood is accelerated by extreme yang heat, a rapid pulse may be seen.

9-2-3 Identification of cold and hot syndromes

When identifying cold and hot syndromes, a correct diagnosis should be made not just according to isolated symptoms, but according to observation of all the symptoms of the disease, particularly thirst (or no thirst), complexion, limbs, urine, tongue coating, pulse, etc. Creeping chills and preference for cold indicate, for instance, heat affection and cold clammy extremities indicate a cold affection. Dark-red scanty urine and constipation indicate a heat affection, while clear profuse urine and loose stools indicate a cold affection. A rapid slippery pulse indicates a heat affection, while a sunken slow pulse indicates a cold affection. A red tongue with a yellow coating indicates a heat affection and a light-coloured tongue with a white coating indicates a cold affection. From the above-mentioned descriptions it may be seen that a cold syndrome pertains to excess yin with deficient yang, and a heat syndrome pertains to excess yang, often a manifestation of consumed yin fluids.

9-2-4 Relation between cold and hot syndromes

Although cold and hot syndromes are different in the flourishing and decline of yin and yang, they are interconnected. They may exist simultaneously in a patient.

9-2-4-1 Intermingling of cold and heat, upper heat and lower cold

The pathological change produced by a combination of pathogenic heat in the upper part of the body and pathogenic cold in the lower in a patient at the same time, e.g., the upper-heat syndrome, such as anxiety and heat in the chest, frequent desire for vomiting and the lower-cold one, such as abdominal pain, preference for warmth and loose stools. It is often caused by intermingling of pernicious cold and heat in pathogenesis and disharmony between yin *qi* and yang *qi*, so that yang is excessive in the upper portion of the body and yin, in the lower.

Exterior cold and internal heat: A sign of intermingling of exogenous pathogenic cold and endogenous pathogenic heat. They are frequently seen in the disease or syndrome when the endogenous heat affection is complicated with the exogenous wind-cold affection or the exogenous pathogenic factor transfers inwardly and exogenous pathogenic cold is not yet resolved. For example, children first suffering from food retention and endogenous pathogenic heat, then affected by exogenous pathogenic wind-cold, have not only abdominal fullness, restlessness, thirst and yellow tongue coating caused by endogenous pathogenic heat and food retention, but also have fever and creeping chills, pain caused by exterior cold that pertains to exterior-cold and interior-heat syndromes.

Exterior heat and interior cold: Also a sign of intermingling exogenous heat and endogenous cold. It is often seen in patients with endogenous cold who suffer from the external affection of pathogenic wind-heat, e.g., the patient who is originally weak and cold in his or her speech and the kidney is externally affected by pathogenic wind-heat, manifesting as an exterior-heat syndrome, such as fever, headache, aversion to cold, swelling and pain in the throat, and an interior-cold syndrome, such as cold limbs, loose stools or dysentery and no thirst.

9-2-4-2 Transformation of cold and heat

This refers to a cold syndrome followed by a heat one and a gradual disappearing of the cold syndrome after the heat, e.g., after the affection of pathogenic cold, fever and creeping chills, general ache, anhidrosis, white tongue coating and superficial taut pulse pertain to an exterior-cold syndrome. Along with the further development of the pathological change, exogenous pathogenic cold invades the deeper part of the body and produces heat with symptoms such as creeping fever, anxiety and thirst, and the continuous appearance of a yellow tongue coating. This indicates that the exterior cold has transformed into interior heat.

It is a transformation of heat into cold when a heat syndrome is followed by a cold one, e.g., high fever, cold clammy extremities, pallor, deep slow pulse appear due to persistent hyperhidrosis, and yang consumed together with body fluids. This is a sign of the transformation of a heat syndrome into a cold one.

Whether cold and heat syndromes transform into each other depends upon the anti-pathogenic and pathogenic factors. A transformation of a cold syndrome into a heat syndrome depends on that the anti-pathogenic factor is enriched and yang *qi* is flourishing, so that the pathogenic factor can produce pernicious heat. When the anti-pathogenic factor fails to conquer the pathogenic factor and yang *qi* is impaired, a heat syndrome will transform into a cold syndrome even if it is a heat syndrome.

9-2-4-3 True and false cold and heat

In a disease process, particularly at the critical stage of a disease, symptoms of true heat and false cold or true cold and false heat may also occur.

True heat and false cold denote that the disease itself is of a cold nature but exhibits some apparently hot signs. Its clinical picture is cold clammy limbs and a deep pulse that are seemingly a cold syndrome, but cold limbs with fever and aversion to heat, not cold, deep, rapid and forceful pulse, and polydipsia and indulgence in cold drinks, dry throat, ozostomia or heat dysentery, dark-red tongue with yellow dry coating. Cold clammy limbs and deep pulse in this case are due to false cold, while internal heat is the essence of the disease. As the syndrome of true heat and false cold is caused by excess internal heat and yang *qi* is blocked so it fails to spread over the four extremities, the cold is excluded from the heat and yin is excluded by the internal excess yang. It is also called "excessive yang hinders yin." It is known as "yang *jue*"[2] or "heat *jue*"[3] according to its characteristics of cold clammy limbs caused by depressed yang and excess heat.

True cold and false heat denote that the disease itself is of a hot nature, but exhibits some apparently cold symptoms caused when yang is forced outward by internal excess yin cold. It is also termed "excessive yin hinders yang." Symptoms include fever, flushed face, thirst, large pulse, apparent heat syndrome, but fever with desire for more clothes and blankets, thirst and indulgence in hot drinks, large forceful pulse, with cold signs such as cold clammy extremities, clear urine, loose stools, and a light-coloured tongue with a white coating.

From the above-mentioned analysis, it may be seen that the so-called true and false cold and heat reflect that the symptoms of disease do not always accord with the essence of the disease. "True" indicates the essence of disease, while "false" is a false sign at a certain stage of the illness.

Identification of true and false cold and heat may be detected from the following:

a. As a false phenomenon occurs at the four extremities, skin or complexion and changes of the viscera, *qi* and blood and body fluids are the essence of disease, a diagnosis should be made according to the interior syndrome, pulse indication and tongue coating during identification of syndromes.

b. False phenomena are, however, different from true ones. A flushed face due to false heat means that only the zygomatic area and cheek of a pale face are sometimes slightly red and delicate and sometimes not, which differ from the whole flushed face. False cold is often manifested in cold clammy extremities, but high fever in the chest and abdomen or coolness in the entire body, but no desire for more clothes and blankets, which differs from the rolling body in bed and preference for warmth and desire for more clothes caused by true cold.

9-2-5 Relation between cold/heat and exterior/interior

A variety of symptoms may occur when cold and heat syndromes and exterior and interior syndromes are interconnected.

9-3 Deficiency and excess

Deficiency and excess are the two guiding principles for identifying the flourishing and decline of pathogenic and anti-pathogenic factors. Deficiency refers to an insufficient anti-pathogenic factor, while excess refers to the violent and substantive pathogenic factor.

Since a disease or syndrome is a deficiency or excess type and deficiency and excess are connected with exterior, interior, cold and heat, symptoms are comparatively com-

Table for Identification of True and False Cold and Heat

		True Cold and False Heat (yin syndrome resembling yang one)	True Heat and False Cold (yang syndrome resembling yin syndrome)
	Face	Delicate red malar flush, light-whitish lips	Shining eyes with Spirit, red and dry lips although complexion is dull
	Mental State	Listlessness and general lassitude although restlessness and signs resembling a yang syndrome may appear	Mental confusion and signs resembling yin syndrome, but sometimes anxiety, strong and forceful body form
	Tongue	Dull tongue, dark-greyish, moist and slippery tongue	Dark-red tongue with yellow or dark, dry and thorny coating
Auscultation-Olfaction		Cold and faint breath, low voice, much excreta with no offensive smell	Hot coarse breath, sonorous voice, foul mouth, much excreta with offensive smell
		Thirst with no desire for drinking, much excreta with desire for more clothes, normal defection or constipation; sore throat without swelling and congestion	Thirst and desire for cold drinking, severe chills with no desire for more clothes, dark yellow urine, constipation, burning hot anus
Palpation of Pulse		Rapid pulse felt forceless, minute and faint; chest and abdomen not burning hot when pressed by hand	Slippery rapid pulse or sudden pulse felt forceful, burning hot chest and abdomen when pressed by hand although hands and feet are cold
Pathogenesis		Yang is excluded externally by internal excess yang	Yin is excluded by yang heat that stagnates internally and fails to spread outward
Treatment		Restore yang for resuscitation, induce fire to clear up and purge internal heat and dissipate yang *qi*	

Table for Exterior, Interior, Cold and Heat Syndromes

	Clinical Picture	Tongue Indication	Pulse Indication	Pathogenesis	Treatment
Exterior-cold Syndrome	Aversion to cold and fever, general ache, no sweat	Thin, whitish coating	Superficial and taut	External affection of pathogenic cold	Diaphoresis with pungent cool drugs
Exterior-heat Syndrome	Fever, slight aversion to wind-cold, slight thirst, perspiration	Red edge and tip of the tongue	Superficial and rapid	External affection of pathogenic heat	Diaphoresis with pungent cool drugs
Interior-cold Syndrome	Cold body and limbs, no thirst or indulgence in less speech, clear urine and loose stools	Light-coloured tongue with white coating	Sunken and slow	Yang deficiency or the internal body attacked by pathogenic cold	Warm yang and dissipate pathogenic cold
Interior-heat Syndrome	Flushed face and bodily fever, dry and thirsty mouth, indulgence in cold drinks, restlessness, irritability and talkativeness, dark-yellow urine, dry stools	Red tongue with yellow coating	Full & rapid	Excess of internal heat	Clear up heat and purge fire

plex. In a disease process, deficiency and excess may transform into each other and symptoms of intermingling deficiency and excess may also appear.

By identifying deficiency and excess the flourishing and decline of pathogenic and anti-pathogenic factors in a patient can be understood and treated accordingly. It is advisable to treat an excess syndrome by purgation and a deficiency syndrome by tonification. Only by identifying syndromes accurately can purgative and tonifying therapies be used correctly.

9-3-1 Deficiency syndromes

Although a deficiency syndrome varies with deficient and impaired yin, yang, *qi* and blood, all the syndromes pertaining to deficiency are symptoms of a deficient anti-pathogenic factor. "The reason why a pathogenic factor succeeds in attacking the body is that its *qi* must be deficient" explains that anti-pathogenic and pathogenic factors and deficiency and excess influence one another. Yet, the syndromes that are fully ascribed to deficient *qi*, blood or deficient yin and yang are frequently seen in clinic and whether the pathogenic factor flourishes or not should be analysed according to clinical practice.

Clinical picture: Since a deficiency syndrome varies with different symptoms and signs of deficient yin, yang, *qi* and blood, its clinical signs are quite different and can hardly be generalized. They are commonly: pallor, withered yellow complexion, listlessness, mental fatigue, and general lassitude, palpitation and short breath, cold limbs and fever in the chest, palms and soles, perspiration and night sweat, incontinence of stools and urine, little or no tongue coating, empty pulse, etc.

Analysis of symptoms: A deficiency syndrome forms due to congenital deficiency and acquired malnourishment, mainly caused by improper diet, weakness of the acquired foundation; the "seven emotions," fatigue and lack of physical exercise, internal injury of the viscera, *qi* and blood, excess sexual activity, consumed primordial *qi* in the kidney, or prolonged illness and affected anti-pathogenic factor due to delayed or wrong treatment, etc.

As yang *qi* is too weak to carry on its warming, transporting and consolidating functions, pallor, cold limbs and trunk, mental fatigue and general lassitude, short breath and spontaneous sweating, incontinence of stools and urine result. As blood is too deficient to restrain yang and fails to perform its nourishing and moistening functions, hot palms and soles, irritability and palpitation, withered yellow complexion, night sweats, etc. may be seen. Since both *qi* and blood are deficient and the meridian cannot be enriched and blood circulation promoted, the pulse feels empty and forceless. Owing to deficient yang's failure to evaporate body fluids and consumed yin's failure to nourish the organs in the upper portion of the body, the tongue has little or no coating.

9-3-2 Excess syndromes

An excess syndrome has symptoms reflecting a violent pathogenic factor. In general, although it is caused by a preponderant pathogenic factor, the anti-pathogenic factor can still resist it and has not yet been impaired. Therefore, the excess syndrome usually exhibits a stage at which pathogenic and anti-pathogenic factors are struggling.

Clinical picture: As the characteristics and location of an excess syndrome vary, its clinical signs are entirely different. They are chiefly: fever, abdominal distension and pain aggravated by pressure, chest distress and restlessness, even mental confusion and delirium, coarse and asthmatic breath, profuse sputum and saliva, constipation, difficulty in urination, full forceful pulse, thick glossy coating of tongue, etc.

Analysis of symptoms: An excess syndrome is formed by the invasion of an exogenous pathogenic factor and visceral dysfunction and obstructed metabolism so that pathological products, such as *tan-yin* (phlegm and excess exudates), aqueous damp, stagnant blood, etc. are retained within the body.

As the pathogenic factor is violent, the anti-pathogenic factor vies with it and yang heat is in excess, fever occurs as the substantive pathogen disturbs the mind or mists the heart, and restlessness or even mental confusion results. Since the pathogenic factor blocks the lung, the lung fails to perform its dispersing and descending functions, causing chest distress, asthmatic breath and excess phlegm with a rattling throat. Since the substantial pathogen accumulates in the intestine and stomach and *qi* in the yang viscera is blocked, abdominal distension and pain aggravated by pressure and constipation appear. Because of internal retention of aqueous liquid and stagnation of *qi* activities, difficulty in urination may result. Since the blood is influenced by the struggle between the anti-pathogenic and pathogenic factors, the pulse is full and forceful. As pathogenic damp and turbid matter spread, a thick glossy tongue coating is frequently seen.

9-3-3 Relation between deficiency and excess syndromes

Deficiency and excess syndromes are quite different in the interconnection between the pathogenic and anti-pathogenic factors.

9-3-3-1 Intermingling between deficiency and excess

This denotes that there are pathological changes of deficient anti-pathogenic and pathogenic factors.

The symptoms of intermingling of deficiency and excess are: The main excess syndrome intermingled with the deficiency syndrome; the main deficiency syndrome intermingled with the excess one. For example, profuse sputum and saliva, asthmatic breath, cough and fullness in the chest intermingled with the deficiency syndrome of asthmatic breath aggravated by exertion, cold limbs and body, incontinence of urine, etc. The condition of deficiency and excess and whether an excess syndrome is the main one or not and which factor is the chief one, must be cleared up in clinic. Then, therapeutic principles, such as the major elimination, or the prior reinforcement and post elimination, or simultaneous elimination and reinforcement can be adopted in treatment.

9-3-3-2 Transformation of an excess syndrome into a deficient syndrome

An excess syndrome transforms into a deficient syndrome due to delayed or wrong treatment, etc., so that the duration of the illness is prolonged, and the anti-pathogenic factor is still impaired even though the pathogenic factor has been eliminated. For instance, the excess-heat syndrome of high fever, thirst, perspiration and large pulse causes consumed and impaired body fluids and *qi* due to improper treatment and prolonged duration of recovery, with emaciation, pallor, no appetite, general weakness and shortness of *qi*, little or no tongue coating, minute, weak pulse, etc., which indicates that the syndrome has transformed from an excess syndrome into a deficient one and the therapy should be changed accordingly and mainly tonification adopted.

9-3-3-3 Excess syndrome caused by deficiency syndrome

This denotes that in a deficient syndrome there are various excess symptoms due to a deficient anti-pathogenic factor, producing substantive pathogen. For example, splenic *qi* and pulmonary *qi* are so weak that they fail to carry on their digesting, dispersing and descending functions, resulting in such substantive pathogens as *tan-yin* (phlegm and excess exudates) or aqueous damp, etc. It is chiefly treated by tonifying splenic and pulmonary *qi*. Aqueous damp and *tan-yin* would disappear spontaneously when the lung resumes its dispersing and descending functions to full capacity and the spleen resumes its transforming and digesting functions.

9-3-3-4 The true and false deficiency and excess

When identifying syndromes, the true and false deficiency and excess syndromes should be carefully identified:

a. The true excess and false deficiency: The disease is originally an excess syndrome, with pathogenic heat retained in the intestine and stomach and blocking phlegm and food that obstruct the meridians and make *qi* and blood flow unsmoothly, with the signs of a deficiency syndrome, such as listlessness, cold limbs and trunk, deep slow pulse, etc. simultaneously seen. But, if the patient who has a sonorous voice and coarse breath is carefully examined, the forceful pulse is felt when pressed heavily even if it is deep and slow, which indicates that phlegm, food and heat stagnating internally are the true essence of the pathological change, but deficient signs are false. It is a true-excess and false-deficiency syndrome.

b. The true deficiency and false excess: A deficiency syndrome is characterized by insufficient and hypofunctional visceral *qi* and blood, resulting in abdominal fullness, distension and pain, stringy pulse, etc., which resembles an excess syndrome. But, abdominal fullness is sometimes relieved, and the abdominal pain is relieved by pressure and a stringy pulse is weak when pressed heavily. Judging from these conditions insufficient and hypofunctional *qi* and blood are the essence of the pathological change, but abdominal fullness and pain are false signs. It is a true-deficiency and false-excess syndrome.

The true excess and false deficiency is the "appearance of deficiency in extreme excess" and the true deficiency and false excess, is a "sign of excess in extreme deficiency." To identify true and false deficiency and excess syndromes the pulse, tongue and symptoms should be carefully examined to find the true nature of the pathological change.

9-3-4 Relation between deficiency and excess, exterior and interior, cold and heat

Deficiency and excess are often reflected by exterior and interior and cold and heat, forming a variety of symptoms. Those that are frequently seen in clinic are exterior-deficiency, exterior-excess, interior-deficiency (including the deficiency-cold and deficiency-heat), interior-excess (including the excess-cold and excess-heat), etc.

9-3-4-1 Exterior-excess and exterior-deficiency

a. An exterior-excess syndrome: A type of exterior syndrome with clinical characteristics of chills, no sweating, superficial taut pulse besides symptoms of the exterior-cold syndrome caused by the affection of exogenous pathogenic cold.

b. An exterior-deficiency syndrome: A variety of the exterior syndrome clinically characterized by sweating, aversion to wind, superficial slow pulse besides symptoms and signs of an exterior syndrome: the skin is loose, sweating and weak in defensive *qi* and easily affected by exogenous pathogenic factors because of weak spleen and lung *qi*. An exterior-excess syndrome should be treated with warm, pungent and mild diaphoretics and the exterior deficient syndrome should be treated by nourishing *qi* and relieving the exterior of the body (a diaphoretic therapy). Diaphoresis can relieve an exterior syndrome.

9-3-4-2 Deficiency-cold and excess-cold

A deficiency-cold syndrome formed by endogenous pathogenic cold produced by deficient yang within the body. An excess-cold syndrome is caused by the destruction of yang *qi* by excessive pathogenic cold.

9-3-4-3 Deficiency-heat and excess-heat

A deficiency-heat syndrome generally refers to fever caused by insufficient yin, yang, *qi* and blood, but is most frequently caused by deficient yin. The excess-heat syndrome results from extreme pathogenic heat.

Table for Identification of Excess-cold and Deficiency-cold Syndromes

	Clinical Picture	Pathogenesis	Treatment
Excess-cold	Aversion to cold and cold limbs, abdominal pain aggravated by pressure, constipation, profuse phlegm and asthmatic breath, white, thick and glossy tongue coating, deep, hidden, stringy, forceful pulse	Obstruction of yang *qi* due to excess pathogenic cold	Warmly unobstruct and dissipate pathogenic cold
Deficiency cold	Fear of cold and cold limbs, abdominal pain alleviated by pressure, low spirits and watery loose stools, clear profuse urine, shortage of *qi* and lassitude, minute or deep, slow and forceful pulse	Inability of deficient yang *qi* to warm the body	Warmly tonify yang *qi*

Table for Identification of Excess-heat and Deficiency-heat Syndromes

Symptoms	Clinical Picture	Pathogenesis	Treatment
Excess-heat	Strong fever and polydipsia, mental confusion and delirium, distension, full and painful abdomen aggravated by pressure, dark-red urine, dry stools, yellow tongue coating, full, rapid, slippery and substantive pulse	Excess pathogenic heat	Clear up pernicious heat and purge pernicious fire
Deficiency heat	Tidal fever, night sweat, emaciation, fever in the chest, palms and soles, dry mouth, dry throat, red tongue with less coating, minute rapid pulse	Consumption of yin fluid and internal generation of fever caused by deficiency	Replenish yin and clear up pernicious heat

9-4 Yin and yang

Yin and yang is the key principle among the eight guiding principles. In diagnosis, all diseases can be divided into two main aspects, yin and yang, according to the pathological features of symptoms. *Plain Questions* states, "One who is good at diagnosing a disease by inspecting the patient's complexion and feeling the patient's pulse first identifies yin and yang." Zhang Zhongjing, an eminent medical expert, classified febrile diseases into yin and yang syndromes with three yin and three yang characteristics as their general guiding principle. Zhang Jingyue of the Ming Dynasty (1368-1644) also stressed, "It is the key principle that yin and yang must be first examined whenever feeling the patient's pulse and planning treatment." Yin and yang occupy an important position in the identification of syndromes.

9-4-1 Yin and yang syndromes

9-4-1-1 Yin syndrome

It is called a yin syndrome when all the symptoms and signs possess the general feature of "yin," e.g., interior, cold and deficiency syndromes belong to the category of a yin syndrome.

Clinical picture: Dull complexion, listlessness, sensation of heavy body and rolling body in bed, cold trunk and limbs, general lassitude and weakness, low voice with fear, dyspepsia, tasteless mouth with no thirst, foul-smelling stools, profuse watery urine, light-coloured flabby and delicate tongue, deep, slow, weak or minute irregular pulse.

Analysis of symptoms: Listlessness, general lassitude and low voice with fear are signs of an interior-cold syndrome. A light-coloured, flabby and delicate tongue and a deep slow, faint weak, minute and irregular pulse are both caused by deficiency and cold.

9-4-1-2 Yang syndrome

It is called a yang syndrome when all the symptoms possess the general features of "yang," e.g., exterior, heat and excess syndromes pertain to a yang syndrome.

Clinical picture: Flushed face, fever, burning skin, mental anxiety, restlessness, coarse voice, rough breath, asthmatic breath and rattling throat, dry mouth and indulgence in drinking, constipation, or foul stools, dark-red scanty urine, dark-red tongue with dark yellowish coating and superficial, rapid, full, large slippery and substantive pulse.

Analysis of symptoms: A yang syndrome is a summary of exterior, excess and heat syndromes, characterized by the exterior syndrome with aversion to cold and fever seen simultaneously. Slightly flushed face, mental anxiety and restlessness, burning skin, dry mouth and indulgence in drinking are manifestations of a heat syndrome. Coarse voice, rough breath, asthmatic breath, constipation, etc. are manifestations of an excess syndrome. A dark-red tongue with a dark-yellowish thorny coating and a full, large, slippery and substantive pulse are both signs of an excess heat syndrome.

9-4-1-3 Identification of yin and yang syndromes

Yin and yang syndromes are compared according to the four diagnostic techniques as follows:

Table for Identification of Yin and Yang Syndromes

Four Diagnostic Techniques	Yin Syndrome	Yang Syndrome
Inspection	Pale or dull complexion, heavy and rolling body in bed, general lassitude, listlessness, with moist slippery coating	Flushed face, fever and preference for coolness, mania, dry lips, dark-red tongue, yellowish or yellow, even dry cleft or dark thorny coating
Auscultation-olfaction	Low voice, calmness and little speech, weak, perspiration with fear, short breath	Sonorous voice, rough breath, asthmatic breath, rattling throat, moodiness and crying

Inquiry	Foul stools, decreased appetite, listlessness, no polydipsia, or preference for hot drinks, profuse thin or scanty urine	Hard stools or constipation, or extremely foul stools, anorexia, dry mouth, polydipsia, with desire for drinking, dark red scanty urine
Palpation	Abdominal pain relieved by pressure, cold body and feet, deep, faint, minute, irregular, slow, weak and forceless pulse	Abdominal pain aggravated by pressure, fever and warm feet, a superficial, full, rapid, large, slippery and forceful pulse

The balance of yin and yang is relative. Excess yang leads to deficient yin and vice versa. The treatment is to balance them. For instance, if a full large pulse and a red tongue with dry coating accompanied by thirst, strong fever, etc. are diagnosed, the flourishing yang and declining yin may be treated by restraining the yang and replenishing the yin; if a deep slow pulse and a white tongue with moist coating accompanied by abdominal pain, diarrhea, etc. are diagnosed, it means flourishing yin and declining yang and may be treated by warming the yang and restraining the yin. However, in certain diseases only yin is deficient, but yang is not excessive or only yang is excessive, but yin is not deficient. In this case, the yin and yang can also be balanced only by treating the deficient yin or excess yang. Take a tidal fever as an example. If the symptoms of a minute, rapid and weak pulse and a red tongue with little or no coating accompanied by malar flush and red lips, fever in the chest, palms and soles, cough, night sweats, etc. are diagnosed, it is a tidal fever due to deficient yin and may be treated by replenishing the yin (that is restrain yang); if a deep forceful pulse with a yellow, dry and thorny coating accompanied by anxiety and asthmatic breath, constipation, delirium, mania, etc. are observed, it indicates a tidal fever due to excessive yang and may be treated by replenishing the yin (i.e., to preserve the yin).

9-4-2 Insufficiencies of true yin and yang

Insufficiencies of true yin and yang are insufficiencies of kidney yin and kidney yang. Since the kidneys are the congenital foundation, whether yin and yang are sufficient or not is determined by the patient's constitution. Insufficient congenital endowment leads to comparative weakness of the kidney yin and yang and because of different conditions of the invasion of disease insufficient yin or yang may result.

Insufficiency of true yin: Frequently blazing fire due to deficiency, pallor and malar flush, red lips, dry mouth, dry red tongue with no coating, dry throat, anxiety, dizziness, blurred vision, tinnitus, sore and weak loins and legs, "steaming of bones," night sweat, nightmares and spermatorrhea, anuria and constipation, hot palms and soles and rapid forceless pulse, etc. may be seen.

Insufficiency of true yang: Pallor, light-coloured lips and tongue, normal taste, anorexia, enlarged abdomen and asthmatic breath, cough, puffiness, spontaneous sweating, vertigo, anorexia, enlarged abdomen and swollen legs, cold muscles and loose stools, or diarrhea before dawn, impotence and cold semen, atrophic and weak feet, large weak pulse, etc.

The pulse indications and symptoms of insufficiencies of true yin and yang have been mentioned above. Shen Jinao, a famous medical expert, stressed their pulse indications and supplemented their treatment. He said, "Both deficient yin and yang are ascribed to the kidney. Yang deficiency is caused by deficiency of true yang in the kidney. It is deficient fire when the pulse at the *chi* section of the right hand is weak, and it is advisable to tonify true yin (kidney yin), but not to attack yang *qi*. Yin deficiency is caused by deficiency of true yin in the kidney. If there is deficient kidney water and the pulse is minute and faint, it is advisable to tonify true yin but not to injure yang *qi*."

Table for Identification of Depletion of Yin and Yang

	Sweats	Four Limbs	Tongue	Pulse	Others
Depletion of Yin	Hot and salty	Warm	Red	Full, substantive or hasty, forceless by press	Hot skin, rough breath, thirst, indulgence in cold drinks
Depletion of Yang	Cold and tasteless	Cold	White and moist	Superficial, rapid and vacant, or minute faint	Cold skin, faint breath, no thirst, indulgence in hot drinks

9-4-3 Depletion of yin and yang

Depletion of yin and yang is a critical sign of disease. If they are wrongly identified or the treatment is somewhat delayed, death would result. Depletion usually occurs when there is a high fever and hyperhidrosis or vomiting and diarrhea, and severe blood loss, particularly hyperhidrosis. Sweat is yin fluid, and so is blood. Hyperhidrosis and hemorrhea would lead to depletion of yin fluid together with blood and sweat. Since yin and yang are interdependent and yang *qi* usually spreads due to consumed blood, hyperhidrosis and hemorrhoea would lead to depletion of yin fluids together with blood and sweat. Since yin and yang are interdependent and yang *qi* usually spreads due to consumed yin fluids, yang *qi* spreads in the case of depletion of yin, and yin fluids are impaired in the case of depletion of yang.

In his *Treatise on Depletion of Yin and Yang,* Xu Lingtai stated how to distinguish the depletion of yin from that of yang. In the case of hyperhidrosis due to depletion of yin, there is aversion to heat, hot hands and feet, hot skin and muscles, hot and salty sweating, thirst and indulgence in cool drinks, rough breath, deep substantive pulse. In the case of hyperhidrosis due to the depletion of yang, there is aversion to cold, cold hands and feet, cold skin, cold, tasteless and slightly mucoid sweat, no thirst and indulgence in hot drinks, superficial, rapid and empty pulse.

To sum up, the ebb and flow of yin and yang are relative. In the case of the depletion of yin, a series of hot signs occur because deficient yin leads to excessive yang, but it pertains to a deficiency syndrome, so the pulse is weak, although it seems to be full, substantive, restless and heavy. In the case of the depletion of yang, a series of cold signs appear because declining yang leads to cold, and as deficient yang spreads outward, the pulse feels superficial, rapid and empty, even minute and faint. With depleted yin, the tongue is red and dry, with depleted yang, it is white and moist.

Notes

[1.] The four stages of a febrile disease.
[2. 3.] Cold limbs due to excessive pathogenic heat which impairs tissue fluid and interferes with the circulation of yang *qi* to the limbs.

10. IDENTIFICATION OF SYNDROMES ACCORDING TO *ZANG-FU* (VISCERA)

Identification of syndromes according to *zang-fu* (viscera) is to analyse and identify symptoms of disease. *Zheng* differs from the symptoms, but is a pathological generalization of the cause, location and characteristics of disease at a certain stage and balance between pathogenic and anti-pathogenic factors after an analysis of various symptoms. Identification of syndromes is the analysis of clinical data, obtained through the four techniques of diagnosis and then the interrelation of various pathological changes are differentiated according to basic theories, such as the *zang-fu* (visceral) theory, meridian theory, etiology and pathology, etc. in order to make a diagnosis.

Bianzheng and *lunzhi* (planning treatment according to diagnosis) are a key link in the clinical application of the theories and general rules of treatment. *Bianzheng* is recognizing disease and *lunzhi* is the therapeutic method adopted according to diseases or syndromes. *Bianzheng* is the premise and reason that decide the treatment, while therapeutic effects are the standard to identify whether the identification of the syndrome was correct or not. The identification of syndromes according to the eight guiding principles is mainly used for miscellaneous diseases and is also the basis for other identifications; the identifications of syndromes according to the meridians, according to *wei* (defence), *qi* (vital energy), *ying* (nutrition) and *xue* (blood) phases and according to the triple energizer are chiefly applied in exogenous febrile diseases. The identification of syndromes according to *qi*, blood and body fluids is closely related to the identification of syndromes according to viscera and they supplement each other.

10-1 Identification of syndromes according to etiology

The cause of disease varies. It can be caused by the six excesses, seven emotions, fatigue, lack of physical exercise and external injuries. There is no symptom without reason. A symptom is a pathological reaction of the patient affected by a pathogenic factor. Identification of syndromes according to etiology means that pathological reactions (symptoms) of the patient are analysed and the disease is determined according to pathogenic characteristics of various causes of disease for the purpose of treatment.

10-1-1 Identification of syndromes according to the "six excesses" and pestilential factor

The six excesses and pestilential factors are the causes of exogenous disease. The six excesses include pathogenic wind, cold, summer-heat, damp, dryness and fire (intense heat). The pestilential factor is a highly-infectious pathogenic factor.

10-1-1-1 Symptoms of pathogenic wind

Wind is the primary pathogenic factor for hundreds of diseases. It is light, easily moving, changeable and invades the body rapidly.

Clinical picture: Fever and aversion to wind, headache, perspiration, cough, stuffy nose and nasal discharge, thin white tongue coating and superficial and slow pulse. Or numbness of the trunk and body, stiffness, spasm and convulsions of the four extremities, opisthotonos and itchy skin.

Analysis of the symptoms: As exogenous pathogenic wind attacks the body surface and injures the defensive *qi* of the body and the junction between the skin and muscle becomes loose and defensive *qi* weak, fever and aversion to wind, headache and perspiration result. Exogenous pathogenic wind is likely to invade the upper part of the body. If it invades the lung, *qi* will fail to perform its dissipating function. Since the trachea, throat and nose all belong to the "pulmonary connection"[125] cough, stuffy nose and nasal discharge appear. A superficial slow pulse and thin white tongue coating are symptoms caused by invasion of the lung by exogenous pathogenic wind. The invasion of the body surface by exogenous pathogenic wind leads to numbness. If it invades the meridians, stiffness, spasm, convulsions and opisthotonos may result. Stasis of exogenous wind in the skin arouses an intolerable itch.

10-1-1-2 Symptoms of pathogenic cold

Cold is a yin pathogen and is clear, cold, stagnant and contracting in nature. It is likely to injure yang *qi* and obstruct the circulation of *qi* and blood.

Clinical picture: Creeping chills and fever, anhidrosis, headache, general ache, cough and asthmatic breath, white thin tongue coating and superficial taut pulse, or rigid hands and feet, cold clammy extremities and faint pulse, or abdominal pain and borborygmi, diarrhea, vomiting, etc.

Analysis of symptoms: As exogenous pathogenic cold invades the exterior of the body, the pores are obstructed, the defensive *qi* fails to spread so fever and creeping chills and anhidrosis result. Congealed exogenous cold in the meridian leads to headache and general ache. Since the lung is concerned with skin and hair which influence the lung when they are affected, and lung *qi* fails to spread, cough and asthmatic breath and stuffy nose result. A superficial taut pulse and white thin tongue coating are the signs that exogenous cold has invaded the exterior of the body. If exogenous cold stagnates in the meridian, yang *qi* can be impaired and the *qi* mechanism is obstructed, and rigid hands and feet may appear. When exogenous cold stagnates and yang *qi* fails to reach the four extremities, cold clammy extremities occur. When stagnant cold cools *qi* and tendons and vessels contract, a faint pulse appears. If cold directly attacks the interior of the body, it impairs spleen and stomach yang in performing their transporting and digesting functions, and abdominal pain, borborygmi, vomiting and diarrhea may result.

10-1-1-3 Symptoms of exogenous pathogenic summer-heat

Summer-heat is hot, ascending and spreading. Hot signs will be seen if it produces disease. Pathogenic summer-heat is most likely to consume body fluids and is often associated with pathogenic damp which causes disease.

Clinical picture: Injury due to pathogenic summer-heat, aversion to heat, perspiration, thirst, fatigue, yellow urine, red tongue, white or yellow tongue coating, and empty rapid pulse. Heatstroke, fever, sudden fainting, persistent sweating, thirst, hasty breath, even coma and epileptiform convulsion, dark-red tongue and soft, weak and rapid pulse.

Analysis of symptoms: Injury due to pathogenic summer-heat is caused by the affection of pathogenic summer-heat and damp, hyperhidrosis and consumed body fluids and *qi*. Consumption of body fluids by summer-heat leads to aversion to heat, hyperhidrosis, thirst, and yellow urine. As *qi* is excreted together with sweat in a summer-heat disease, fatigue and empty rapid pulse appear. As pathogenic summer-heat is associated with pathogenic damp that spreads over the upper energizer, a white or yellow tongue coating results. Heatstroke is due to prolonged labour in the sun in summer so that the blazing summer-heat upwardly disturbs the sense organs and inwardly affects the Spirit, resulting in sudden fainting. As *qi* and body fluids are consumed by pathogenic summer-heat, fever, thirst, perspiration and hasty breath appear. If pathogenic summer-heat mists the sense organs in association with pathogenic damp and inwardly sinks to the pericardium, mental convulsions will result. If it consumes body fluids and *qi* so that liver wind moves internally and yang *qi* fails to reach the limbs, epileptiform convulsion will occur. When nutritional yin is consumed by violent pathogenic summer-heat, a dark-red dry tongue and soft, weak and rapid pulse result.

10-1-1-4 Symptoms of pathogenic damp

Damp is heavy, lingering, mucoid and congealed. Pathological change caused by damp is often lingering and stubborn and is not easily cured.

Clinical picture: Distension and pain in the head, chest distress, no thirst, sensation of heaviness and pain in the body, fever and bodily fatigue, clear profuse urine, white slippery tongue coating, soft, weak and slow pulse appear. If the body is affected by pathogenic damp, there is an excruciating pain as if the head is tightly bandaged, general discomfort, lassitude of the limbs and soft weak pulse will result. When pathogenic damp injures the joint, soreness and sensation of painful and heavy joints that fail to flex and extend freely occur.

Analysis of symptoms: When pathogenic damp invades the body, it is most likely to injure the skin, muscles, tendons and bones. Damp injury can cause distension of the head, chest distress and soft, weak and slow pulse.

Pathogenic affection is usually caused by mountainous plague of the steaming of damp after cloudy and rainy weather becomes sunny. An excruciating pain as if the head is tightly bandaged may appear. Damp is a turbid pathogenic factor in the earth, but the head is the sea of all yang, higher in position, clear in its *qi* and weak in substance. As clear yang *qi* gathers to the head, distension and pain, as if the head were tightly bandaged is a typical damp disease. Since pathogenic damp has invaded the joints and *qi* and blood are blocked, a sensation of bodily heaviness results, called damp *bi* (blockage) syndrome[126] in clinic.

10-1-1-5 Symptoms of pathogenic dryness

Pathogenic dryness can consume body fluids and is classified into cool-dry[127] and warm-dry.[128]

Clinical picture: In cool-dryness, slight headache, creeping chills, anhidrosis, cough, itchy throat, stuffy nose, white dry tongue and superficial pulse occur; in warm-dryness, fever with sweating, thirst, dry throat, cough and chest pain, even bloody sputum, and dry nose when expiring, a dry tongue with yellow tongue coating and superficial rapid pulse occur.

Analysis of symptoms: Cool-dryness occurs when the weather becomes cool in late autumn. The weather is cold and dry and exogenous pathogenic cold and dryness invade the protecting lungs. It is manifested by slight headache, creeping chills in association with symptoms and signs of a dry tongue, and superficial pulse, etc. Warm-dryness occurs when the weather is still hot in early autumn, and summer-heat has not yet disappeared.

Pathogenic dryness and heat invade the protecting lung and consume body fluids, resulting in fever with perspiration, thirst, and dry throat. If they injure the lung, cough and dry nose may occur; if pathogenic dryness injures the collateral meridians of the lung, and transforms body fluids into phlegm, blood sputum may appear.

10-1-1-6 Symptoms of pathogenic fire

As both fire (intense heat) and heat belong to the same classification, and are signs of excess yang, they are often mistaken for one another. In general, heat is milder than fire. Pathogenic warmth and heat have the same nature, but fire is intense heat, while warmth is mild heat. Since pathogenic warmth is also the cause of exogenous pathogenic disease, it is often mentioned together with pathogenic heat. To sum up, as pathogenic fire, heat and warmth are scorching and rapid and consume body fluids, they may frequently make tendons and vessels dry, exogenous pathogenic wind move, and blood extravasate.

Clinical picture: Strong fever, thirst, flushed face, restlessness, delirium, epistaxis, hemoptysis, maculopapule or mania, purulent carbuncle, dark-red tongue and a rapid or minute pulse.

10-1-1-7 Symptoms of epidemic pestilential diseases

An epidemic pestilential disease is caused by infection of a pestilential factor.

a. Symptoms of pestilential disease are caused by the affection of pestilential factor and characterized by rapid onset, a serious condition and infection.

Clinical picture: At the initial stage, creeping chills are followed by fever and then fever without creeping chills occurs. During the second or third day of the initial stage, the pulse is not superficial and deep, but rapid, with headache, pain in the body and fever occurring day and night. The fever is higher in the daytime, and the tongue coating is white.

Analysis of symptoms: As the pathogenic factor is situated between the exterior and interior of the body, and influences the *wei* (defence) phase outwardly, chills, fever and bodily pain, etc. occur. When the pestilential factor is turbid and stagnant, the tongue coating is white. When occurring it is similar to external symptoms and signs of the *taiyang* and *yangming* diseases caused by cold injury. Yet, headache in *yangming* disease is not so excruciating as in pestilential disease. In cold injury there is no sweating, whereas in this case sweating can be seen on the upper part of the body, particularly at the head because the head is where all the yang meridians gather. Fire is flaring up in nature, toxic fire is entrenched internally, the "five fluids"[129] are consumed and hot *qi* spreading upward makes the head perspire profusely. Thus, attention should be paid to differentiate perspiration although headache is the same.

b. Disease and symptoms of epidemic infectious rashes are caused by the affection of epidemic noxious disease and heat.

Clinical picture: At the initial stage, there is high fever, excruciating headache, red or dark-red, or purple or black maculopapule and rapid pulse. It is "depressed pestilence" if a minute, rapid, deep and hidden pulse, dull complexion, coma, cold clammy extremities, profuse sweating at the head, excruciating headache, twitching intestine with desire for vomiting and diarrhea, and shaking head appear.

Analysis of symptoms: Toxic pestilential factor invades the lung and stomach via the skin or mouth and nose. All the meridians meet at the lung and the stomach is the sea of the twelve meridians. Both of them can nourish tissues and organs via the meridian. The pestilential factor invades the meridian, affects the tissues and organs, resulting in fever, headache, and maculopapule. A rapid pulse in pestilential rashes is a sign of stagnant, steaming and toxic heat. The type with a superficial, large and rapid pulse is ascribed to a drastic toxic factor; that with a deep, minute and rapid pulse implies that the toxic factor has already entered the deep body. A rapid pulse signifies toxic heat is trapped in the area between the exterior and interior of the body. "Depressed pestilence" with a minute, rapid, deep and hidden pulse at the initial stage is caused by the inability of the deep-rooted toxic pulse to spread outwardly.

c. Infectious jaundice is caused by the epidemic noxious factor associated with pathogenic damp and heat.

Clinical picture: At the early stage, fever and aversion to cold, sudden jaundice of the entire body, teeth and sclera, which is called acute jaundice, appear. In severe cases varieties of complications of cold clammy extremities or mental disturbance and delirium, or straight fixation of the eye, or enuresis, even rolling tongue and withdrawing scrotum and carphologia result.

Analysis of symptoms: Both infectious jaundice and infectious "toxin" are associated with pathogenic damp-heat. If the damp-heat congeals between the skin and muscle, chills and fever and sudden jaundice will occur; if pestilential "toxin" affects the five yin viscera and makes yin and yang dissociate, cold clammy extremities may result; if it inwardly disturbs the heart (mind), mental disturbance and delirium may appear; if it upwardly affects the "cerebral connection"[130] and mists the sense organs, straight fixation of the eye may appear; if it invades the liver and kidney, the lower energizer is weakened and enuresis and withdrawing scrotum appear; if the vital principle of the *shaoyin* meridian is exhausted, a rolling tongue and carphologia may appear. All of these are serious signs that the infectious "toxin" is imprisoned in the five yin viscera and the vital principle is exhausted.

10-1-2 Symptoms of the "seven emotions"

The "seven emotions" refer to joy, anger, anxiety, worry, grief, apprehension and fright. They can cause miscellaneous diseases of internal injury. Because of different environmental stimuli, emotions change and become excited or restrained, so that the five yin viscera may be injured resulting in disease. The pathogenesis of the seven emotions is chiefly manifest in changes of yin and yang, *qi* and blood, e.g., overjoy injures yang, overanger injures yin, depressed *qi* produces pernicious fire, regurgitating *qi* results in the aberration of blood and then directly injures the five yin viscera, manifested by the symptoms of the five yin viscera.

Clinical picture: Injury by overjoy leads to mental restlessness or incoherent speech and an abnormal manner. Injury by overanger leads to regurgitation of liver *qi*, and in severe cases, blood stagnation in the upper part of the body, leading to mental disturbance and sudden *jue* (fainting) syndrome. Injury by anxiety leads to emotional depression, mental fatigue and lassitude and poor appetite; injury by worry leads to somnolence; palpitation of a vigorous heart, disturbed sleep and emaciation; injury by grief leads to pallor and lack of Spirit; injury by apprehension leads to palpitation, desire to be alone and fear; injury by fright leads to abnormal speech and manner.

Analysis of symptoms: Overjoy can injure the heart and induce sluggish *qi*, even incoherent speech, etc. Extreme anger can injure the liver, and rage causes regurgitation of *qi* and aberration of blood, even rapid *jue* (fainting) syndrome due to the blood congealing in the upper part of the body. Excessive anxiety can injure the lung and spleen because the person with anxiety has obstructed *qi*, depressed mood and poor appetite. Excessive worry can injure the spleen and cause palpitation of a vigorous heart, somnolence, insomnia and emaciation. Grief can injure the lung and cause *qi* to disappear with pallor seen. Excessive apprehension can injure the kidney and result in deficient kidney *qi*, manifested as palpitation with fright and fear to be captured. Excessive fright can cause disorder of *qi* which can disturb the heart (mind) and cause emotional restlessness, even mental disorder. Since the symptoms of the seven emotions are closely related to those of internal injuries, they must be distinguished in association with *zang-fu* (viscera), *qi* and blood.

10-1-3 Injuries due to improper diet, fatigue and lack of physical exercise and excessive sexual activity

Injuries due to improper diet, overfatigue, lack of physical exercise and excessive sexual activity can be determined by examination and their syndromes may also be distinguished according to specific clinical symptoms.

10-1-3-1 Injury due to improper diet

Clinical picture: Stomachache due to injury of the stomach by improper diet, aversion to smelly food, poor appetite, fullness and distension of the chest, acid regurgitation, emaciation, thick glossy tongue coating and slippery forceful pulse. Abdominal pain and diarrhea may appear if the intestine is injured by food. In common injury due to improper diet, a slippery rapid or deep substantive pulse and thick glossy or yellow tongue coating are seen. If poisonous food is taken, vomiting, nausea or alternate vomiting and diarrhea and colical pain in the abdomen may result.

Analysis of symptoms: The diet is the source of nutrients. If one eats too much food, the spleen and stomach might fail to perform their transporting and digesting functions, and the symptoms of injury due to improper diet may form. The stomach receives and carries food downward. If the diet injures the stomach and stomach *qi* fails to descend, so that it cannot receive food, stomachache, fullness and distension of the chest, etc. may appear. If the small intestine fails to receive food and the large intestine fails to carry on its transmitting function, food can accumulate and stagnate, and abdominal pain and diarrhea may occur. As food stagnates internally, pulse *qi* is constrained and a rapid slippery or deep substantive pulse may be seen. Since stagnant food and turbid *qi* have not yet been processed, a thick glossy tongue coating or ozostomia may result. Poisonous food injuries the stomach and intestine and disturbs the *qi* mechanism, leading to alternate vomiting and diarrhea.

10-1-3-2 Injuries from fatigue and lack of physical exercise

Clinical picture: Fatigue leads to general lassitude, preference for lying down, disinclination to talk, poor appetite and slow large, superficial or minute pulse. Lack of physical exercise leads to puffiness, asthmatic breath and thirst after exertion, palpitation and shortness of breath and weak limbs.

Analysis of symptoms: Both fatigue and lack of physical exercise cause disease because then *qi* and blood, tendons bones and muscles fail to carry on their normal physiological functions and produce pathological problems.

Fatigue leads to impaired primordial *qi*, resulting in mental dullness, lassitude and preference for lying down; an easy and comfortable life leads to *qi* stasis and the unsmooth circulation of blood leads to palpitation, asthmatic breath and thirst after exertion, etc. Injuries from fatigue and lack of physical exercise must be distinguished, e.g., prolonged lying injures *qi*, prolonged sitting injures muscles, prolonged standing injures bones, prolonged walking injures tendons, and hyperhidrosis by overexertion consumes body fluids and *qi*. Aging and overworked lungs damage *qi*; an overworked heart damages the Spirit; an overworked spleen damages digestion; an overworked liver damages blood; an overworked kidney consumes *jing* (vital principle) etc. All of these must be carefully distinguished.

10-1-3-3 Injury from excessive sexual activity

Clinical picture: Deficient yin, cough and hemoptysis, "steaming of bone"[131] and tidal fever, palpitation and night sweat; deficient yang, impotence and prospermia, cold hands and limbs, lumbago and weak legs, night emission and spermatorrhea.

Analysis of symptoms: Excessive sexual activity and consumed *jing* are likely to cause a deficiency syndrome. Since the acquired vital principle is the foundation of life after birth, the sufficient vital principle produces high Spirit, whereas the deficient one makes *qi* deficient. Deficient yin *qi* can lead to excessive yang, which consumes yin, resulting in blazing fire and phlegm accumulation which causes cough and hemoptysis, "steaming of bone" and tidal fever, etc. Deficient yang *qi* leads to night emission and spermatorrhea and fails to nourish tendons and vessels. Impotence, weak loin and bones, cold hands and feet will appear in this condition. To sum up, injury from excessive sexual activity must be distinguished from the patient's constitution, severity of injury and other accompanying symptoms.

10-1-4 External injuries

External injuries refer to local symptoms and the reaction of the whole body caused by trauma, such as wounds, injuries from falls, fractures, sprains and strains, animal bite and poisonous insect stings.

10-1-4-1 Incised wound

This refers to the trauma caused by injury to the body by sharp metal instruments. A stab wound caused by a sharp metal instrument can become infected, suppurative and ulcerated.

Clinical picture: Local rupture and hemorrhage, pain, congestion and swelling; if the tendons are injured and bones fractured with persistent bleeding, the pain will be excruciating. Signs of collapse, such as pallor, dizziness, dull vision, etc. are caused by hemorrhoea. The invasion of the affected area by pathogenic wind and toxic factors are manifested in chills and fever, muscular twitching, lockjaw, paroxysmal convulsions of tendons and muscles, opisthotonos, profuse phlegm and saliva, etc. which are ascribed to tetanus.

Analysis of symptoms: Hemorrhage is caused by local injury by sharp metal instruments which results in the rupture of the skin, muscles and vessels, and injury of the vessel leads to extravasation of blood. As the vessel is broken, the *qi* in it is affected, particularly if *qi* and blood congeal outward the vessel, a local pain, congestion and swelling occur. Injury of tendons, fracture and injury of the vessels lead to extravasation of *qi* and persistent bleeding. Hence, the pain is excruciating. In severe cases, hemorrhea and exhausted *qi* together with blood usually cause collapse. When pathogenic wind and toxic factors invade the meridian via the local wound, causing tetanus, the pathogenic factors first lie in the superficial part of the body, resulting in chills and fever and muscular twitching. When they invade the area between the exterior and interior of the body, lockjaw, convulsions of tendons and muscle, and opisthotonos result.

10-1-4-2 Insect or animal bites

Clinical picture: In mild cases, there is local congestion, swelling, pain and numbness or rashes. In severe cases, numbness or severe pain in the limb, dizziness and chest distress may appear. There is also ecchymosis and bleeding. If a person is bitten by a mad dog, hydrophobia, photophobia, phonophobia, etc. may appear.

10-1-4-3 Injuries from falls, fractures, sprains and strains

Clinical picture: Pain, swelling and distension, injured tendons, skin rupture, hemorrhage, fracture, etc. usually occur at the wound; falling from a high place may lead to hemoptysis and bloody stool; if the bone and brain are injured, dizziness, upward fixation of the eye, aphasia, even fainting, etc. may result.

Analysis of symptoms: Injuries from falls, fractures, sprains and strains cause congealed *qi* and blood in the meridian and thus can lead to pain, swelling and distension around the wound. The rupture of skin and muscle, injury of the meridian and hemorrhage, injury of tendons, fracture, bleeding joint and obstructed blood circulation due to swelling *qi* can cause distension, pain, congestion and swelling around the wound. If the internal organ is injured due to falling from a high place, hemoptysis and bloody stool will result. If the brain is injured due to a concussion to the skull which is the residence of primordial Spirit and injury to the brain, the primordial Spirit can lose its dwelling place and ominous signs such as upward fixation of the eye, aphasia, fainting, etc. will appear.

10-2 Identification of syndromes according to *qi*, blood and body fluids

Identification of syndromes according to *qi*, blood and body fluids includes analysis of pathological changes of *qi*, blood and body fluids and differentiation of their symptoms.

Qi, blood and body fluids are not only the basis for the functions of the viscera, but also products of these activities. Therefore, pathological changes of the viscera may influence those of *qi*, blood and body fluids while pathological changes of *qi*, blood and body fluids will affect certain viscera. Hence, pathological changes of *qi*, blood and body fluids are closely related with *zang-fu* (viscera).

10-2-1 Identification of *qi* disorder

Varieties of pathological changes of *qi* are *qi* deficiency, trapped *qi*, *qi* stasis and *qi* regurgitation.

10-2-1-1 *Qi* deficiency syndrome

They are symptoms of visceral hypofunction.

Clinical picture: Dizziness and blurred vision, shortage of *qi* and indolent disinclination to talk, fatigue and general lassitude, spontaneous sweating aggravated after exertion, tasteless tongue and weak pulse.

Analysis of symptoms: Prolonged illness, weak constitution because of senility and improper diet, etc., shortage of *qi*, indolent disinclination to talk, fatigue and general lassitude are caused by insufficient primordial *qi* and hypofunctional viscera. Inability of deficient *qi* to nourish the upper portion of the body leads to dizziness and blurred vision, weak defensive *qi* fails to perform its function of protecting the body surface, and spontaneous sweating results. As exertion consumes *qi*, the above-mentioned symptoms are aggravated by exertion. A light-coloured tongue appears since nutritional *qi* is too weak to ascend to reach the tongue. A lack of motive force to promote blood circulation causes an emptying weak pulse.

Treatment: Tonify *qi* with prescription, such as the Decoction of Four Noble Ingredients.[1]

10-2-1-2 Trapped *qi* syndrome

Trapped *qi* stands for a variety of pathological changes of *qi* deficiency, chiefly characterized by failure of *qi* to ascend.

Clinical picture: Dizziness and blurred vision, shortage of *qi* accompanied by lassitude, sensation of dropping and distending abdomen, rectal prolapse or prolapse of uterus, pale tongue with white coating and weak pulse.

Analysis of symptoms: Shortage of *qi* and lassitude result from *qi* deficiency. Hypofunction, dizziness and vertigo are caused by the failure of clear yang *qi* to rise. Trapped *qi* leads to the viscera's failure to hold them up, with a dropping and distending abdomen, visceroptosis as prolapse of rectum, prolapse of uterus or gastroptosis, etc.

Treatment: Nourish *qi* and hold up the viscera with prescriptions, such as Gastrosplenic *Qi* Reinforcing Decoction.[2]

10-2-1-3 *Qi* stasis syndrome

This refers to the symptoms of *qi* blockage of a certain portion of the body or a certain viscus.

Clinical picture: Local fullness, distension and pain are caused by abnormal emotions, improper diet, external affection or overexertion, sprains and strains, etc. Local fullness, distension and pain are caused by an obstructed *qi* mechanism. The distension and pain are sometimes severe, but sometimes mild, often indefinite in location and pain is relieved after eructation or passing gas and always related to an emotional factor.

Treatment: Promote *qi* circulation with prescriptions, such as Decoction of Five Grand Ingredients,[3] Powder of *Fructus Meliae Toosendan*.[4]

10-2-1-4 *Qi* regurgitation syndrome

This refers to the abnormally ascending and descending *qi* and *qi* regurgitation. It generally refers to regurgitation of pulmonary and gastric *qi* and regurgitation of liver *qi* caused by the excessively-flourishing growth of liver *qi*.

Clinical picture: Chiefly characterized by cough and asthmatic breath. In regurgitation of gastric *qi*, hiccup, eructation, nausea and vomiting can be seen. Excess liver *qi* can lead to headache, vertigo, fainting, hematemesis, etc.

Analysis of symptoms: The regurgitation of lung *qi* is caused by the affection of an exogenous pathogenic factor or stagnation of phlegm and the turbid matter, so that lung *qi* cannot be purified and sent downward, with cough and asthmatic breath appearing. A cold affection to the stomach and accumulating excess fluid or blocked *qi* mechanism by phlegm and food or the invasion of exogenous pathogenic factor to the stomach may cause the regurgitation of stomach *qi*, with hiccup, eructation, vomiting, acid regurgitation, etc. The injury to the liver by depressed anger and excess liver *qi* and regurgitation of *qi* fire can lead to headache, vertigo, fainting and even hematemesis.

Treatment: Check regurgitating *qi* with prescriptions, such as Decoction of *Perilla fructescens*[5] and Decoction of *Inula japonica* and *Inula* and *Haematitum*.[6]

10-2-2 Identification of blood disease

Blood disease or syndrome varies greatly and can be generalized as deficient blood, congealed blood and hot blood.

10-2-2-1 Blood deficiency syndrome

Symptoms caused by insufficient blood's failure to nourish *zang-fu* (viscera) and meridians.

Clinical picture: Pale or withered-yellow complexion, light-coloured lips, dizziness and blurred vision, palpitations and insomnia, numb hands and feet, scanty menstruation and irregularity of menstrual cycle or amenorrhea, light-coloured tongue and minute forceful pulse.

Analysis of symptoms: Pathological changes of deficient blood are frequently caused by hemorrhoea or the weak spleen and stomach, excess of "seven emotions" and persistent consumption of yin blood, etc. As deficient blood fails to nourish the head, eyes and face, dizziness and blurred vision, pale or yellow complexion and light-coloured lips may appear. Inability of blood to nourish the heart leads to palpitations and insomnia. Malnourishment of the meridian leads to numb hands and feet. Since the "sea of blood" is empty, the tongue is not nourished by blood, it becomes light-coloured. Since the meridian (vessel) is not enriched with blood, the pulse is minute and forceless.

Treatment: Tonify blood with the prescriptions, such as Four-ingredient Decoction.[7]

10-2-2-2 Blood stagnation syndrome

It is called extravasating blood when blood stagnates at a certain area or accumulates in the meridian or an organ due to its unsmooth circulation. The disease or syndrome caused by stagnant blood is blood stagnation syndrome. It pertains to an excess syndrome because the pathogenic factor is substantive and generally treated by promoting blood circulation and dispersing congealed blood. It can also be divided into different types.

a. Blood stagnation syndrome associated with *qi* deficiency

Clinical picture: General weakness and lassitude, shortage of *qi* and spontaneous sweating, pain aggravated by pressure, dull tongue or dull tongue with ecchymosis, etc.

Analysis of symptoms: Because of the inability of weak *qi* to promote blood circulation, blood circulates unsmoothly, with symptoms of stagnant blood, such as dark-purplish tongue or tongue with ecchymosis and symptoms of *qi* deficiency, such as general lassitude, shortage of *qi* and spontaneous sweating, etc.

Treatment: Tonify *qi* and promote blood circulation with prescriptions, such as Decoction of Tonifying Yang and Promoting Blood Circulation.[8]

b. Blood stasis syndrome with blood deficiency

Clinical picture: Dizziness and blurred vision, palpitation and insomnia, light-coloured tongue with ecchymosis, minute irregular pulse or painful masses aggravated by pressure at a definite site.

Analysis of symptoms: Because of the obstruction of congealed blood and lack of new blood, the blood is deficient; blood deficiency is associated with blood stasis due to other causes; the accumulation and stagnation of the extravasating blood within the vessel after a variety of hemorrhages are the causes of blood stasis syndrome with blood deficiency frequently seen in clinic. As deficient blood cannot enrich and nourish the whole body, vertigo, palpitation and insomnia, light-coloured tongue and minute pulse result. Ecchymosis on the tongue, irregular pulse or masses with pain aggravated by pressure, and immobility are caused by obstructed blood circulation.

Treatment: Nourish and promote blood circulation with prescriptions, such as Four-ingredient Decoction with *Persia Davidim* and *Carthamus Tinctorius*.[9]

c. The syndrome of blood affected by pathogenic cold: It is also called the blood-cold syndrome. Its main manifestations are stagnant blood and pain. It is discussed in the blood stagnation syndrome.

Clinical picture: Pain and preference for warmth, the pain relieved by warmth, cold limbs and trunk, light-coloured and dull tongue and deep, slow and irregular pulse.

Analysis of symptoms: It is often caused by the direct affection of exogenous pathogenic cold and obstructed yang *qi* in the body, e.g., frostbite, *tuo-ju*,[132] etc. As pathogenic cold is yin and contracting, it causes blood stagnation when it invades the blood vessel, resulting in a blood stagnation syndrome with cold affection. It is commonly seen in women. If they suffer from a cold during menstruation or labour and pathogenic cold attacks the blood vessel and the uterus is cold and blood stagnant, cold and pain on either side of the abdomen, fear of cold and cold limbs, irregularity of menstrual flow, pale menstrual flow with blood clots, etc. may be seen.

Treatment: Warm the meridians and promote blood circulation with prescriptions, such as Angelica Sinensis Decoction for cold limbs[10] and Meridian-warming Decoction.[11]

d. The blood-heat syndrome is a blood stagnation syndrome associated with the heat syndrome. Its pathological changes are located in different areas, such as the intestine and stomach, or the lower energizer, and pathogenic heat entering the blood chamber in women. Its symptoms and signs belong to the excess syndrome and are also manifested as the intermingling of deficiency and excess syndromes.

Clinical picture: Pain and preference for cold, fever or hemorrhage or masses, rapid pulse, dark-red tongue, etc. If pathogenic heat is excessive in the body and blood combines with pernicious heat in the intestine and stomach or lower energizer, delirium, somnolence, abnormal distension, fullness and pain aggravated by pressure, dry, dark red, easily excreted stools, or contraction or rigidity on either side of the lower abdomen, normal urination, mania, etc. may also be seen. If the heat enters the blood chamber and combines with blood in women, firmness and fullness in the lower abdomen or thoracic and hypochondriac region, chills and fever resembling those in malaria, delirium at night, menopause, etc. may also be seen. And if blood and pernicious heat combine and the blood is exhausted by burning heat, "steaming of bone" and fever due to consumptive disease, scaly skin, menopause, etc. may also be seen.

Analysis of symptoms: Combination of blood and pathogenic heat may be caused by external affection, emotional injury, visceral dysfunction or stagnant blood which produces pernicious heat. Fever may be seen because of combined blood and heat. Injury to the blood vessel by pernicious heat may cause hemorrhage. Combined blood and heat in the intestinal blood may cause bloody stools, and it is easily cured if the *qi* phase has not yet been impaired. If the heat stagnates in the lower energizer and at the *xue* (blood) phase, rigidity on either side of the lower abdomen may result; urination is normal because it does not interfere with *qi* activities. As stagnant heat upwardly disturbs the mind along the meridian, mania results. Since pernicious heat enters the blood chamber and mental restlessness and blood pertains to yin, delirium at night occurs. As the heat stagnates internally and persistently and *qi* and fire (intense heat) combine, blood is severely consumed and fails to nourish the body, and "steaming of bone" and consumptive fever, scaly skin, menopause, etc. may be seen.

Treatment: The case due to combined blood and heat in the intestine and stomach is treated by clearing up the pernicious heat and dispersing stagnant blood, dissipating stagnation and swelling with prescriptions, such as *Qi*-tonifying Decoction of *Persica*

Davidian,[12] Decoction of Removing Stagnant Blood[13] or Decoction of *Pheum Officinale* and *Paeonia Suffruticosa*,[14] etc. The case due to the pernicious heat entering the blood chamber is treated by harmonizing and clearing up the heat and promoting blood circulation with prescriptions, such as Minor *Radix Bupleuri* Decoction with additives of *Persica Davidian, Carthamus tinctorius*, Chinese Angelica (root), and *Nepeta japonica*.[15] The case due to the exhaustion of blood by burning heat is treated by clearing up the heat and harmonizing the middle energizer, eliminating ecchymosis and promoting granulation with prescriptions, such as *Pheum Officinale* and *Eupolyphaga Sinensis* Pills.[16]

10-2-2-3 Blood-heat syndrome

The symptoms of pernicious heat invade the *xue* (blood) phase.

Clinical picture: Anxiety or restlessness and mania, thirst with no desire for drinking, fever aggravated at night, minute rapid pulse or varieties of hemorrhage, menstruation ahead of schedule with a large amount of menstrual flow.

Analysis of symptoms: Blood heat syndrome is constantly caused by the affection of exogenous pathogenic heat or production of pathogenic fire by a depressed liver. As blood heat is intense, and disturbs the mind, anxiety or even restlessness with mania may be seen. Since pathogenic heat enters the *xue* (blood) phase and blood pertains to yin, fever is aggravated at night. The consumed yin blood leads to a dry mouth. No desire for drinking is due to pathogenic heat in the *xue* (blood) phase. As the blood is consumed by heat, the pulse is minute and rapid. Since heat is excessive at the *xue* (blood) phase, the blood is affected by it and the blood vessel is easily injured, with epistaxis, hematemesis, hematuria, subcutaneous bleeding and polymenorrhea seen.

Treatment: Clear up pathogenic heat and cool blood with prescriptions, such as Ying-clearing Decoction,[17] *Cornu Rhinoceri* and *Radix Rehmanniae* Decoction.[18]

10-2-3 Identification of syndromes according to *qi* (vital energy) and *xue* (blood) phases

Qi is yang and blood is yin. Being interdependent, *qi* warms, produces, promotes and governs blood. Therefore, blood is often deficient due to failure of deficient *qi* to produce it. Blood is often stagnant because *qi* is too cold to warm it. It is often obstructed because *qi* is too weak to promote it. Blood often extravasates because *qi* fails to control it. Blood nourishes and transports *qi*. Hence, *qi* decreases because blood is too deficient to transport it. Various diseases caused by pathogenic dryness and heat occur because *qi* is not nourished by the blood, particularly exhausted blood can make *qi* fail to append to it, resulting in the scattering of yang *qi* or even the collapse of *qi* and exhaustion of yang. The blood stagnation syndrome with *qi* deficiency and the syndrome of *qi* and blood deficiency introduced previously belong to the category of *qi* and blood disease.

10-2-3-1 The obstructed *qi* and blood syndrome

This refers to the obstruction of blood circulation due to *qi* stasis with stagnant blood.

Clinical picture: Distension, full and indefinite pain in the chest and hypochondria, irascibility associated with masses with stabbing pain aggravated by pressure, dark-purplish tongue, or ecchymosis on the tongue. In women, amenorrhea or dysmenorrhea, dark-purplish menstrual flow with clots, distension and pain in the breasts, etc. may be seen.

Analysis of symptoms: It is caused by depressed emotions and traumatic wounds such as sprains or strains. Since the liver is concerned with dispersion and discharge and stores blood, depressed emotion can cause stagnant liver *qi* and the liver fails to perform its dispersing and discharging functions, with anxiety, irascibility, distension, fullness and indefinite pain in the chest and hypochondria and dysmenorrhea, amenorrhea, menstrual flow with blood clots, distension and pain in the breasts, etc.

Treatment: Promote the circulation of *qi* and blood with prescriptions, such as *Xiaoyao* Powder with additives of *Persica Davidian, Carthamus Tinctorius* and *Sparganium Stoloniferum Caesalpinia Sapan.*[19]

10-2-3-2 Deficient *qi* and blood syndrome

This refers to symptoms of both deficiencies of *qi* and blood.

Clinical picture: Shortage of *qi* and indolent disclination to talk, general lassitude and spontaneous sweating, pallor or withered yellow complexion, palpitation and insomnia, light-coloured delicate tongue, minute weak pulse, etc.

Analysis of symptoms: Prolonged illness and injuries of both *qi* and blood or blood loss that cause consumed *qi* together with blood or deficient blood that results in insufficient blood.

Treatment: Tonify both *qi* and blood with prescriptions, such as Decoction of Eight Precious Ingredients[20] or Blood-tonifying Decoction with Chinese Angelica Root.[21]

10-2-3-3 Deficient *qi* and blood loss syndromes

Symptoms of blood loss due to deficient failure of *qi* to control blood appear. The blood is discharged from the lower portion of the body (metrorrhagia, hematuria, melanemia, etc.) because *qi* becomes insubstantial and descending.

Clinical picture: The deficient *qi* syndromes, such as shortness of breath, general lassitude, pallor, a soft, weak and faint pulse and light-coloured tongue are simultaneously seen when bleeding.

Analysis of symptoms: Deficient *qi* can lead to extravasating blood, with hemorrhage. As blood circulates together with *qi*, deficient *qi* and blood escaping from the lower portion of the body, manifesting as hemorrhage from the lower portion such as metrorrhagia are most frequently seen in women.

Treatment: Tonify *qi* to induce blood to control the meridians (vessels) with prescriptions, such as *Gui-pi* Decoction.[22]

10-2-3-4 The exhausted *qi* syndrome with severe hemorrhage

The symptoms of abrupt exhaustion of *qi* due to hemorrhoea appear.

Clinical picture: Pallor, cold clammy extremities, profuse sweating, even fainting, faint minute or hollow pulse are seen simultaneously during hemorrhoea.

Analysis of symptoms: The exhausted *qi* syndrome is often caused by trauma or metrorrhagia and postpartum hemorrhoea. *Qi* fails to rely on blood due to hemorrhoea, resulting in exhausted *qi*. Since *qi* and yang are exhausted and fail to warm and consolidate the body surface, profuse cold sweats may occur; cold clammy extremities; as *qi* and blood cannot ascend to nourish the head and eyes, fainting may be seen. As blood vessels are not enriched by *qi* and blood, a faint minute or hollow pulse may result.

Treatment: Tonify *qi* to check its exhaustion with prescriptions, such as Single Ginseng Decoction[23] or Ginseng and *Aconiti* Decoction[24] according to the principle of "replenish *qi* if severe hemorrhage occurs."

10-2-4 Identification of body fluids disease

Pathological changes of body fluids disease vary, but they can be generalized to insufficient body fluids and stagnant aqueous liquid.

10-2-4-1 Insufficient body fluids

Since deficient body fluids fail to nourish and moisten the body, they cause a dryness syndrome. Thus, a variety of the dryness syndrome appears.

Clinical picture: Dry throat, lips and tongue, thirst, dry mouth, dry or withered skin, scanty urine, constipation and minute rapid pulse.

Analysis of symptoms: Insufficient body fluids is often caused by profuse sweating, severe hemorrhage, blood loss, vomiting and diarrhea, polyuria, and injury of body fluids by pathogenic dryness and heat. Since the mouth, lips, skin and blood vessels are not enriched and nourished by body fluids, a dry throat and thirst and dry or withered skin and minute pulse may result. Since body fluids, the resource of urine, are in deficiency, scanty urine may appear. As the large intestine is not moistened by body fluids, constipation results.

Treatment: Supplement body fluids with prescriptions, such as Body Fluid Supplementing Decoction.[25]

10-2-4-2 Stagnant aqueous liquid

This is caused by dysfunctions of the lung, spleen, and kidney, and often forms *tan-yin* (phlegm and excess exudes) and edema, etc. *Tan-yin* syndromes commonly seen are differentiated as follows:

a. The common *tan* (phlegm) syndrome

a) Wind-phlegm: A disease or syndrome of the movement of endogenous pathogenic wind caused by excess phlegm.

Clinical picture: Dizziness and vertigo, rattling throat, sudden fainting, facial paralysis, stiff tongue, numb limbs, paraplegia, etc. caused by deficient yin and excess yang and internally accumulated phlegm and saliva. The wind-phlegm disturbs the upper portion of the body resulting in dizziness and blurred vision and rattling throat: If it affects the meridian, numb limbs, paraplegia and facial paralysis may result; if it obstructs sense organs, mental disturbance and sudden fainting and stiff tongue may appear.

Treatment: Clear up endogenous pathogenic wind and eliminate phlegm with prescriptions, such as Major *Gentiana Nacrophy* Decoction.[26]

b) Heat-phlegm: The combination of pathogenic phlegm and heat

Clinical picture: Fever with anxiety, yellow mucoid expectoration, sore throat, constipation, or mania, and slippery rapid pulse.

Analysis of symptoms: Heat-phlegm results from the affection of pathogenic heat or consumption of body fluids by excess yang *qi* in the body. The internal disturbance of heat-phlegm leads to fever with anxiety. Constipation of body fluids by yang heat results in expectoration of yellow sputum. As phlegm and heat combine to obstruct the *qi* mechanism, a sore throat may be seen. Since phlegm-heat stagnates in the stomach and intestine, dry stools appear. Disturbance of phlegm-heat by pathogenic wind may cause mania. The combination of phlegm and heat results in a slippery rapid pulse.

Treatment: Clear up pathogenic heat and subdue phlegm with prescriptions, such as *Qi*-clearing and Phlegm-subduing Pills[27] and Phlegm-eliminating Pills.[28]

c) Cold-phlegm: The symptoms due to the combination and stagnant pathogenic cold and phlegm or excess phlegm with cold signs are cold-phlegm syndromes.

Clinical picture: Aversion to cold and cold, clammy extremities, expectoration of whitish sputum, or bone *bi* (blockage) syndrome[133] with stabbing pain, immovable limbs, deep slow pulse, etc.

Analysis of symptoms: Cold-phlegm is caused by the affection of exogenous pathogenic cold, excess yin and deficient yang of the body and retention of aqueous liquids. The impairment of yang and stagnant cold and phlegm leads to aversion to cold and cold clammy extremities. Owing to the obstructed meridian and depressed *qi*, the bone *bi* syndrome with stabbing pain, immovable limbs and deep slow pulse may result. As cold aqueous liquid is in excess, expectoration of thin whitish sputum may be seen.

Treatment: Warmly subdue phlegm and saliva with prescriptions, such as *Sanzi Yangqin* Decoction[29] or *Erchen* Decoction with additives of *Zingiber officinale, Asarum Sie Boldi* and *Fructus Schizandrae.*[30]

d) Damp-phlegm: Phlegm formed by accumulating damp and excess phlegm sputum, sensation of a heavy body and lassitude, soft slippery pulse and thick glossy coating of tongue.

Analysis of symptoms: It is caused by the production of endogenous pathogenic phlegm and damp due to a weak spleen, or the affection of exogenous pathogenic cold-damp so that the lung is restrained and the spleen obstructed. Aqueous damp is retained internally and accumulates to form phlegm. The weak spleen and obstructed endogenous damp lead to poor appetite. The obstruction of the upper energizer by pathogenic phlegm-damp leads to regurgitation of gastric *qi* (vomiting). The obstruction of clear yang (*qi*) by phlegm-damp arouses the sensation of a heavy body and lassitude.

Treatment: Remove endogenous pathogenic damp and subdue phlegm with *Erchen* Decoction.[30]

e) Dry-phlegm: Phlegm syndrome with dry signs.

Clinical picture: Mucoid sputum like a lump or bloody, dry mouth and nose, dry sore throat, dry stools, dry tongue (with less fluid) and a stringy, slippery and rapid pulse.

Analysis of symptoms: With the affection of exogenous pathogenic dryness or formation of phlegm due to the consumption of body fluids by pathogenic dryness, a small amount of expectoration of sticky mucoid sputum may appear with difficult expectoration. Pernicious dryness injures the collateral meridian of the lung, causing bloody sputum. Dry mouth, nose and throat and constipation are caused by injuries of the lung and large intestine by harmful dryness.

Treatment: Moisten the body and subdue phlegm with prescriptions, such as Dryness-relieving and Lung-saving Decoction[31] and Kidney-reinforcing Decoction with Lily Bulb.[32]

b. Common yin (excess exudates) syndrome: "Yin" is derived from stagnant aqueous liquid due to the dysfunctional viscera. It refers to the disease or syndrome caused by *shui-yin* (excess watery fluid). As "*yin*" is similar to phlegm and water and they are closely connected in a pathological process, a *yin* syndrome is often termed *yan-yin* or *shui-yin*. It is caused by a weak spleen and stomach yang complicated with the affection of exogenous pathogenic cold and damp and injuries from overfatigue and lack of physical exercise. *Yin* can be divided into *tan-yin, xuan-yin, yi-yin, zhi-yin*, etc. according to different locations of retaining *shui-yin*. But this is caused by deficient yang and excess yin and abnormal water metabolism. It should be treated by using drugs of a warm and nourishing nature.

a) *Tan-yin* (phlegm and excess exudates)

Clinical picture: Fullness and distension of the chest and epigastrium, stomach discomfort, vomiting up clear thin sputum and saliva, no thirst or thirst with no desire for drinking, vertigo, palpitation and shortness of breath, white slippery tongue coating, stringy slippery pulse.

Analysis of symptoms: Hypoactivity of spleen yang and stomach yang and internal retention of *shui-yin* cause fullness and distension in the chest and hypochondria, retention of *shui-yin* (excess exudates) in the epigastric region creates stomach discomfort; regurgitation of *shui-yin* leads to vomiting up clear thin sputum and saliva; water retention in the middle energizer causes no thirst or thirst with no desire for drinking; obstruction of ascending clear yang by water leads to vertigo; the upward affection of the heart and lung by *shui-yin* results in palpitation and shortness of breath.

Treatment: Warmly subdue *tan-yin* with prescriptions, such as Decoction of Poria, Cinnamon Bark, *Atractylodes macrocephala* and *Glyeyrrhiza*.[33]

b) *Xuan-yin* is the *shui-yin* retained in the area below the chest and above the abdomen.

Clinical picture: Hypochondriac pain aggravated by cough and spitting and induced by breathing. Distension and fullness in the intercostal region, short, hasty breath and deep stringy pulse.

Analysis of symptoms: The epigastric region is a pathway through which *qi* ascends and descends. When water is retained and blocked, the ascending and descending movements of *qi* will be disturbed, resulting in a pain in the epigastric region and intercostal pain caused by cough, spitting and breathing. As *shui-yin* presses the lung, distension and fullness appear in the intercostal region causing short and hasty breath. As *shui-yin* stagnates internally, the pulse is deep and stringy.

Treatment: Expel *shui-yin* with prescriptions, such as Ten-date Decoction,[34] Saliva-controlling Pills,[35] etc.

c) *Yi-yin* is *shui-yin* retained in the muscles of the four extremities, the same as the common aqueous-*qi* disease.

Clinical picture: Painful and heavy limbs, even puffy limbs and trunk, difficulty in urination, or fever, aversion to cold and no sweat, frothy expectoration, white tongue coating and stringy, taut pulse.

Analysis of symptoms: As the spleen and lung *qi* fail to be distributed, *shui-yin* is retained in the muscles of the limbs, resulting in a painful and heavy sensation in the limbs and trunk, even puffiness. If exogenous pathogenic wind-cold affects the body surface and the defensive *qi* is blocked, fever, aversion to cold and anhidrosis will result. Since cold *yin* (excess fluid) stagnates in the lung, and the lung fails to perform its dissipating and descending functions, cough and asthmatic breath and frothy sputum may be seen.

Treatment: Warmly eliminate excess fluid. It is advisable for the case associated with exogenous cold to remove the pathogenic factor from the superficial part of the body and subdue *yin* (excess exudates). The prescriptions used are Five-Poria Powders[36] associated with Five-bark Cold Decoction,[37] Minor Dark-blue Dragon Decoction,[38] etc.

(d) *Zhi-yin* symptoms and signs of retention of *shui-yin* in the thoracic and epigastric regions.

Clinical picture: Cough and asthmatic breath, fullness in the chest and shortness of breath, difficulty in lying flat, facial puffiness, white frothy sputum, white glossy tongue coating and stringy taut pulse.

Analysis of symptoms: As *shui-yin* and lung *qi* descend, cough and asthmatic breath and difficulty in lying flat may result. As aqueous liquid overflows due to its failure to transmit downward, facial puffiness is frequently seen. Since concealing *yin* (excess fluids) exists inside the body with the affection of exogenous cold in the outside, it reoccurs frequently and lasts many years.

Treatment: Quench pernicious fire in the lung and expel excess fluid. For the case associated with exterior syndrome, diaphoretic and *yin*-subduing therapies should be applied with Decoction of *Decuraini Sophia* and Dates[39] and Minor Dark-blue Dragon Decoction.[38]

10-3 Identification of syndromes according to *zang-fu* (viscera)

Identification of syndromes according to *zang-fu* (viscera) is a syndrome identification in which symptoms and signs of the disease are analysed and summed up according to physiological functions and pathological manifestations of the viscera, in order to explore the pathogenesis and judge the location, feature of pathological changes and flourishing and decline of anti-pathogenic and pathogenic factors, as well as an important component of the syndrome-identification system.

Syndrome identification varies and must be applicable to the viscera if the location and feature of disease are to be accurately identified and the treatment determined, e.g., as to the eight guiding principles, there are different yin deficiencies of the heart, lung, liver, kidney and stomach, etc. Only by identifying them can the treatment be accurate and favourable effects obtained. Another example, although identification of syndrome with the names of the six meridians and according to the *wei* (defence), *qi* (vital energy), *ying* (nutrition) and *xue* (blood) phases and the triple energizer are mainly used for exogenous febrile diseases, pathological processes of the disease that are identified with them are related to disorders of the yin, yang, *qi* and blood of the viscera. Pathological processes may even lie in the viscera concerned. Thus identification of syndromes according to the viscera is a basic procedure in clinical diagnosis, particularly of miscellaneous syndromes in internal medicine as well as a basis for other syndrome identification.

A disease or syndrome reflects the dysfunction of the internal organ. The yin or yang property of the pathogenic factor is ascertained with identification of syndromes according to the etiology and cold and heat, deficiency and excess. Pathological changes are distinguished by identification of syndromes of the visceral symptoms.

There is a connection between the five yin and six yang viscera and between the viscera and various tissues and organs. Therefore, not only the pathological change of a yin or yang viscus should be considered, but attention must be paid to the interconnection and influence between the yin and yang viscera. Only in this way can the whole pathological process be grasped.

Identifications of syndromes according to viscera includes identification of the yin viscera diseases, yang viscera diseases and yin-yang viscera diseases. Since a simple yang viscera disease is rare and is often related to a yin viscus, it is described together with the yin viscera disease concerned. Some commonly seen symptoms and signs of the viscera are introduced in this section since pathological changes of the viscera are rather complex and these symptoms and signs vary greatly.

10-3-1 Identification of heart and small intestine disorders

As the heart controls blood vessels, stores the mind, opens to the tongue and is concerned with the small intestine, all the symptoms and disorders of blood vessels and emotions, such as palpitation, insomnia, mental disturbance, mania, etc. are regarded as a heart disease or syndrome.

A heart disease or syndrome is either deficient or of an excess nature. The deficient type is due to insufficient *qi*, blood, yin and yang while the excess is due to the invasion of pathogenic fire, heat, phlegm and stagnant matter, etc.

10-3-1-1 Deficiencies of heart *qi* and heart yang

Clinical picture: The common symptoms are palpitations and shortness of breath aggravated by exertion and minute weak or irregular or regularly intermittent pulse. If the symptoms are accompanied by pallor, mental fatigue and general lassitude, spontaneous sweating and shortage of *qi* and light-coloured tongue with white coating, it is deficient heart *qi*; if accompanied with aversion to cold, cold limbs, dull complexion, chest distress or pain and tasteless and delicate tongue, it is deficient heart yang. If accompanied by prolonged sweating, cold, clammy extremities, dark-purplish lips, weak breath, faint pulse, semi-consciousness, or even coma, it is a critical sign of exhausted heart yang.

Analysis of symptoms: Deficient heart yang and *qi* is caused by a weak constitution due to a prolonged illness, consumed yang or *qi* due to an abrupt disease, senile weakness of visceral *qi*, congenital deficiency, etc. Blood is not promoted and enriched by heart yang, causing palpitations, shortness of breath and a minute, weak pulse. Weak *qi* and yang fail to strengthen the body surface, resulting in spontaneous sweating. *Qi* in the meridian flows discontinuously, causing an irregularly or regularly intermittent pulse. As *qi* is consumed by exertion, all the symptoms are aggravated by exertion. Since heart *qi* and blood fail to nourish the upper portion of the body, a pallor and light coloured tongue may appear. Owing to deficient yang's failure to warm the body and limbs, cold limbs and fear of cold result. Since heart yang is not vigorous and yang *qi* in the chest is blocked, chest distress or pain occurs. Because of deficient and declining yang *qi* and abnormal blood circulation, dark-purplish lips and tongue may be seen. As heart yang is declining and abruptly exhausted and chest *qi* is severely consumed, cold extremities, profuse sweating, short and faint breath, semi-consciousness, even coma and faint pulse result.

Treatment: For deficient heart *qi*, tonify and nourish it with Heart-nourishing Decoction[40] or by puncturing *Xinshu* (B. 15), *Daling* (P 7) and *Fuliu* (K 7) with tonifying manipulation or do moxibustion on them with a moxa stick; for deficient heart yang, tonify it with Primordial *qi* Protecting Decoction[41] or by doing moxibustion on *Tongli* (H 5), *Fuliu* (K 7), *Yongquan* (K 1) and *Tanzhong* (CV 17) with a moxa stick; for exhausted yang, revive the yang with Ginseng and Aconite Decoction.[24]

10-3-1-2 Deficiencies of heart blood and heart yin

Clinical picture: Common symptoms of deficiencies of heart blood and heart yin are palpitations, somnolence, insomnia and dreaminess. If they are accompanied by vertigo, dull complexion, light-coloured lips and tongue and minute weak pulse, it is deficient heart blood. If accompanied by fever in the chest, palms and soles, night sweat, dry mouth and throat, dry red tongue with minute rapid pulse, it is deficient heart yin.

Analysis of symptoms: Deficiency of heart blood and heart yin is due to the blood's lacking its resource or blood loss or injury of yin in febrile disease or internal injury by the "seven emotions" or prolonged consumption of yin blood. As yin blood is insufficient and the heart is not nourished, palpitations occur. Since blood does not nourish the heart and *shen* (Spirit) storing in the heart (Mind), insomnia and dreaminess result; as deficient blood cannot nourish the upper portion of the body, vertigo and amnesia, dull complexion, light-coloured lips and tongue appear. As blood is too deficient to enrich the vessel, the pulse is minute and weak. As heart yin is deficient and pernicious fire due to deficiency disturbs the body internally, fever in the chest, palms and soles, night sweat, dry mouth and throat, dry red tongue and minute rapid pulse may appear.

Treatment: It is advisable for deficient heart blood to nourish blood and soothe the nerves with prescriptions, such as the Four-ingredient Decoction[1] with additives of Jujube Nut, *Semer Thujae*, Poria Cocos, etc.; or by puncturing *Xinshu* (B 15), *Shenmen* (H 7), *Tongli* (H 5), *Neiguan* (P 6) and *Sanyinjiao* (Sp.6) with tonifying manipulation; for deficient heart yin to replenish yin and soothe the nerves with prescriptions, such as Heart-reinforcing Pills[42] or by puncturing *Daling* (P 7), *Tongli* (H 5) with moderate manipulation and *Taixi* (H 5) with tonifying manipulation.

10-3-1-3 Excess heart fire

Clinical picture: Anxiety, insomnia, flushed face and thirst, sores in the mouth and tongue, red tongue, rapid pulse, even mania and delirium, or accompanied by dark-red urine and irregular urination with stabbing pain, hematuria, etc.

Analysis of symptoms: Excess heart fire is caused by internal production of emotional fire, or transformation of depressed *qi* into fire, or overeating pungent and hot food and tonics of a warm nature. Internal burning of heart fire leads to anxiety. Disturbance of the heart (Mind) by fire leads to insomnia, even mental disorders. Blazing heart fire causes sores in the mouth and tongue and flushed face. The consumption of body fluids by pathogenic fire (intense heat) results in thirst. Since the heart transfers pernicious fire to the small intestine, dark-red urine with burning pain appears and hematuria results from the injury of the blood vessel by pernicious heat.

Treatment: Clear up heart fire with Heart-fire-clearing Decoction[43] or by puncturing *Daling* (P 7), *Laogong* (P 8) and *Zhongchong* (P 9) with purging manipulation. For mania, add *Dazhi* (GV 14) and *Taichong* (Liv 3), *Xuehai* (Sp 10) and *Yanglingquan* (GB 34) with moderate manipulation. It is advisable for the heart transferring its heat to the small intestine to purify the heart by clearing heart fire with Daochi Powders.[44]

10-3-1-4 Phlegm confusing the mind and phlegm-fire disturbing the heart

Clinical picture: In phlegm confusing the mind, idiocy, mental depression or mental disturbance, abnormal manner, muttering to oneself, fainting, unconsciousness, rattling throat, white glossy tongue coating and moderate slippery pulse may appear. In phlegm-fire disturbing the heart (Mind), anxiety and thirst, disturbed sleep with dreams, flushed face and coarse voice, constipation and dark-red urine may be seen; in severe cases, mental disturbance, delirium, abnormal crying and laughing, mania, excitability, red tongue with yellow glossy coating and stringy, slippery and substantive pulse result.

Analysis of symptoms: Phlegm confusing the heart (Mind) is due to injuries of the "seven emotions," such as depression, rage, etc. or affection of pathogenic damp and the turbid matter that block *qi* so that *qi* and phlegm stagnate in the heart (Mind). If depressive *qi* transforms itself into pernicious fire that consumes body fluids and forms phlegm and phlegm-fire disturbs the heart (Mind) or pathogenic factor in exogenous febrile disease inwardly affects the pericardium together with phlegm, phlegm-fire will disturb the mind.

Pathogenic phlegm and the turbid matter are yin that is concerned with calmness. Mental confusion will result if the heart (Mind) is blocked by the phlegm and turbid matter. Fire pertains to yang that is concerned with motion. Mania will result if phlegm-fire upwardly disturbs the heart (Mind).

Treatment: For phlegm confusing the heart (Mind), expel stubborn phlegm for resuscitation with prescriptions, such as Phlegm-eliminating Decoction[45] in association with Storax Pills[46] or by puncturing *Dazhui* (GV 14), *Xinshu* (B 15), *Baihui* (GV 20), *Neiguan* (P 6), *Renzhong* (GV 26), and *Fenglong* (S 40) with moderate manipulation; for phlegm-fire disturbing the heart (Mind), dispel pathogenic heat from the heart and break through phlegm with Phlegm-eliminating *Chlorite-schist* Pills[28] or by puncturing *Renzhong* (GV 26), *Zhongchong* (P 9), *Laogong* (P 8), *Tongquan* (K 1), *Dazhui* (GV 14) and *Taichong* (Liv 3) with purging manipulation.

10-3-1-5 Stagnant and obstructed heart blood

Clinical picture: Heart palpitations, chest distress or stabbing pain in the shoulder, back and medial aspect of the upper arm at intervals, dark-purplish tongue sometimes with petechae and ecchymosis, minute irregular or regularly intermittent pulse. In severe cases excruciating pain, dark-purplish mouth and lips, cold, clammy extremities and mental disturbance and faint pulse may be seen.

Analysis of symptoms: It is often secondary to the diseases (or syndromes) of deficient heart *qi* or heart yang. As yang *qi* is too deficient to warmly promote blood circulation, stagnant blood blocks the heart vessel. It is induced or aggravated by fatigue and lack of physical exercise, cold affection, internal injury of overjoy or rage or accumulated phlegm and the turbid matter.

As heart yang is inactive and blood stagnates in the heart vessel, chest distress with stabbing pain occurs; since the Heart Meridian of Hand-*shaoyin* runs along the shoulder and back, pain in the shoulder, back and medial aspect of the upper arm results. As deficient yang and stagnant blood cause abnormal heartbeat, palpitations may occur. An irregular or regularly intermittent pulse leads to a dark-purplish tongue with petechae and ecchymosis, which is a sign of stagnant *qi* and blood. Since heart yang is abruptly exhausted and blood is stagnant and vessels blocked, an excruciating pain in the heart, dark-purplish complexion, even fainting and faint weak pulse result.

Treatment: Unblock yang and subdue stagnant blood with Decoction of Immature, Bitter Orange, *Allium Mascrotemon* and Cassia Twig[47] associated with Sense-organ-unblocking and Blood-invigorating Decoction.[48] For the abrupt exhausted heart yang, restore the yang for resuscitation with Ginseng and Aconite Decoction[24] or by puncturing *Tongli* (H 5), *Neiguan* (P 6), *Ximen* (P 4), *Shaohai* (H 3), *Xinshu* (B 15) and *Jueyinshu* (B 14) with moderate manipulation. For the case with cold clammy extremities and mental disturbance, add *Qihai* (CV 6), *Zusanli* (S 36) and *Neiguan* (P 6) by moxibustion with a moxa stick.

As to identification of small intestine disorder, there is excess heat in the small intestine, deficiency cold in the small intestine, *qi* pain in the small intestine, etc. The first has been mentioned in "excess heart fire," the second two are related to the syndromes of "deficient spleen yang" and "obstruction of the Liver Meridian by cold."

10-3-2 Identification of lung and large intestine disorders

Difficulty in breathing, asthma and shortage of *qi*, expectoration of bloody sputum, etc. are mainly ascribed to the pathological processes of the lung because the lung is concerned with air, respiration, purification, descendance and flow of fluid, and is closely related to skin and hair, open to the nose and closely connected with the large intestine.

The pathological changes of the lung are of the deficiency and excess types. The deficiency type is commonly seen in impaired *qi* and deficient yin fluid and the excess type is due to the invasion of pathogenic wind, cold, dryness and heat or to the invasion of the lung by phlegm and the turbid matter.

10-3-2-1 Deficient lung *qi*

Clinical picture: Mental fatigue and shortage of *qi*, cough and asthmatic breath and general lassitude, short breath by exertion, low voice, spontaneous sweating and fear of cold, pallor, light-coloured tongue and weak pulse.

Analysis of symptoms: Deficient lung *qi* is mainly caused by the consumption and impairment of lung *qi* by prolonged cough or asthmatic breath or deficient *qi*. Consumed and deficient lung *qi* leads to shortness of breath, cough, asthmatic breath, general lassitude, and low voice. As lung *qi* cannot make defensive *qi* spread to the body surface and the junction between the skin and muscle is weak, spontaneous sweating, fear of cold and susceptibility to cold may result. Since both *qi* and blood fail to upwardly nourish the face, pallor results.

Treatment: Tonify and nourish lung *qi* with prescriptions, such as the Four Noble Ingredient Decoction with the additive of Atraglus Root, etc. or nourish *qi* and strengthen the body surface with prescriptions, such as Jade-screen Powders[49] or by puncturing *Feishu* (B 13), *Taiyuan* (L 9) and *Fuliu* (K 7) with tonifying manipulation and doing moxibustion with a moxa stick.

10-3-2-2 Deficient lung yin

Clinical picture: A dry cough and short breath, less mucoid sputum or bloody sputum, dry mouth and throat, coarse voice, emaciation, tidal fever in the afternoon, fever in the chest, palms and soles, night sweat and malar flush, dry red tongue and minute rapid pulse.

Analysis of symptoms: Deficient lung yin is caused by internal injury from strain or the consumption of lung yin by a prolonged cough.

Since yin fluid in the lung is insufficient so that the lung cannot carry on its clearing, moistening and descending functions, a dry mouth and throat, coarse voice, dry cough, short breath and some mucoid sputum may appear. The internal steaming of pernicious heat due to deficiency caused by yin deficiency leads to tidal fever, fever in the chest, palms and soles, night sweat and malar flush. The lung collateral meridians are injured by pathogenic heat, with bloody sputum or hemoptysis.

Treatment: Replenish the yin and moisten the lung or replenish the yin and clear up pernicious fire with prescriptions, such as Lung-reinforcing Decoction with Lily Bulb[32] or by puncturing *Chize* (L 5), *Kongzui* (L 6), *Yuji* (L 10) and *Sanyinjiao* (Sp 6) with moderate manipulation.

10-3-2-3 Invasion of the lung by exogenous pathogenic cold

Clinical picture: Cough and asthmatic breath, thin white sputum, no thirst, watery nasal discharge; or accompanied by creeping chills, fever, pain in the head and body, white tongue coating and taut pulse.

Analysis of symptoms: It is caused by the affection of exogenous pathogenic cold that stays in the lung. That associated with the exterior syndrome is ascribed to the affection of the body surface by exogenous pathogenic wind-cold, but that associated with no exterior syndrome is due to the invasion of the lung by pathogenic cold.

As exogenous pathogenic wind-cold affects the body surface and the lung cannot carry on its dispersing function, aversion to cold, fever, pain in the body, watery nasal discharge result; since exogenous pathogenic wind-cold invades the lung that cannot perform its dispersing and descending functions, body fluids are concentrated as *tan-yin* (phlegm and excess exudates) which blocks the respiratory tract, a cough, asthmatic breath and thin white sputum occur. A white tongue coating and taut pulse are ascribed to pathogenic cold and the body surface affected by exogenous pathogenic wind-cold causes a superficial taut pulse.

Treatment: Ventilate a troubled lung and dissipate pathogenic cold with prescriptions, such as Almond and Perilla Leaf Powders[50] and *Huagai* Powders[51] or by puncturing *Hegu* (LI 4), *Taiyuan* (L 9) and *Dingchuai* (Extra 17), *Fengchi* (GB 20) and *Dazhui* (GV 14) with moderate manipulation and do moxibustion on them with a moxa stick.

10-3-2-4 Obstruction of the lung by pathogenic heat

Clinical picture: Cough, asthmatic breath, rough breath, yellow mucoid expectoration, sore throat and thirst, or fever, slight aversion to wind and cold or chest pain, expectoration of foul sputum mixed with purulent blood, constipation, dark-scanty urine, red tongue with yellow coating and rapid pulse.

Analysis of symptoms: Caused by the affection of exogenous pathogenic warm-heat or invasion of the lung by exogenous pathogenic wind-cold. That associated with the exterior syndrome is ascribed to the invasion of the lung by exogenous pathogenic wind-heat, but that associated with no exterior syndrome is ascribed to the affection of the lung by pathogenic heat, even prolonged stagnant phlegm-fire that forms *feiyong*.[134]

Since pathogenic heat invades the lung so that the lung cannot carry on its clearing functions, cough, asthmatic breath, hasty and rough breath and yellow mucoid sputum occur; as body fluids are consumed by the burning heat, thirst results. Since the throat is the door of the lung, the blockage of the lung by pathogenic heat would lead to a sore throat. If exogenous pathogenic wind-cold affects the body surface and lung *qi* can carry on its dispersing function, fever, aversion to wind and cold may be seen. If pathogenic heat stagnates in the lung for long, then body fluids are concentrated as phlegm, which blocks the lung together and the heat and nutritional blood are impaired and pus forms and lung abscess and gangrene of the lung will be caused, with chest pain and foul expectoration with purulent blood.

Treatment: Clear up the lung heat, relieve cough and asthmatic breath with prescriptions, such as Mulberry Leaf and Chrysanthemum Flower Cold Decoction,[52] Decoction of *Herba Ephedra*, Almond Licorice and Gypsum[53] for lung abscess and gangrene of the lung, clear up pathogenic heat and drain pus with *Phramites Comminis Trin* Decoction with a Thousand Gold[54] or by puncturing *Neiguan* (P 6), *Chize* (L 5), *Fengchi* (GB 20), *Feishu* (GB 13) and *Fenglong* (S 40) with purging manipulation. For the case with sore throat and thirst, add *Shaoshang* (L 11) to cause bleeding with a triangular needle.

10-3-2-5 Invasion of the lung by pathogenic dryness

Clinical picture: A dry cough with less mucoid sputum that is hardly expectorated, or asthmatic breath and white frothy expectoration, dry nose and throat, chest pain induced by severe cough, dry tongue with thin dry coating and minute rapid pulse; or accompanied by the exterior syndrome, such as fever, aversion to wind and cold, headache, etc.

Analysis of symptoms: The lung is invaded by pathogenic dryness due to the consumption and impairment of lung fluid by exogenous pathogenic dryness or consumption of body fluids and production of pernicious dryness by pathogenic wind-warmth.

Since pathogenic dryness invades the lung, body fluids are severely consumed and the lung cannot perform its moistening, clearing and descending functions and then cough and asthmatic breath with no or little mucoid sputum, dry mouth, nose and skin and a dry tongue with thin dry coating appear. As lung *qi* becomes abnormal due to the injury of the lung by pathogenic dryness, chest pain results. As the body surface is affected by pathogenic dryness and lung *qi* cannot carry on its dispersing function, fever and aversion to cold are also seen. A minute, rapid pulse occurs when body fluids are consumed by pathogenic dryness; in the case associated with an exterior syndrome, the pulse is also superficial.

Treatment: Ventilate the troubled lung by moistening it with prescriptions, such as Mulberry Leaf and Almond Decoction[55] and Dryness-relieving and Lung-saving Decoction[31] or by puncturing *Neiguan* (P 6), *Chize* (L 6), *Yuji* (L 10) and *Hegu* (LI 4) with purging manipulation.

10-3-2-6 Lung blocked by pathogenic phlegm-damp

Clinical picture: A cough with profuse thin, white sputum easily expectorated, chest distress or asthmatic breath and scratchy throat, a light-coloured tongue with white glossy coating and a stringy slippery or soft moderate pulse.

Analysis of symptoms: It is caused by the affection of exogenous pathogenic wind-cold-damp or prolonged cough and asthmatic breath so that the lung fails to distribute body fluids that accumulate to form phlegm-damp or pathogenic damp accumulates to form sputum due to the prolonged deficient spleen *qi*, which affects the lung.

As the phlegm-damp blocks the lung and the lung fails to perform its dispersing and descending functions, a profuse, thin and whitish expectoration appears; the obstructed respiratory tract results in asthmatic breath and scratchy throat. Since the phlegm-damp is yin and turbid, the tongue is light-coloured and its coating white and glossy, stringy slippery and soft moderate pulse are the signs of phlegm-damp.

Treatment: Remove pathogenic dryness and expel phlegm with prescriptions such as *Erchen* Decoction[30] in association with *Sanzi Yangqin* Decoction[29] or by puncturing *Taiyuan* (L 9), *Fenglong* (S 40), *Feishu* (GB 13) and *Pishu* (B 20) with moderate manipulation and do moxibustion on them with a moxa stick.

10-3-2-7 Affection of the large intestine by exogenous pathogenic damp-heat

Clinical picture: Abdominal pain, dysentery with purulent blood and tenesmus; or fulminating watery diarrhea, burning sensation in the anus, dry mouth with no desire for drinking and dark-red scanty urine, or accompanied by chills, fever and thirst, red tongue with yellow glossy coating and slippery rapid pulse.

Analysis of symptoms: It is frequently seen in the summer and autumn when pathogenic summer-heat and damp invade the stomach and intestine. It is also seen when stagnant pathogenic damp-heat accumulates in the large intestine due to improper diet and eating unripened or contaminated food.

As pathogenic damp and heat accumulate and stagnate, the lung and large intestine and the heat forces *qi* to stagnate and abdominal pain and tenesmus result; as the large intestine fails to perform its transporting function, diarrhea occurs. Since pathogenic damp and heat impair *qi* and blood and the heat produces pus, diarrhea with purulent blood appears. Since the damp-heat affects the lower portion of the body, fulminating watery diarrhea and a burning sensation in the anus appears. Owing to the consumption and body fluids by the heat, thirst results. That by an exterior syndrome is often associated with fever and aversion to cold, while that due to endogenous pathogenic heat is only associated with fever.

Treatment: Clear up pathogenic damp-heat with prescriptions, such as Decoction of *Pueraria* Root, *Stellaria* Root and *Coptis* Root[56] or *Pulstilla* Root Decoction[57] or by puncturing *Tianshu* (S 25), *Dachangshu* (B 25), *Quchi* (LI 11) and *Shangjuxu* (S 37) with purging manipulation.

10-3-2-8 Consumption of the large intestine fluid

Clinical picture: Dry stools excreted once every several days, red dry tongue with yellow dry coating and minute irregular pulse, dizziness and ozostomia, etc. may be seen.

Analysis of symptoms: Body fluids consumed by pathogenic dry-heat in the large intestine or deficient stomach yin's failure to descend to the large intestine. It is frequently seen in the aged or women after delivery or at the late stage of febrile disease.

As the large intestine fluid is consumed and the intestinal tract is not moistened and fails to perform its transporting function, stools are dry or excreted once every several days. The obstruction of *qi* of the yang viscera in the large intestine would influence the descendance of stomach *qi* and the stomach fails to perform its descending function and the turbid matter regurgitates and ozostomia and dizziness result. As body fluids are consumed by pathogenic dry-heat, the pulse is minute, irregular and the tongue coating yellow and dry.

Treatment: Moisten the intestine and promote bowel movements with prescriptions, such as Hemp Seed Pills[58] or by puncturing *Tianshu* (S 25), *Dachangshu* (B 25), *Zigou* (TE 6) and *Shangjuxu* (S 37) with moderate manipulation.

10-3-3 Identification of spleen and stomach disorders

The spleen is concerned with transmission and digestion and governs blood and the stomach. The spleen sends the clear (nutrient) upward and the stomach propels it downward. They jointly complete digestion, absorption and distribution of nutrients and are the resource of *qi* and blood and acquired foundations. Therefore, varieties of damp and swelling and fullness caused by disordered digestion and absorption of food or vomiting and diarrhea, caused by abnormally ascending and descending spleen and stomach *qi* or visceroptosis, a variety of hemorrhages caused by deficient *qi* and various syndromes of insufficiencies of *qi* and blood caused by the above-mentioned causes are pathological changes of the spleen and stomach.

Gastrosplenic diseases or syndromes are either a deficient type or an excess type. The spleen disease of the deficient type and the stomach disorder of the excess type are commonly seen. Deficiencies are often caused by consumed and impaired yang and *qi* and yin fluids, while their excesses are often caused by disturbance of pathogenic cold, damp, dryness and heat and food retention.

10-3-3-1 Deficient spleen and stomach *qi*

Clinical picture: Poor appetite and dyspepsia, distension and fullness in the epigastric and abdominal regions after meals, loose thin stools, shortage of *qi* and disinclination to talk, general lassitude, emaciation, withered, yellow and dull complexion, light-coloured tongue with white coating and slowed pulse.

Analysis of symptoms: Deficient spleen and stomach *qi* is caused by improper diet or fatigue and lack of physical exercise or severe vomiting and diarrhea or the influence of other disorders, e.g., a liver (wood) trouble counteracts upon the spleen (earth) and invades the stomach.

Insufficient gastrosplenic *qi* leads to spleen hypofunction, resulting in poor appetite, dyspepsia, distension and fullness after meals and loose thin stools. Deficient *qi* and blood lead to malnutrition of the four extremities, resulting in shortage of *qi* and indolent disinclination to talk, general lassitude, emaciation, withered, dark-yellowish complexion, light-coloured tongue and slow weak pulse.

Treatment: Nourish *qi* and reinforce the spleen with prescriptions, such as the Four Noble Ingredients Decoction[1] or the Six Noble Ingredients Decoction[59] or by puncturing *Zusanli* (S 36), *Pishu* (B 20), *Weishu* (B 21) and *Dadu* (Sp 2) with tonifying manipulation and do moxibustion on them with a moxa stick.

10-3-3-2 Deficient spleen yang

Clinical picture: Dyspepsia and abdominal distension, epigastric pain relieved by pressure and warmth, tasteless mouth and no thirst, cold limbs, loose stools, general puffiness, difficulty in urination or clear, thin and profuse leukorrhea, a light-coloured delicate tongue with white slippery coating and deep minute or slow weak pulse.

Analysis of symptoms: Deficient spleen yang often develops from deficient gastrosplenic *qi* as well as improper diet, overeating unripened or cold food or injury to spleen yang by taking too many cold-cool drugs. It is also called a deficient cold spleen syndrome because deficient yang may produce cold.

Deficient spleen yang leads to the spleen's failure to perform its function, resulting in dyspepsia, abdominal distension and loose thin stools. As it is due to deficiency and cold, epigastric and abdominal pain relieved by pressure and warmth occurs. Since the middle energizer is weak and cold, a tasteless mouth and no thirst result. As yang is deficient, cold limbs occur. As aqueous liquid cannot be transmitted, urination may be difficult and puffiness of the limbs and trunk may appear and clear, thin and profuse leukorrhea when it escapes from the lower portion of the body.

Treatment: Warmly reinforce spleen yang with prescriptions, such as Decoction of Regulating Spleen and Stomach[60] or warm the spleen and promote water metabolism with Spleen-reinforcing Cold Decoction[61] or by puncturing *Zusanli* (S 36), *Pishu* (B 20), *Weishu* (B 21), *Dachangshu* (B 25) and *Shuifen* (Ren 9) with tonifying manipulation and do moxibustion on them with a moxa stick.

10-3-3-3 Blocked spleen *qi*

Clinical picture: Dizziness, low voice, short breath, epigastric distension immediately after meals, sensation of heaviness and dropping of epigastric and abdominal regions, desire for frequent urination or prolapse of rectum due to prolonged diarrhea or uteroptosis, etc.

Analysis of symptoms: Blocked spleen *qi* is also called a "trap of the middle *qi*" or "trap of deficient *qi*." It is from a weak spleen and insufficient gastrosplenic *qi* and also from prolonged diarrhea or fatigue and lack of physical exercise.

Since spleen *qi* descends abnormally, rather than ascending and clear yang *qi* cannot ascend to the head, vertigo results; as gastrosplenic *qi* is weak and chest *qi* deficient, shortness of breath, low voice and general lassitude may be seen; because the spleen cannot carry on its transporting function, epigastric distension appears immediately after eating; as weak *qi* fails to strengthen the body surface, spontaneous sweating appears;

owing to abnormal descent of gastrosplenic *qi*, a sensation of heavy and dropping epigastrium and abdomen, frequent urination, or prolapse of anus or uteroptosis result.

Treatment: Nourish *qi* to check an abnormally ascending spleen *qi* with Gastrosplenic Qi Reinforcing Decoction[2] or by puncturing *Zusanli* (S 36) and *Pishu* (B 20), *Qihai* (Ren 6), *Baihui* (GV 20) and *Changqiang* (GV 1) with tonifying manipulation and do moxibustion on them with a moxa stick.

10-3-3-4 The spleen's failure to govern blood.

Clinical picture: Bloody stools, muscular epistaxis or polymenorrhea, metrorrhagia and other hemorrhages, etc. possibly accompanied by symptoms of deficient spleen *qi* or spleen yang.

Analysis of symptoms: The spleen's failure to govern blood is caused by weak and impaired spleen *qi* due to a prolonged illness or injury of the spleen by overfatigue and lack of physical exercise.

Spleen *qi* governs blood. If weak, it will fail to control blood, so that the blood cannot circulate along the meridian, but exudes through the skin, causing subcutaneous bleeding; if it exudes through the bladder, bloody urine results. Deficient *qi* leads to the weak Strategic Vessel Meridian and Conception Vessel Meridian, causing polymenorrhea or metrorrhagia, etc.

Treatment: Nourish *qi* and check extravasating blood with *Guipi* Decoction[22] or by puncturing *Pishu* (B 20), *Xuehai* (Sp 10), *Yinbai* (Sp 1) *Sanyinjiao* (Sp 6) with moderate manipulation.

10-3-3-5 Pathogenic cold-damp stagnating in the spleen

Clinical picture: Fullness and distension of the epigastrium and abdomen, anorexia, nausea and desire for vomiting, tasteless mouth with no thirst, abdominal pain and diarrhea, sensation of heavy head; heaviness or swelling of the body, dark yellowish complexion, flabby tongue with glossy coating and soft slow pulse.

Analysis of symptoms: Indulgence in cold drinks and overeating unripened and cold fruit result in pathogenic cold-damp stagnating in the middle energizer of the body. Exposure to rain or wading or living in a humid place causes the inward invasion of pathogenic cold-damp or prolonged excessive endogenous pathogenic damp and obstructed spleen yang and even production of endogenous pathogenic cold-damp.

Since the spleen is obstructed by endogenous pathogenic cold-damp and fails to perform its transporting and digesting functions and its *qi* fails to move the purified (nutrient) upward, epigastric distension and fullness, poor appetite, nausea and vomiting, abdominal pain and loose stools result; as the cold-damp stagnates in the meridian and obstructs *qi*, the sensation of a heavy head and body result; pathogenic damp exuding through the skin leads to edema. When the spleen is obstructed by damp and cannot perform its functions and *qi* and blood cannot nourish the exterior of the body, the skin is internally blocked with no body fluids consumed, there is a tasteless mouth with no thirst.

Treatment: Warm the middle energizer (spleen and stomach) and remove pathogenic damp with *Weiling* Decoction[62] or by puncturing *Zhongwan* (Ren 12), *Weishu* (B 21), *Zusanli* (S 36), *Gongsun* (Sp 4) and *Neiguan* (P 6) with moderate manipulation and do moxibustion on them with a moxa stick.

10-3-3-6 Pathogenic damp-heat stagnating in the spleen and stomach

Clinical picture: Fullness and distension of the epigastrium and abdomen, vomiting and anorexia, sensation of heavy trunk and limbs, loose stools, dark-red scanty urine with heavy trunk and yellow face, eyes and skin or itchy skin, or rising or falling fever still persistent after sweating, yellow glossy tongue coating and soft rapid pulse.

Analysis of symptoms: The affection of pathogenic damp-heat or improper diet, overeating and drinking too much alcohol forms pernicious damp-heat that stagnates in the spleen and stomach.

Pathogenic damp-heat stagnating in the spleen and stomach results in their dysfunction, with epigastric fullness, distension of the abdomen, vomiting and anorexia. As the damp-heat obstructs and acts upon the intestine, there are loose stools, dark-red scanty urine with dysuria; since the damp-heat in the spleen and stomach severely affects the liver and gallbladder and bile is discharged, itchy skin, icteric face, eyes and skin occur; as pathogenic damp is mucoid and glossy, and it combines with pathogenic heat, an undulating fever not relieved by sweating results. A yellow glossy tongue coating and soft, rapid pulse are the signs of pathogenic damp-heat.

Treatment: Clear up pathogenic heat and remove pathogenic damp with Detoxicating Pills for General Relief[63] or by puncturing *Zhongwan* (Ren 12), *Weishu* (B 21), *Pishu* (B 20), *Yinlingquan* (Sp 9) and *Xuehai* (Sp 10) with purging manipulation.

10-3-3-7 Stomach cold syndrome

Clinical picture: Persistent epigastric coldness and pain which becomes rigid and excruciating in severe cases, and is aggravated by pernicious cold and alleviated by warmth. Tasteless mouth and no thirst, overflowing clear liquid in the mouth, or vomiting after meals and borborygmi, light-coloured tongue with white slippery coating and stringy or slow pulse appear.

Analysis of symptoms: Stomach cold syndrome is due to a prolonged weak stomach associated with contaminated food and overeating unripened cold food or the affection of epigastric and abdominal regions by exogenous pathogenic cold so that pathogenic cold is retained in the stomach.

Since pathogenic cold lies in the stomach and stomach yang is obstructed, epigastric cold and pain occur; as warmth can dissipate pathogenic cold, the cold and pain are relieved by it; as stomach yang is affected by pathogenic cold and pernicious *yin* (excess exudates), clear aqueous liquid overflowing in the mouth results. Borborygmi arouses if *yin* is retained in the stomach and intestine. Since pathogenic cold stagnates in the middle energizer and stomach *qi* is regurgitated, vomiting after meals may appear.

Treatment: Warm the middle energizer and dissipate pathogenic cold with Decoction for Warming the Spleen and Stomach with Magnolia Bark[64] or by puncturing *Zhongwan* (Ren 12), *Zusanli* (S 36), *Gongsun* (Sp 4), *Neiguan* (P 6) with tonifying manipulation and do moxibustion on them with a moxa stick.

10-3-3-8 Stomach fire syndrome

Clinical picture: A burning pain in the epigastrium, acid regurgitation and *cao-za*[141] thirst and indulgence in cold drinks, insatiable hunger[142] or vomiting immediately after meals or stomachache after eating or drinking, ozostomia, or swelling and pain in the gums, bleeding gums, constipation, red tongue with yellow coating and slippery rapid pulse are seen.

Analysis of symptoms: Stomach fire syndrome is formed due to a combination of the relative-excess stomach heat and depressed fire because of emotional factors or invasion of the stomach by pathogenic heat and overeating pungent food (or drugs) of a hot nature.

As pathogenic heat stagnates in the stomach, a burning pain in the epigastrium results; if depressed fire in the liver enters the stomach together with regurgitating *qi*, there may be acid regurgitation and *cao-za*; as pathogenic fire has the action of digesting food, there is ozostomia and swelling and pain in the gums and bleeding gums and extravasating blood due to injury of blood vessels by burning fire. As pernicious heat is excessive in the yangming meridian and consumes body fluids, thirst and indulgence in cold drinks and constipation result.

Treatment: Clear up the stomach and purge pathogenic fire with Heart-fire Clearing Decoction[43] or *Yunü* Decoction[65] or by puncturing *Zhongwan* (Ren 12), *Neiguan* (P 6), *Zusanli* (S 36) and *Gongsun* (Sp 4) with purging manipulation.

10-3-3-9 Food retention in the epigastrium

Clinical picture: Epigastric distension and pain, anorexia, thick glossy tongue coating and slippery pulse.

Analysis of symptoms: Food retention is ascribed to improper diet, voracious eating and drinking so that food is retained and is not digested. As the food is retained in the stomach and the stomach is obstructed and the stomach fails to receive food, epigastric distension, fullness and pain and anorexia result. Since the accumulated food is not digested but becomes erosive, and stomach *qi* regurgitates, helitosis or vomiting up sour foul food occurs.

Treatment: Promote digestion with Stomach-harmonizing Pills[66] or by puncturing *Zhongwan* (Ren 12), *Taichong* (Liv 3), *Neiguan* (P 6) and *Zusanli* (S 36) with purging manipulation.

10-3-3-10 Insufficient stomach yin

Clinical picture: A dry mouth and tongue, hunger but no desire to eat or retching and hiccup, uncomfortable epigastrium, constipation, scanty urine, bright red tongue with little fluid and minute rapid pulse.

Analysis of symptoms: It is usually caused by the consumption of yin fluid by fire. As stomach yin is deficient, body fluids fail to ascend, so that the lips and tongue become dry and the stomach is not moistened, resulting in poor appetite. Owing to failure of the stomach *qi* to propel downward, retching and hiccup occur. Since deficient body fluids produce heat that disturbs the stomach, epigastric fullness and discomfort result, and the intestinal tract is not moistened due to a dry stomach caused by injury of body fluid with constipation. As stomach fluid is too deficient to ascend, a red and dry tongue appears.

Treatment: Replenish stomach yin with Stomach-nourishing Decoction[67] or by puncturing *Zusanli* (S 36), *Neiguan* (P 6), *Gongsun* (Sp 4), *Dachangshu* (B 25), *Weishu* (B 21), *Pishu* (B 20) with purging manipulation.

10-3-4 Identification of liver and gallbladder disorders

Identification of liver and gallbladder disorders

The liver performs its dispersing and discharging functions, stores blood and should flourish and not be restrained. It governs muscles and opens to the eye. It is reflected by the nail and is closely related to the gallbladder. Therefore, vertigo, rigid tendons and vessels caused by the movement of endogenous pathogenic wind, stagnant *qi* and blood, distension, fullness and pain, depression and discomfort or restlessness and irascibility caused by the liver and gallbladder's failure to perform their functions and varieties of eye troubles, etc. are mainly pathological changes of the liver. As the liver and gallbladder affect digestion, their dysfunction often influences the spleen and stomach, manifested as the abnormal reception, digestion and absorption of food.

A liver disease (or syndrome) is of the deficient or excess type. The deficient one is often seen in deficient liver yin and liver blood and the excess type is often an excess of *qi* fire or invasion and disturbance of pathogenic damp-heat. The syndrome caused by the movement and upward disturbance of endogenous yang wind is a deficiency disease with excess symptoms.

10-3-4-1 Stagnant liver *qi*

Clinical picture: Emotional depression, irascibility, chest distress and preference for sighing, distension and pain in the chest and hypochondria or breasts and on either side of the lower abdomen, dysmenorrhea, irregular menstruation and stringy pulse, plum-stone syndrome[135] or goiter in the neck and nape or abdominal masses.

Analysis of symptoms: Stagnant liver *qi* is caused by an emotional depression or injury of the liver by depressed anger or the liver's failure to perform its functions due to other reasons.

Since the liver fails to perform its dispersing and discharging functions, mental depression occurs; as the *qi* flow is obstructed, chest distress and sighing appear with prolonged mental depression and irascibility. As liver *qi* is stagnant and the meridian is obstructed, distension and pain appear in the chest, hypochondria, or breasts and on either side of the lower abdomen where the Liver Meridian traverses. Since the *qi* disorder affects blood and stagnant *qi* causes blood stasis and disharmony between the Strategic Vessel Meridian and the Conception Vessel Meridian, irregular menstruation or abdominal pain during the menstrual period is seen. As liver *qi* regurgitates and combines with phlegm in the throat, a plum-stone syndrome results; the accumulating phlegmatic *qi* leads to goiter; a prolonged depression and stagnant *qi* and blood may cause abdominal masses.

Treatment: Relieve stagnant liver *qi* with Liver-soothing Powders with Buplerum Root.[68] It is advisable to treat a plum-stone syndrome by regulating *qi* and subduing phlegm with *Si Qi* Decoction with Buplerum Root,[69] Goiter Seaweed Decoction,[70] and abdominal masses, by promoting blood circulation and softening the firm with Turtle Shell Pills[71] or by puncturing *Neiguan* (P 6), *Xingjian* (Liv 2), *Sanyinjiao* (Sp 6), *Taichong* (Liv 3), *Ganshu* (B 18) and *Qimen* (Liv 14) with moderate manipulation.

10-3-4-2 Blazing liver fire

Clinical picture: Headache, vertigo, tinnitus, flushed face and congestive eyes, bitter mouth and dry throat, burning pain in the hypochondria and intercostal regions, restlessness and irascibility, insomnia, nightmares or hematemesis and epistaxis, constipation and dark-red urine, red tongue with yellow rough coating, and stringy rapid pulse.

Analysis of symptoms: Blazing liver fire is caused by pernicious fire produced by a depressed liver and the adverse fire induced by excess *qi*.

As liver fire is likely to flare up and attack the head, headache, vertigo, tinnitus, flushed face and congestive eyes result; the depression of the Liver Meridian by fire leads to burning heat in the hypochondria and intercostal region; if it ascends together with gallbladder *qi*, a bitter mouth and dry throat may be seen; if it still flares up, a hot temper and irascibility and even mania will appear; since the disturbing fire causes mental restlessness, dreaminess and insomnia occur; if it injures blood vessels and causes the extravasated blood, hematemesis and epistaxis may result, when it consumes body fluids, constipation and dark-red scanty urine will appear.

Treatment: Clear up liver fire with Pills of Chinese Angelica Root, Chinese Gentian and Aloes[72] or Decoction of Reducing Liver Fire with Chinese Gentian[73] or by puncturing *Taichong* (Liv 3), *Xiaxi* (GB 43), *Qiuxu* (GB 40), *Neiguan* (P 6), *Zhigou* (TE 6) and *Ganshu* (B 18) with purging manipulation.

10-3-4-3 Insufficient liver blood

Clinical picture: Dull complexion, vertigo, dreaminess, tinnitus, dry and uncomfortable eyes, blurred vision or night blindness, numb trunk and limbs, or rigid tendons and vessels, twisting muscles, pale nails, oligomenorrhea or amenorrhea, light-coloured tongue and minute pulse.

Analysis of the symptoms: Insufficient liver blood is caused by insufficient blood, or excessive blood loss or consumption of liver blood by a prolonged illness.

Insufficient liver blood cannot nourish the head and face, so pallor, vertigo, tinnitus and light-coloured tongue may result; as blood cannot nourish the eye, dry and uncomfortable eyes, blurred vision or night blindness appear. Since the musculofascia meridian is not nourished by nutritional blood, the nails are not bright; since deficient blood induces the movement of endogenous wind, numb limbs, spasmotic tendons and twisting muscles are seen. As insufficient blood cannot enrich blood vessels, a minute pulse occurs. Since the "sea of blood"[136] is empty, oligomenorrhea and amenorrhea result. As blood is not sufficient enough to soothe the nerves, dreaminess is likely to appear.

Treatment: Replenish and tonify liver blood with Liver-tonifying Decoction[74] or by puncturing *Ququan* (Liv 8), *Ganshu* (B 18), *Pishu* (B 20), *Xuehai* (Sp 10) and *Sanyinjiao* (Sp 6).

10-3-4-4 Excess rise of liver yang

Clinical picture: Vertigo and tinnitus, distension and headache, flushed face and congestive eyes, irascibility, insomnia, dreaminess, amenorrhea, palpitation, weak loin and knees, dark-red tongue and minute rapid pulse.

Analysis of symptoms: Excess rise of liver yang is caused by the failure of deficient liver and kidney yin to restrain liver yang or depressed anger and anxiety, transformation of depressed *qi* into fire, consumed yin blood and the failure of yin to restrain yang. The disease is due to yin deficiency and its symptoms are an excess of yang or a yin deficiency and hyperactive liver.

As liver yin and kidney yin are insufficient and yang *qi* is in excess, vertigo and tinnitus, aching and distending head, flushed face and congestive eyes and irascibility result. Since yin deficiency would cause unrestrained yang, and malnourished *shen* (Spirit) palpitation and amnesia, insomnia and dreaminess may appear. As the liver governs tendons, the kidney controls bones and deficient yin leads to overactive fire and malnourished tendons and bones. The loin and knees are weak. A dark-red tongue and a stringy, minute and rapid pulse are the signs of vigorous fire induced by deficient yin and the excessive rise of liver yang.

Treatment: Replenish the yin, check the overactive liver and restrain the yang with Pills of Wolfberry Fruit, Chrysanthemum Flower[75] and Prepared Rythmannia Root or Cold Decoction of *Gastrodia Tuber* and *Uncaria Rhynchophyla*[76] or by puncturing *Taichong* (Liv 3), *Xingjian* (Liv 2), *Waiguan* (TE 5), *Sanyinjiao* (Sp 6) and *Taixi* (K 3) with tonifying manipulation.

10-3-4-5 Liver wind moving internally

Tremor, vertigo, and convulsions, etc. appearing in a pathological process are known as liver wind. Those that are commonly seen are endogenous pathogenic wind derived from liver yang, endogenous pathogenic wind due to extreme heat and endogenous pathogenic wind due to deficient blood. It is treated by puncturing *Taichong* (Liv 3), *Yanglingquan* (GB 34), *Baihui* (GV 20) and *Fengchi* (GB 20).

a. Endogenous wind derived from liver yang

Clinical picture: Vertigo, headache, numbness and tremor of limbs, peristalsis of hands and feet, incoherent speech, a floating way of walking, red tongue and stringy and minute pulse. If sudden fainting, stiff tongue, facial paralysis and hemiplegia occur, there will be windstroke (apoplexy).

Analysis of symptoms: As liver yin and kidney yin are severely consumed, yang *qi* is not restrained but overactive and produces endogenous pathogenic wind.

As wind yang is overactive and fire rises excessively, headache and vertigo with immediate fainting occur; numb and twitching limbs and peristalsis of hands and feet, incoherent speech are all signs of the movement of endogenous pathogenic wind. The wind moves in the upper portion of the body indicating the excess in the upper portion of the body; the yin is consumed in the middle, and deficiency is consumed in the lower body. Since excess wind yang consumes body fluids, changes them into phlegm and disturbs the upper portion of the body together with phlegm and mists the mind, sudden fainting occurs. As wind-phlegm affects the meridian and blood is disharmonious, facial paralysis, hemiplegia and stiffness of the tongue may result.

Treatment: Cultivate the yin, check the overactive liver and expel endogenous pathogenic wind with Decoction of Checking Overactive Liver and Eliminating Wind.[77] For *bi* (blockage) syndrome of apoplexy, treat with Treasure Pills[78] or Storax Pills[46]: for the *yun* (collapse) syndrome, give first aid with Ginseng and Aconiti Decoction[24] or Rehmannia Root Cold Decoction[79] or puncture the above-mentioned acupoints plus *Quchi* (LI 11), and *Hegu* (LI 4). For sudden unconsciousness, add *Renzhong* (GV 4); for stiff tongue, add *Lianquan* (Ren 23), for facial paralysis, add *Jiache* (S 6) and *Dichang* (GB 30) and *Yanglingquan* (GB 34).

b. Extreme heat producing wind

Clinical picture: It is mainly caused by the affection of the Liver Meridian and pericardium by excess pathogenic heat.

As extreme heat consumes body fluids, high fever and thirst occur. As the heat affects the Liver Meridian and the tendons and vessels are malnourished with the movement of endogenous wind, convulsions and stiffness at the nape of the neck, opisthotonos and upward fixation of the eye result; since the heat enters the pericardium and disturbs the heart (mind), restlessness results; if it obstructs the heart (mind), there will be coma.

Treatment: Clear up pathogenic heat in the liver and expel endogenous pathogenic wind with Antelope's Horn and *Uncaria Rhynchophylla* Decoction.[80] It is advisable to treat a coma patient by resuscitation with Bezoar Resurrection Pills,[81] or by puncturing the above-mentioned acupoints plus *Renzhong* (GV 26) with moderate manipulation, *Zhongchong* (P 9) causing a little bleeding and *Dazhui* (GV 14) with moderate manipulation, causing a little bleeding.

c. Wind produced by deficient blood: Insufficient blood and malnourished tendons and vessels would lead to the movement of endogenous pathogenic wind due to asthma. As to its pulse and symptoms and treatment, refer to "The Deficient Liver Blood

Syndrome." Or treat it by puncturing the above-mentioned acupoints plus *Pishu* (B 20), *Ganshu* (B 18) and *Xuehai* (Sp 10) with moderate manipulation.

10-3-4-6 Cold stagnating in the Liver Meridian

Clinical picture: Dropping, distension and pain on the bilateral side of the lower abdomen that affects the testes, or contraction of the scrotum aggravated by cold, but relieved by heat, accompanied by cold trunk and limbs, white slippery coating of the tongue, deep stringy or slow pulse, etc.

Analysis of symptoms: Stagnant *qi* and blood in the Liver Meridian reach the bilateral side of the lower abdomen by running around the external genitalia and *qi* and blood in the meridian are stagnant due to retention of cold in the meridian, dropping, distension and pain on the bilateral side of the lower abdomen that affects the testes; since cold is concerned with contraction, coldness and contraction of the scrotum are seen. As heat helps to unblock and cold leads to stagnation, the pain is aggravated by cold, but relieved by heat. Owing to cold stagnating in the Liver Meridian and yang *qi* failing to distribute, cold trunk and limbs result, while a slippery tongue coating and deep stringy or slow pulse are all cold and painful signs.

Cold stagnating in the Liver Meridian is often seen in cold hernia. As it is characterized by dropping, distension and pain of *qi* in the small intestine that spreads from the lower abdomen to the Scrotum, it is also known as *qi* pain in the small intestine.

Treatment: Warm the liver and dissipate pathogenic cold with prescriptions, such as Liver-warming Decoction[82] or by puncturing *Chengjiang* (Ren 24), (moderate manipulation), *Taichong* (Liv 3), (moderate manipulation), *Qihai* (Ren 6) (moxibustion with a moxa stick) and *Guanyuan* (Ren 4) (moxibustion with a moxa stick).

10-3-4-7 Pathogenic damp-heat stagnating in the liver

Clinical picture: Distension and pain in the hypochondriac and intercostal region, bitter mouth and dyspepsia, nausea and abdominal distension, irregular bowel movements, dark-red scanty urine, yellow greasy tongue coating and stringy, rapid pulse; or yellow body and eyes, alternate chills and fever, eczema of the scrotum, swelling, distension, heat and pain in the testes, yellow, foul leukorrhea in women, itching external genitalia, etc.

Analysis of symptoms: Pathogenic damp-heat stagnating in the liver is caused by pathogenic damp affection or too much alcohol and rich food which produces pernicious damp-heat or dysfunctions of the spleen and stomach that produce pernicious damp and turbid matter. Depressed damp turns into pernicious heat and both damp and heat stagnate in the liver and gallbladder.

As pernicious damp-heat is stagnant and the liver and gallbladder cannot perform their functions, distension and pain in the hypochondriac and intercostal regions result; regurgitation of gallbladder *qi* leads to a bitter taste; as the damp-heat is obstructed, the spleen fails to send the purified matter upward, so dyspepsia, nausea, abdominal pain and irregular bowel movements result; as the damp and heat steam each other and the bile overflows outward, yellow skin and eyes may be seen; as the pathogenic factor stagnates in the *shaoyang* meridian, alternate chills and fever may occur; as the damp and heat descend, dark-red scanty urine may be seen; since the Liver Meridian winds around the genital organs, the damp-heat descends, with eczema of the scrotum or a swelling, distension, hotness and pain in the testes, or itchy external genitalia and yellow foul leukorrhea seen in women.

Treatment: Clear up and expel pathogenic damp-heat and soothe the liver and gallbladder with Oriental Wormwood Decoction[83] or *Xiegan* Decoction with Chinese Gentian[73] or by puncturing *Qiuxu* (GB 40), *Neiguan* (P 6) and *Yanglingquan* (GB 34), *Sanyinjiao* (Sp 6).

10-3-4-8 Stasis of gallbladder *qi* and disturbance of phlegm

Clinical picture: Vertigo, bitter mouth, nausea, restlessness and insomnia, palpitation with fear, chest distress and preference for sighing, yellow glossy tongue coating and stringy slippery pulse.

Analysis of symptoms: It is caused by emotional factors, production of phlegm by depressed *qi*, internally disturbing phlegm-heat, gallbladder dysfunction and the stomach being disposed to propel downward.

As the Gallbladder Meridian connects with the head and eyes and the phlegm and turbid matter disturb the upper portion of the body along the meridian, vertigo results; since the gallbladder is a clearing organ, phlegm-heat disturbs it internally disrupting *qi* and restlessness, insomnia and palpitation with fright may be caused. Because of the obstruction by phlegm and the turbid matter, the gallbladder's dysfunction, blocked *qi*, chest distress and preference for sighing result. When the stomach propels downward, nausea and vomiting result.

Treatment: Clear up pernicious phlegm-heat, depress the upward adverse flow of stomach *qi* with Gallbladder-warming Decoction with Coptis Root[84] or by puncturing *Qiuxu* (GB 40), *Zulingqi* (GB 41), *Neiguan* (P 6), *Xingjian* (Liv 2) with purging manipulation.

10-3-5 Identification of kidney and bladder disorders

The kidney, the congenital foundation, stores *jing* (vital principle), governs bones and produces medulla. Linked with the brain, it controls body fluid, absorbs *qi*, opens to the ears and external genitalia and the anus, reflects on the hair and is closely related to the bladder. Therefore, the abnormal growth, development, genital function water metabolism and pathological process of the brain, medulla, bones and respiration, hearing and defecation and micturation are all ascribed to it.

Primordial yin and yang stored in the kidney is the foundation of human growth and development. Primordial yin pertains to water and primordial yang, fire, so it is said that "the kidney is the residence of water and fire." Primordial yin and yang should be stored, but not consumed and excreted. Although pathological changes of the kidney vary, they are mainly deficient kidney yang, deficient kidney yin, consumed kidney *jing* (vital principle) and deficient kidney *qi*.

10-3-5-1 Deficient kidney yang

It is also termed a decline of *mingmen* (vital portal) fire. As the foundation of yang *qi* of the entire body, kidney yang has the function of warming the body, consuming aqueous liquid and promoting growth and development. If it is deficient and declines, it will fail to perform its warming function, resulting in disease and fear of cold and cold limbs, sexual hypofunction and overflowing water, etc.

a. Insufficient kidney yang

Clinical picture: Pallor, cold limbs and trunk, listlessness, sore and cold loin and kidney, impotence, cold uterus and infertility, light-coloured tongue with white coating, deep, minute and weak pulse, particularly at the *chi* section of the wrist.

Analysis of symptoms: Insufficient kidney yang is caused by deficient yang, a weak kidney or impairment and consumption of kidney yang by a prolonged illness or excessive sexual activity.

Since deficient yang cannot warm the body and invigorate Spirit, cold limbs and trunk, pallor, mental fatigue and lassitude may appear. As the loin is the residence of the kidney, declining kidney yang and deficient yang in the lower portion of the body would lead to a sore loin and knees. Since the kidney is concerned with production, declining fire due to yang deficiency and genital hypofunction would cause impotence, cold uterus and infertility. As the pulse at the *chi* section corresponds to the kidney, deficient yang's failure to invigorate the pulse would result in a deep minute pulse, especially at the *chi* section.

Treatment: Tonify kidney yang with kidney-*qi* Pills[85] or *Yougui* Cold Decoction[86] or by puncturing *Shenshu* (B 23), *Guanyuan* (Ren 4), *Fuliu* (K 7) and *Zusanli* (S 36) with tonifying manipulation and do moxibustion on them with a moxa stick.

b. Overflowing water due to yin deficiency

Clinical picture: Fear of cold, cold limbs, oliguria and swelling in the body that is severe below the loin, distension in the abdomen, sore loin and cold limbs, or palpitation and short breath, asthmatic breath, cough and rattling throat, light-coloured flabby and indented tongue with white slippery coating and deep stringy pulse.

Analysis of symptoms: This problem is mainly due to the disharmony of the body caused by a prolonged illness, a weak constitution, or consumed kidney yang that cannot warm aqueous liquid. As deficient yang and declining fire fail to warm the body, cold limbs and trunk result.

Since the bladder cannot evaporate body fluids due to deficiency caused by deficient and declining kidney yang, dysuria and oliguria occur. As aqueous liquid cannot be smoothly excreted but stagnates internally and overflows in the skin, general edema appears. As aqueous liquid cannot ascend but descends, severe swelling below the loin is seen. Water retention due to deficient yang and blocked *qi* leads to abdominal distention and fullness. Since pernicious water overflows and regurgitates affecting the heart and lung, palpitation, asthmatic breath, cough and short breath results. As overflowing water forms and phlegm and *tan-yin* (phlegm and excess exudates) invade the lung, a rattling throat may occur. A flabby, delicate and indented tongue with white slippery coating and deep stringy pulse are the signs of yang deficiency with water.

Treatment: Warm the yang and remove excessive fluid through diuresis with *Zhenwu* Decoction[88] and Kidney-*qi* Pills for Saving Lives[89] or by puncturing *Shenshu* (B 23), *Guanyuan* (CV 4), *Shifen* (CV 9), *Sanyinjiao* (Sp 6) and *Zusanli* (S 36) with tonifying manipulation and do moxibustion on them with a moxa stick. For the case with asthmatic breath, add *Feishu* (B 13), *Dingchuan* (Extra 17) and *Fuliu* (K 7).

10-3-5-2 Deficient kidney yin

Deficient kidney yin is also termed insufficient kidney water. As the foundation of yin fluid for the entire body, kidney yin has the function of moistening the superficial body and viscera, enriching the brain and bones, restraining overactive yang and fire, so as to maintain normal growth and development and functions such as reproduction, etc. If it is consumed and impaired, the superficial body and marrow will be insufficient and *mingmen* (vital portal) fire and kidney yang will not be restrained, but often do harm with its hyperactivity.

Clinical picture: Vertigo, tinnitus, decreased vision, amnesia, and insomnia, sore and weak loin and knees, emaciation, dry throat and tongue aggravated at night, fever in the chest, palms and soles or tidal fever in the afternoon, night sweat and malar flush, spermatorrhea, oligomenorrhea and amenorrhea, or metrorrhagia in women, red tongue with less dry coating and minute rapid pulse.

Analysis of symptoms: Injury of the kidney by a prolonged illness, or excessive sexual activity, or consumed blood or too much warm food or drugs harmful to yin or internal injury from emotional factors and prolonged consumption of kidney yin.

As kidney yin is deficient, the brain and bones are malnourished, so vertigo, amnesia, tinnitus and sores and weak loin and knees may result; as the vital principle of yin fails to ascend to nourish the eyes, decreased and blurred vision result; as the body, mouth and tongue are not replenished by yin fluid, a dry throat and mouth and emaciation occur. Since deficient yin fails to restrain yang and pernicious fire (intense heat) due to deficiency moves internally, fever in the chest, palms and soles, or tidal fever in the afternoon, malar flush and night sweat result; as pernicious fire disturbs the heart (mind), insomnia appears; as the fire disturbs the *jing* (vital principle) chamber (kidney), spermatorrhea occurs. Since *jing* and blood are deficient, oligomenorrhea or amenorrhea appears. If fire due to deficiency disturbs the interior of the body and blood heat is in aberration, metrorrhagia may be seen.

Treatment: Replenish and tonify kidney yin with Six-ingredient Pills with Rehmannia Root[90] or replenish yin and remove pernicious fire with Pills of Anemarhena Rhizome, Phellodendron Bark and prepared Rehmannia Root[91] or by puncturing *Shenshu* (B 23), *Pishu* (B 20), *Rangu* (K 2), *Sanyinjiao* (Sp 6), *Tongli* (H 5) and *Shenmen* (H 7) with moderate manipulation. For the case of nocturnal emission and abnormal menstruation, add *Guanyuan* (CV 4) (moderate manipulation).

10-3-5-3 Weak kidney *qi*

Clinical picture: Mental fatigue, sore and weak loin and knee, frequent and clear urine that dribbles after urination, or enuresis and incontinence of urine, frequent night urination, spermatorrhea and prospermia, clear thin leukorrhea, moving fetus that is easily delivered, etc.

Analysis of symptoms: Weak kidney *qi* due to senility, or insufficient infant kidney *qi* or impairment of the kidney by prolonged illness and overexertion may weaken kidney *qi*. As kidney *qi* is weakened and its functions decline, mental fatigue and sore and weak loin and knee may appear. Since the kidney is weak and the bladder is not controlled by it, frequent clear urine, dribbling urine after micturation, frequent night urination and even enuresis result. Deficient kidney *qi* and the uncontrolled *jing* chamber lead to spermatorrhea and prospermia; declining and deficient yang *qi* fails to strengthen and protect the Strategic Vessel Meridian and the Conception Vessel Meridian which leads to clear thin leukorrhea and miscarriage.

Treatment: Tonify the kidney and arrest spermatorrhea with Pills of Enriching Kidney *jing*[87] or by puncturing *Shenshu* (B 23), *Mingmen* (GV 4), *Guanyuan* (CV 4) and *Zhongji* (CV 3) with tonifying manipulation and do moxibustion with a moxa stick.

10-3-5-4 Insufficient kidney *jing* (vital principle)

Clinical picture: Infertility due to spermatorrhea in men and amenorrhea in women, delayed development of infants, retardation of intelligence and movement, atrophy and weakness of bones, delayed closing of the fontanel. Presenility, hair loss and loose teeth, amnesia and trance, atrophic and weak feet, retardation of movement, etc.

Analysis of symptoms: Congenital deficiency, prenatal maldevelopment or postnatal malnutrition, fatigue, lassitude and injury of the kidney by prolonged illness.

The function of kidney *jing* is for reproduction and development. If it is insufficient, infertility due to spermatorrhea in men or amenorrhea in women will result. The kidney is the congenital foundation. If its *jing* is deficient, the bone marrow is not enriched and the bones and brain are malnourished, the Five Delays[137] and Five Softnesses[138] in young children and presenility in adults and atrophic and weak feet, mental dullness, retardation of movement, etc. may be seen.

Treatment: Tonify and nourish kidney *jing* with *Dazao* Pills of Human Placenta[92] or by puncturing *Shenshu* (B 23), *Taixi* (K 3), *Xuanzhong* (GB 39) and *Mingmen* (GV 4) with tonifying manipulation; for the case of delayed closing of the fontanel and dullness, add *Baihui* (GV 20) and *Sishencong* (Extra 6) with moderate manipulation.

10-3-5-5 Exogenous pathogenic damp-heat stagnating in the bladder

Clinical picture: Hasty urination, frequent urination, oliguria and dysuria, yellow dark-red and cloudy urine or hematuria, or scanty urine. It may be associated with fever and lumbago, yellow glossy tongue coating and rapid pulse.

Analysis of symptoms: As exogenous pathogenic damp-heat stagnates in the bladder so that *qi* function is abnormal, urine and difficulty and dribbling in urination result; as the damp-heat descends affecting the urinary tract, owing to the obstructed damp-heat, dysuria occurs; if the yin collateral meridians are injured, hematuria may result and calculus forms due to a prolonged affection of damp-heat, which can be excreted together with urine. Fever may be seen if the damp-heat is stagnant and steaming. The bladder is closely related with the kidney and the yang viscera disorder involves the yin one. Therefore, the blockage of the kidney by damp-heat may cause lumbago.

Treatment: Clear up pathogenic heat, remove pathogenic damp and regulate urination with *Bazheng* Pills[93] or by puncturing *Zhongji* (Ren 3), *Yinlingquan* (Sp 9), *Pangguangshu* (B 28), *Xuehai* (Sp 4) and *Shenshu* (B 23) with purging manipulation.

10-3-6 Identification of visceral disorders

As there is a close connection between the functions of the viscera, they often influence one another when pathological changes occur. It is called a viscera disorder when more than two internal organs are affected successively or simultaneously.

Although the symptoms of viscera disorder are rather complex, they are general disorders of a yin viscus complicated by the disorder of another viscus.

10-3-6-1 Disharmony between the heart and kidney

Heart yang descends to warm kidney water; kidney yin ascends to support the heart and nourish heart fire. Harmony between the two yin viscera leads to mutual support between water and fire. If kidney yin is deficient, but heart fire is excessive, or heart fire fails to descend and harmonize with kidney yin and kidney yang, water and fire of the heart and kidney do not support each other, and disharmony between the heart and kidney may result.

Clinical picture: Anxiety due to deficiency and insomnia, palpitation and amnesia, dizziness and tinnitus, dry throat, sore and weak loin and knees, nocturnal emission or tidal fever and night sweat, or sore, obstructed and cold loin and knees.

Analysis of symptoms: Injury of heart yin and kidney yin, prolonged illness, fatigue and lack of physical exercise, excessive sexual activity, or five extreme emotions, extreme heart fire downwardly affecting kidney yin or extreme heart fire's failure to harmonize with the kidney.

As kidney water fails to ascend, heart fire is not restrained, and anxiety due to deficiency and insomnia and palpitation result. When yin *jing* (vital principle) is deficient and consumed, the head and eyes are malnourished and the bone marrow is not enriched, so amnesia, dizziness, tinnitus, dry throat and mouth, sore and weak loin and knees appear. When yin is deficient and yang excessive and the fire goes wild due to deficiency, tidal fever, night sweat, nocturnal emission occur. When heart fire is excessive in the upper portion of the body and kidney water stagnates in the lower, sore weak and cool loin and knees are seen.

Treatment: Harmonize the heart and kidney by replenishing the yin and removing pathogenic fire with Coptis Root and Donkey-hide Gelatin Decoction[94] and *Jiaotai* Pills,[95] or by puncturing *Tongli* (H 5) with moderate manipulation, *Shenmen* (H 7) with moderate manipulation, *Taixi* (K 3) with tonifying manipulation, *Fuliu* (K 7) with tonifying manipulation, *Fengchi* (GB 20) and *Zusanli* (S 36) with moderate manipulation.

10-3-6-2 Deficient heart and kidney yang

As heart and kidney yang both warm the viscera, promote blood circulation and evaporate body fluids, deficient heart and kidney yang often cause pathological changes, such as internal excess yin cold, obstructed blood circulation and aqueous retention, etc.

Clinical picture: Cold body and limbs, palpitations, oliguria and general edema, dark-purplish lips and nails, dark-purplish dull tongue with white slippery coating and deep faint pulse.

Analysis of symptoms: Prolonged illness or fatigue and lack of physical exercise.

As declining yang fails to warm and nourish the body, the body feels cold as heart yang and kidney yang are deficient, cold water cannot evaporate. Since aqueous liquid affects the heart, heart palpitations appear; because aqueous liquid is retained internally, oliguria and general edema are seen. As deficient yang cannot promote blood circulation and blood stagnates, dark-purplish lips and nails and a dark-purplish tongue result. As aqueous damp is stagnant, a white slippery tongue coating may appear.

Treatment: Tonify the heart and kidney with *Zhenwu* Decoction[88] in association with Primordial *Qi* Protecting Decoction[41] or by puncturing *Xinshu* (B 15), *Shenshu* (B 23), *Neiguan* (P 6), *Shuifen* (CV 9) and *Guanyuan* (CV 4) with tonifying manipulation.

10-3-6-3 *Qi* deficiencies of the lung and kidney

The lungs are concerned with gases, and the "lung is the master of *qi* (gases) and the kidney, the root of *qi*." Therefore, deficient kidney *qi* often causes abnormal respiration. It is caused by the kidney's failure to absorb *qi*. This syndrome is a yang deficiency or is immediate exhausted yang *qi* as well as deficient yin which fails to restrain yang.

Clinical picture: Exhaustion and little inhalation, asthmatic and short breath aggravated by exertion and low voice, or spontaneous sweating and enuresis, cold limbs and dark-purplish complexion, light-coloured tongue, cold sweat and an empty, superficial and rootless pulse, or flushed face and restlessness and a red tongue, minute rapid pulse.

Analysis of symptoms: Asthmatic breath and cough due to a prolonged illness, kidney *qi* consumed by overexertion, and impaired lung and kidney.

As lung *qi* and kidney *qi* are deficient, *qi* cannot return to *Guanyuan* (Ren 4) (the kidney cannot absorb *qi*), much exhalation and little inhalation. Asthmatic and short breath aggravated by exertion result. Since lung deficiency leads to faint chest *qi*, a low voice due to shortage of *qi* appears; as *qi* is deficient and defensive yang *qi* is weakened, spontaneous sweating often occurs; because the bladder is out of control, urine discharged along with cough or enuresis and incontinence of urine result. As deficient yang cannot nourish the trunk and limbs, cold limbs, dark-purplish complexion and a light-coloured tongue may be seen.

Immediate exhaustion of yang *qi* leads to cold sweats. As *qi* floats exteriorly, the pulse is empty, superficial and rootless. If it is due to consumed yang, asthmatic breath may occur, frequently accompanied by flushed face and restlessness, dry throat and mouth, red tongue and minute rapid pulse.

Treatment: Tonify the kidney to absorb *qi* with Ginseng and Walnut (*Juglans regia*) Decoction,[96] *Helixi* Pills,[97] Kidney *qi* Replenishing Pills of Seven Ingredients[98] in association with *Shengmai* Powders[99] or by puncturing *Taiyan* (L 9), *Feishu* (B 13) and *Shenshu* (B 23) with tonifying manipulation and do moxibustion on them with a moxa stick.

10-3-6-4 Deficient lung and kidney yin

Yin fluids of the lung and kidney nourish each other and the kidney yin is the foundation of yin fluids of the entire body. If lung yin and kidney yin are deficient and not nourished and moistened, endogenous pathogenic dryness and heat may occur. So regurgitation of *qi* due to the lung's failure to perform its functions and endogenous pathogenic fire due to the kidney not being replenished are the characteristics of pathological changes of deficient lung yin and kidney yin.

Clinical picture: Cough with little sputum, or blood sputum, dry mouth and throat, or coarse voice, sore and weak loin and knees, anxiety and disturbed sleep, "steaming of bone" and tidal fever, night sweat and malar flush, spermatorrhea, irregular menstruation in women, red tongue with little coating and minute rapid pulse.

Analysis of symptoms: Deficient lung and kidney yin is caused by prolonged injury of the lung, so that the weak lung cannot distribute body fluids to replenish the kidney, or overexertion and deficient and exhausted kidney yin make yin fluids ascend or fire due to deficiency affects the lung, forming the syndrome of deficient lung and kidney yin.

As deficient yin causes dryness of the lung, body fluids fail to ascend and the lung is not purified and cough, even coarse voice results. As pernicious fire due to deficiency flares up to affect the lung collateral meridians, hematemesis or bloody sputum result; as deficient yin produces endogenous heat, "steaming of bone" and tidal fever, malar flush and night sweat may appear. Since pathogenic fire disturbs the mind, anxiety and insomnia occur. As yin *jing* (vital principle) is insufficient, fire due to deficiency occurs, disturbing the inside of the body. Spermatorrhea in men, oligomenorrhea and amenorrhea in women or polymenorrhea may be seen.

Treatment: Moisten and tonify the lung and kidney with Lung-reinforcing Decoction with Lily Bulb[32] or by puncturing *Kongzui* (L 6), *Chize* (L 5), *Yuji* (L 10), *Taixi* (K 3), *Fuliu* (K 7) and *Sanyinjiao* (Sp 6) with moderate manipulation.

10-3-6-5 Deficient liver and kidney yin

Liver yin and kidney yin promote each other. Deficient kidney yin often leads to deficient liver yin and vice versa. Since deficient yin results in excess yang, the pathological change of the deficient liver yin syndrome is characterized by consumed and deficient yin fluid and excess yang and aberration of pernicious fire.

Clinical picture: Vertigo, amnesia, tinnitus, dry throat and mouth, hypochondriac pain, sore and weak limbs and knees, fever in the chest, palms and soles, malar flush and night sweat, spermatorrhea, oligomenorrhea in women, red tongue with less coating and minute rapid pulse.

Analysis of symptoms: Internal injury from the "seven emotions" and impaired *jing* (vital principle) and blood by overexertion or liver yin and kidney yin consumed and impaired by prolonged illness.

As liver yin and kidney yin are insufficient, pernicious fire due to deficiency disturbs the upper portion of the body and the head and eyes are not replenished by yin *jing*, a hypochondriac pain results; since fire due to deficient yin is produced internally, fever in the chest, palms and soles, night sweat and malar flush occur; the disturbance of the mind by fire leads to insomnia and affection of the *jing* chamber by fire, and spermatorrhea. The Strategic Vessel Meridian and the Conception Vessel Meridian pertain to the liver and kidney and the weak liver and kidney lead to the vacancy of the two meridians and oligomenorrhea appears. As deficient yin causes endogenous heat, a red tongue with less coating and minute rapid pulse are seen.

Treatment: Replenish and tonify the liver and kidney with Pills of Wolfberry, Chrysanthemum Flower and Prepared Rehmannia Root[75] or by puncturing *Qiuxu* (G 40), *Fuliu* (K 7), *Zhongdu* (Liv 6), *Taichong* (Liv 3), *Shenshu* (B 23) and *Ganshu* (B 18) with moderate manipulation.

10-3-6-6 Deficient spleen and kidney yang

The spleen is the postnatal foundation, while the kidney is the prenatal foundation. Yang *qi* of the spleen and kidney work in coordination with each other to warm the trunk and limbs, and transport and digest food and evaporate body fluids. Therefore, deficient spleen and stomach yang can cause excess internal yin cold and spleen dysfunction.

Clinical picture: Cold trunk and limbs, pallor, coldness and pain in the loin, knees or either side of the lower abdomen, aqueous grainy diarrhea, diarrhea before dawn or puffy face and limbs, difficulty in urination, ascites, light-coloured delicate tongue with a white slippery coating and deep weak pulse.

Analysis of symptoms: *Qi* is consumed and yang is impaired by a prolonged illness or pathogenic water retained during long or persistent diarrhea so that kidney yang is too deficient to nourish spleen yang. Spleen yang becomes weak so that it cannot enrich kidney yang.

As deficient spleen yang and stomach yang do not nourish the body, pallor and cold trunk and limbs result. Since the meridians are obstructed due to deficiency and endogenous pathogenic cold, coldness and pain in the bilateral lower abdomen and loin and knees appear. Since food cannot be digested and transported, aqueous-grainy diarrhea and diarrhea before dawn result; as the yang is too deficient to transport and evaporate aqueous damp, puffy face and limbs occur and internally-accumulating pathogenic water would lead to difficulty in urination and ascites.

Treatment: Tonify the spleen and kidney. For edema, Spleen-reinforcing Cold Decoction[61] is prescribed; for diarrhea, Decoction of Regulating the Spleen and Stomach with Prepared Aconite Root[100] or Four-spirit Pillets[101] is prescribed, or puncture *Yinlingquan* (B 23), *Dadu* (Sp 2), *Fuliu* (K 7), *Qihai* (CV 6), *Guanyuan* (Ren 4), *Pishu* (B 20), *Shenshu* (B 23), *Shuifen* (Ren 9) with tonifying manipulation and do moxibustion on them with a moxa stick.

10-3-6-7 Deficient heart and lung *qi*

The lung is concerned with air, the heart governs the blood vessel, *qi* controls blood and the blood carries *qi*. The reason why deficient heart blood and lung *qi* often influence each other pathologically is that all the blood passes through the lung and the heart and lung are closely related physiologically. If lung *qi* is weak and chest *qi* lacks its resources, blood circulation will not be normally promoted; insufficient heart *qi* and unsmooth blood circulation may also influence the functions of lung *qi*. Hence, deficient heart and lung *qi* causes abnormal respiration and obstructed blood circulation.

Clinical picture: Palpitation and short breath, asthmatic breath due to shortage of *qi*, chest distress, spontaneous sweating and general lassitude aggravated by exertion, pale and dull complexion, even dark-purplish mouth and lips, dull tongue possibly with ecchymosis and minute weak pulse.

Analysis of symptoms: Heart and lung *qi* consumed and impaired by fatigue and lack of exercise or cough and asthmatic breath due to a prolonged illness.

As heart *qi* and lung *qi* are too weak to promote blood circulation, palpitation occurs. Since lung *qi* is so weak that normal respiration is not possible, short breath and a shortage of *qi* appear. If the lung fails to carry on its purifying and descending function, and lung *qi* ascends adversely, cough, asthmatic breath and chest distress will result. Since *qi* is insufficient and the body surface is not strengthened, general lassitude and spontaneous sweating results. As *qi* and blood are not flourishing, pallor and dull complexion may be seen. If the blood is stagnant in its circulation, dark-purplish mouth and lips and tongue with ecchymosis may be seen.

Treatment: Tonify and nourish the heart and lung with Decoction of Protecting Primordial *Qi*[41], or by puncturing *Xinshu* (B 15), *Feishu* (B 13), *Tanzhong* (CV 17), *Neiguan* (P 6), *Fuliu* (K 7) and *Taiyuan* (L 9) with tonifying manipulation.

10-3-6-8 Deficient spleen and lung *qi*

"The spleen is the source of *qi* and the lung, the pivot of *qi*." The lung will be weak and impaired if the spleen fails to distribute *jing* (vital principle); the latter will be dull if the lung fails to perform its dissipating and descending functions. Insufficient spleen and lung *qi* would lead to difficulty in distributing aqueous liquid, producing phlegm-damp. Deficient spleen and lung *qi* cause pathological changes, such as spleen dysfunction, the failure of aqueous liquid to be distributed and obstruction of the middle energizer by phlegm-damp.

Clinical picture: Short breath and general lassitude, cough with much thin and whitish sputum, anorexia, abdominal distension and loose stools, even puffy face and feet, light-coloured tongue with white coating and a minute, weak pulse.

Analysis of symptoms: A weak lung due to prolonged spleen deficiency or contaminated food and endogenous pathogenic phlegm-damp impair spleen *qi* so that it cannot transport *jing* (vital principle) to the lung.

As the lung is too weak to carry on respiration, short breath results; since the spleen is too weak to nourish the four extremities, general lassitude occurs. Since pathogenic phlegm-damp is stored in the lung and its *qi* cannot carry on its purifying and descending functions, cough and asthmatic breath with thin and clear sputum result. As spleen *qi* is insufficient and fails to perform its transporting and digesting functions, anorexia, abdominal distension and loose stools occur; as the spleen cannot transport pernicious damp, *qi* cannot evaporate excess fluid and aqueous damp overflows and swollen face and feet appear.

Treatment: Tonify and nourish the spleen and lung and warmly subdue phlegm-damp with Six Noble-ingredient Decoction[50] or by puncturing *Feishu* (B 13), *Pishu* (B 20), *Zusanli* (S 36), *Fenglong* (S 40), *Taiyuan* (L 9) and *Yinlingquan* (Sp 9) with tonifying manipulation.

10-3-6-9 Disharmony between liver and spleen

If the liver and spleen are in harmony, the *qi* mechanism and the spleen will function normally. Disharmony between the liver and spleen may result if depressed liver and stagnant *qi* impede the spleen's transporting function or the weak spleen and stagnant damp impede the liver's dispersing and discharging functions.

Clinical picture: Distension, fullness and pain in the chest and hypochondria, sighing, mental depression or irascibility, poor appetite, abdominal distension and loose stool or abnormal bowel movements, borborygmi and passing gas or abdominal pain and diarrhea, white tongue coating and stringy pulse.

Analysis of symptoms: Depressed anger injures the liver. Improper foods, fatigue and lack of exercise injure the spleen so that the liver is depressed and the spleen becomes weak.

As the liver fails to perform its functions, *qi* is blocked in the meridian. Distension, fullness and pain in the chest and hypochondria result. Since the liver should be harmonious and flourishing but not restrained and depressed, stagnant liver *qi* and an abnormal *qi* mechanism would lead to mental depression and preference for long exhalation. When the liver fails to flourish, irascibility easily appears. If the spleen fails to carry on its normal transporting function, poor appetite, abdominal distension and loose or dry thin stools may be seen. Owing to liver depression, *qi* stasis and abnormal spleen *qi*, borborygmi and gas or abdominal pain and diarrhea occur.

Treatment: Soothe the liver and reinforce the spleen with *Xiaoyao* Powders[19] or Powders of White Atractylode Rhizome and Chinese Herbaceous Peony[102] or by puncturing *Xingjian* (Liv 2), *Taichong* (Liv 3), *Neiguan* (P 6), *Zusanli* (S 36) and *Pishu* (B 20) with moderate manipulation. For the case with abdominal bowel movements and diarrhea add *Tianshu* (S 25) with moderate manipulation.

10-3-6-10 Disharmony between liver and stomach

Since the liver has dispersing and discharging functions and the stomach is concerned with reception and propels food downward, stomach *qi* descends if liver *qi* carries on its dispersing function. If the liver fails to perform its dispersing function due to depressed and stagnant *qi*, the stomach will be influenced and fail to propel food downward, causing disharmony between the liver and stomach. It is also termed the invasion of the stomach by liver *qi* that the stomach is influenced by failure of liver *qi* to perform its dispersing function.

Clinical picture: Distension, fullness and pain in the chest, hypochondria and epigastrium, hiccup and emaciation, acid regurgitation and *cao-za* (an unpleasant sensation that mimics pain and hunger), mental depression or irascibility, thin yellow coating and stringy pulse.

Analysis of symptoms: Mental discomfort, depressed liver and weak stomach, and invasion of the stomach by hyperactive liver *qi*.

When the liver is depressed and its *qi* is stagnant and meridian *qi* is blocked, distension and pain in the chest and hypochondria result. Since liver *qi* is hyperactive and stagnates in the epigastric region, epigastric distension and pain occur. As the stomach cannot propel food downward, hiccup and eructation appear. As *qi* is depressed in the stomach and produces pernicious heat, acid regurgitation, *cao-za* and a yellow tongue coating are seen. Mental depression or restlessness and irascibility and preference for sighing are all due to depressed *qi* and the liver's failure to function normally.

Treatment: Soothe the liver and regulate the stomach with Liver-soothing Powders with Buplerum Root[103] in association with *Zuojin* Coptis Root and Evodia Fruit Pills[104] or by puncturing *Neiguan* (P 6), *Zusanli* (S 36), *Zhongwan* (Ren 12), *Taichong* (Liv 3) and *Xingjian* (Liv 2) with moderate manipulation.

10-3-6-11 Weak heart and spleen

The heart can control blood and the spleen produces and governs the blood. If the spleen is too weak to produce and govern the blood, impaired and consumed heart blood results; heart blood consumed and impaired by extreme anxiety may also influence the spleen's transporting and digesting function and control of blood, forming the syndrome of deficient *qi* and blood of the heart and spleen.

Clinical picture: Palpitation and amnesia, insomnia and dreaminess, poor appetite, abdominal distension and loose stool, general lassitude and weakness, withered yellow complexion, subcutaneous bleeding, light-coloured profuse menstrual flow, metrorrhagia or oligomenorrhea and amenorrhea, light-coloured delicate tongue with white coating and minute weak pulse.

Analysis of symptoms: Usually caused by bodily disharmony after an illness, chronic hemorrhage, excessive anxiety or improper diet so that heart blood is consumed and spleen *qi* impaired.

As heart blood is consumed and deficient and the heart (mind) is malnourished, palpitation, amnesia, insomnia and dreaminess result. Since the spleen fails to perform its transporting function, poor appetite, abdominal distension, loose stool, general lassitude and weakness may appear. Since the blood is deficient, a withered yellow complexion occurs. As the spleen is too weak to control blood, polymenorrhea or bleeding appears. If the Strategic Vessel Meridian doesn't flourish due to blood deficiency, oligomenorrhea and amenorrhea may be seen. As both *qi* and blood are severely consumed, a light-coloured delicate tongue and minute weak pulse result.

Treatment: Tonify and nourish the heart and spleen with Decoction of Reinforcing the Heart and Spleen[22] or by puncturing *Shenmen* (H 7), *Tongli* (H 5), *Pishu* (B 20) for the case with subcutaneous bleeding and metropathia, and *Xuehai* (Sp 10) and *Ganshu* (B 18) with moderate manipulation and *Yinbai* (Sp 1).

10-3-6-12 The lung invaded by liver fire

The liver is predisposed to a flourishing growth while the lung is concerned with purification and descendance. Only if they are coordinated is the *qi* mechanism normal. If liver *qi* flourishes and *qi* fire rises excessively to influence the lung, the lung will fail to carry on its purifying function and persisting dry cough will appear, forming the pathological changes of the invasion of the liver by liver fire.

Clinical picture: Burning pain in the chest and hypochondria, irascibility, dizziness and congestive eyes, anxiety and fever, bitter mouth, paraxysmal cough even hematemesis, red tongue with thin yellow coating and stringy rapid pulse.

Analysis of symptoms: Mental depression or transformation of pathogenic heat stagnating in the Liver Meridian into pernicious fire that upwardly invades the lung.

As fire stagnates in the Liver Meridian, causalgia in the chest and hypochondria results. Since *qi* is depressed, pernicious fire flares, and the liver fails to flourish harmoniously and irascibility occurs. As *qi* fire ascends adversely and invades the lung, lung fluid is consumed. If the fire affects the lung collateral meridians (small vessels), hematemesis may be seen. As liver fire flares up, polydipsia, dizziness and congestive eyes may occur.

Treatment: Purify the liver and lung with Natural Indigo Powders[105] associated with Powders for Clearing up Lung Heat[106] or by puncturing *Taichong* (Liv 3) and *Chize* (L 5) with moderate manipulation. For dizziness and congestive eyes, add *Taiyang* (Extra 2) and *Baihui* (GV 20); for anxiety, fever and bitter mouth, add *Neiguan* (P 6); for hematemesis, add *Kongzui* (L 6) and *Geshu* (B 17).

10-4 Identification of syndromes with the names of the six meridians

One of the identifications of syndromes mainly used in exogenous diseases was summed up by Zhang Zhongjing of the Eastern Han Dynasty (A.D. 25-220) in combination with symptoms of febrile diseases and their pathological changes on the basis of the "Treatise on Heat" in *Plain Questions*. It divides general symptoms and signs of exogenous diseases into two major diseases or syndromes with yin and yang as their principles and subdivided into the six patterns; the *taiyang* disease (or syndrome), *yangming* disease (or syndrome) and *shaoyang* disease (or syndrome) collectively termed the "three yang diseases," the *taiyin* disease (or syndrome), *shaoyin* disease (or syndrome) and *jueyin* disease (or syndrome) are collectively termed the "three yin diseases" according to pathological changes at different stages of the disease on the basis of yin and yang diseases. The diseases (or syndromes) with the names of the six meridians generalize pathological changes of the viscera and the twelve meridians. Identification of syndromes with the names of the six meridians stresses the analysis of a series of pathological changes and their transformation and development caused by the affection of exogenous pathogenic cold, and is therefore not the same as that of internal injuries due to miscellaneous diseases.

The classification of syndromes with the names of the six meridians is significant because symptoms and changes of exogenous disease are analysed and summed up according to the strength or weakness of body resistance and the flourishing or declining tendency of the pathogenic factor in order to find out their connection and guide treatment. Classified according to their locations, the diseases (or syndromes) with the names of the six meridians are the *taiyang* disease (or syndrome) in the exterior of the body, the *yangming* disease (or syndrome) are in the interior and the *shaoyang* disease (or syndrome) are between the exterior and the interior. The three yin and yang diseases (or syndromes) in the interior are classified according to the relation between the pathogenic and anti-pathogenic factors and the pathological changes. If body resistance is strong, the diseases tend to be progressive and manifested as heat and excess syndromes, they are the three yang diseases (or syndromes) and should be treated by mainly eliminating the pathogenic factor; if it is weakened and they tend to be retrogressive and manifested as cold and deficient syndromes, they are the three yin diseases and should be treated by mainly reinforcing the anti-pathogenic factor.

Diseases or syndromes with the names of the six meridians are distinguishable and interconnected to a certain extent. It is termed the "concurrent disease" when a disease with the names of two or three meridians occur simultaneously. Complications occur when a meridian disease has not yet been cured, then another appears. The diseases or syndromes with the names of two meridians complicate each other and occur according to different sequences. It is known as the "transference from one meridian to another." It is termed a "direct attack" when an exogenous pathogenic father invades the three yin meridians without undergoing the stage of the three yang diseases (or syndromes).

10-4-1 *Taiyang* diseases

As the *taiyang* meridian governs the whole body surface, controls nutritional and defensive *qi* and resists the invasion of the pathogenic factor, it is known as the "fence of the six meridians."

The main pulse and symptoms of the *taiyang* disease (or syndrome) are superficial pulse, aversion to cold, stiffness and pain in the head and nape of the neck.

As the *taiyang* meridian is the first to be affected by pathogenic wind-cold when it invades the body and the spread of defensive yang *qi* is obstructed, aversion to cold and fever result. Since the *taiyang* meridian runs through the head and nape and *qi* in the meridian is in disorder when the pathogenic factor affects them, stiffness and pain in the head and nape occur. Since *qi* and blood move outward to vie with the pathogenic factor invading the body surface, the pulse is superficial. The above-mentioned pulse and symptoms are common in all the *taiyang* diseases or syndromes. But, as patients' constitutions and pathogenic factors vary, pathological changes and clinical manifestations of the *taiyang* meridian affected by the invasion of the body surface by exogenous pathogenic wind-cold should be treated by diaphoresis with pungent drugs of a warm nature.

10-4-1-1 The *taiyang* syndrome due to wind attack

Clinical picture: Headache, fever, perspiration, aversion to wind and superficial, slow pulse.

Analysis of symptoms: The *taiyang* syndrome is often caused by the loose conjunction between the skin and muscles, injury of defensive *qi* by exogenous pathogenic wind and disharmony between nutritional *qi* and defensive *qi*. The invasion of the body surface by wind and failure of defensive *qi* to resist the internal affection lead to aversion to wind. Defensive yang *qi* struggling against the exogenous pathogenic factor results in fever. Perspiration occurs because defensive *qi* is not strong enough and nutritional yin cannot be kept internally and the pulse is superficial as well as slower due to sweating and loose muscles.

Treatment: Relieve muscles and skin, disperse exogenous pathogenic wind and regulate nutritional and defensive *qi* with Cinnamon Twig Decoction.[107]

10-4-1-2 The *taiyang* syndrome due to cold attack

Clinical picture: Aversion to cold and fever, stiffness and pain in the head and nape, general lumbago, arthralgia, anhidrosis, asthmatic breath and superficial, taut pulse.

Analysis of symptoms: Defensive yang *qi* is blocked and nutritional yin stagnates due to the invasion of the body surface by an exogenous factor. The impairment of defensive yang *qi* by exogenous pathogenic cold leads to aversion to cold. Fever results from obstructed yang *qi* due to the anti-pathogenic factor vying with the pathogenic one. As the cold is yin and stagnant, stagnation and obstruction of nutritional yin cold arouse the disordered *qi* in the meridian, resulting in headache and general ache. As the cold is contracting and the junction between the skin and muscle is closed, anhidrosis may be seen. Since the lung is concerned with the skin and hair, the shutting of skin pores leads to the failure of lung *qi* to spread, with asthmatic breath. A superficial, taut pulse is a sign that exogenous pathogenic wind-cold affects the body surface.

Treatment: Remove exogenous pathogenic factors from the body surface, ventilate the troubled lung and relieve asthmatic breath with Ephedra Decoction.[108]

The above-mentioned syndromes of the *taiyang* meridian affected by exogenous pathogenic wind are called the exterior-deficiency syndrome because there is sweat and a slow pulse, while that of the *taiyang* meridian affected by exogenous pathogenic cold is called the exterior-excess syndrome because there is no sweating and a taut pulse.

10-4-2 *Yangming* disease

A *yangming* disease or syndrome is the late stage during which the anti-pathogenic factor struggles against the pathogenic one. Delayed or wrong treatment of a *taiyang* disease or syndrome allows exogenous pathogenic cold to invade deeply and transform into pernicious heat that consumes body fluids and produces pernicious dryness, resulting in constipation. It may also be formed due to the invasion of the *yangming* meridian by pathogenic dry-heat.

According to different locations and characteristics of the symptoms, the *yangming* disease is divided into those located in the meridian and the others in the yang viscera. The former refers to pathogenic heat in the *yangming* meridian diffusing over the entire body with no dry stool in the intestine and is thus called *yangming* heat syndrome, while the latter refers to pathogenic dry-heat in the stomach and intestines becoming substantive, resulting in constipation and is thus called the interior-heat-excess syndrome.

It is mainly treated by purification whereas the yang viscera syndrome is mainly treated by purgation.

10-4-2-1 The *yangming* syndrome in the meridian

Clinical picture: High fever, hyperhidrosis, extreme thirst with desire for drinking, flushed face and anxiety, yellow-dry tongue coating and full large pulse.

Analysis of symptoms: As pathogenic heat enters the *yangming* meridian and pathogenic dry-heat is excessive in the interior of body, a high fever and flushed face occur. Since pathogenic heat forces body fluids to escape outwardly, hyperhidrosis results. As body fluids cannot be continuously supplied due to sweating, a severe thirst appears. As excessive pernicious heat in the *yangming* meridian upwardly disturbs the heart (mind), anxiety and restlessness follow. Owing to the consumption of body fluids by extreme heat, a yellow dry tongue coating results. The extreme heat and hyperactive yang lead to a full and large pulse.

Treatment: Clear up pernicious heat and produce body fluids with White Tiger Decoction.[109]

10-4-2-2 The *yangming* syndrome in the yang viscera

Clinical picture: Fever, tidal fever every afternoon, persistent perspiration, constipation, abdominal fullness and pain aggravated by pressure, restlessness, delirium, even semi-consciousness or carphologia, anxiety, yellow dry or dark-yellow thorny tongue coating, deep, substantive and forceful pulse.

Analysis of symptoms: A combination of endogenous pathogenic heat in the *yangming* meridian producing dry stool and obstructed *qi* in the yang viscera results in constipation, abdominal fullness and pain aggravated by pressure. The outward spreading of endogenous excess heat leads to fever and perspiration. Tidal fever occurs in the afternoon when *qi* in the *yangming* meridian is flourishing and vies with the pathogenic factor violently. Since pathogenic dryness and heat upwardly attack the heart (mind) together with turbid *qi*, restlessness and delirium even semi-consciousness, carphologia and fright with anxiety appear. As body fluids are consumed by extreme heat, a yellow or dark-yellow, dry and thorny tongue coating and a deep, substantive or deep, slow and forceful pulse may be seen.

Treatment: Cleanse the dry stagnation with Drastic Purgative Decoction.[110]

10-4-3 *Shaoyang* disease

A *shaoyang* disease or syndrome is a pathological process during which the pathogenic factor has not yet been eliminated but the anti-pathogenic factor has been weakened. Thus, the pathogenic factor invades the deeper portion of the body, stagnates in the gallbladder and vies with the anti-pathogenic factor between the exterior and interior of the body. Since the pathological change is situated between the exterior and interior of the body, it is called a semi-exterior-interior syndrome.

Clinical picture: Chills and fevers, fullness and discomfort of the chest and hypochondria, no desire to eat, anxiety and vomiting, bitter mouth and dry throat, blurred vision and stringy pulse.

Analysis of symptoms: *Qi* and blood are weak and the pathogenic factor takes advantage and invades the body or the *taiyang* disease is transmitted inward, or the pathogenic factor invades the *shaoyang* meridian, thus the anti-pathogenic factor struggles against the pathogenic one in the area between the exterior and interior of the body. A stagnant pathogenic factor leads to aversion to cold whereas an excess anti-pathogenic factor is followed by fever. The pathogenic and anti-pathogenic factors vie with each other, resulting in chills and fever. Since the *shaoyang* meridian is located in the chest and hypochondria and *qi* in the meridian is in disorder when the pathogenic factor invades the *shaoyang* meridian, fullness and discomfort of the chest and hypochondria may result. As gallbladder *qi* invades the stomach, the *qi* mechanism is obstructed and the liver's functions become abnormal and dull expression, poor appetite and vomiting due to regurgitation of stomach *qi* may be seen. As pathogenic fire in the *shaoyang* meridian stagnates internally, anxiety appears. When gallbladder fire flares up along the meridian, bitter mouth, dry throat and blurred vision will occur. A stringy pulse may be seen because liver *qi* and gallbladder *qi* are stagnant.

Treatment: Harmonize *shaoyang* with Minor Buplerum Decoction.[15]

10-4-4 *Taiyin* disease

Since the *taiyin* meridian is a protective screen of the three yin meridians, it is the first to be affected when the disease enters them. The *taiyin* disease is a pathological change of deficiency due to pathogenic cold in which spleen yang is weak and pathogenic cold-damp is internally blocked.

The Spleen Meridian of Foot-*taiyin* and the Stomach Meridian of Foot-*yangming* are located in the middle energizer and are closely related, communicating with the spleen and stomach. The pathological processes of the meridians can transform into each other under certain circumstances and are divided into deficiency and excess types. There is a saying, "an excess syndrome occurs in the *yangming* meridian and a deficiency one in the *taiyin*."

Clinical picture: Abdominal fullness and vomiting, poor appetite, diarrhea with pain relieved by warmth and pressure, no thirst, light-coloured tongue with white coating, slow pulse.

Analysis of symptoms: The spleen and stomach are impaired due to improper treatment of the three yang diseases or pathogenic cold attacks the spleen due to prolonged weak spleen *qi*. The yang in the middle energizer is insufficient, so the spleen cannot perform its transporting function, pathogenic cold-damp blocks the interior of the body and the spleen fails to send the purified nutrient upward as well as the stomach, downward, resulting in fullness and pain in the abdomen, diarrhea, vomiting and poor appetite. Since the disease is a cold syndrome of the deficient type, abdominal pain is relieved by warmth and pressure, there is no thirst and a light-coloured tongue with a white coating and slow pulse appear.

Treatment: Warm the middle energizer and disperse pathogenic cold with Lizhong Decoction.[60]

Abdominal fullness and pain are common symptoms of the *taiyin* and *yangming* diseases but they are of different types. Abdominal pain in the *taiyin* disease attacks at intervals, is relieved by warmth and pressure and pertains to the deficiency type, while abdominal fullness, firmness and pain are persistent, aggravated by pressure, and pertain to the excess type.

10-4-5 *Shaoyin* disease

The *shaoyin* disease or syndrome is a pathological process of the hypofunctional heart and kidney. The heart is a fire one and the kidney is a water one. Both of them are the root of yin and yang. When the disease develops into the *shaoyin* meridian, and the heart and kidney become hypofunctional, excessive yin due to deficient yang or deficient yin inducing serious fire appear. The former is present in the syndrome of cold convulsion of *shaoyin* (disease) and the latter, is present in the thermal convulsion of *shaoyin* (disease). The *shaoyin* disease is commonly seen in the syndrome of cold convulsion of *shaoyin* (disease).

10-4-5-1 The syndrome of cold conversion of *shaoyin* (disease)

Clinical picture: Aversion to cold and rolling body in bed, cold clammy extremities, watery diarrhea, vomiting, no thirst or thirst and indulgence in hot drinks, clear urine, light-coloured tongue coating with deep, faint pulse.

Analysis of symptoms: Since heart yang and kidney yang decline, pathogenic cold directly attacks the *shaoyin* meridian or true yang is impaired due to a wrong treatment or excessive diaphoresis. As the yang is too deficient to warm the body, aversion to cold and cold clammy extremities appear. As yang *qi* is not vigorous, listlessness, lassitude and somnolence result. Since the yang in the *shaoyin* meridian is too weak to warm and make the spleen transport and digest, watery diarrhea occurs. A desire for vomiting and anxiety is caused by regurgitation of yin cold and the stomach's failure to propel downward, also nutritional *qi* is restrained by yin cold. As the yin is deficient and cold is excessive, no thirst appears. As yang *qi* is not vigorous, listlessness, lassitude and somnolence result. Since yang in the *shaoyin* meridian is too weak to warm and make the spleen transport and digest, watery diarrhea occurs. A desire for vomiting and anxiety is caused by regurgitation of yin cold and the stomach's failure to propel downward, also nutritional *qi* is restrained by yin cold. As the yin is deficient and cold is excessive, no thirst appears; the case where declining yang in the lower energizer cannot produce *qi* and body fluids with thirst is commonly seen, characterized by preference for a small amount of hot drinks. Clear or clear profuse urine, light-coloured tongue with white coating, and deep faint pulse are all signs of declining yang and excess yin.

Treatment: Restore the yang for resuscitation with Sini Decoction.[111]

10-4-5-2 The syndrome of thermal convulsion of *shaoyin* (disease)

Clinical picture: Anxiety and insomnia, dry throat and mouth, yellow urine, dark-red tip of tongue or dark-red tongue with little coating and minute, rapid pulse.

Analysis of symptoms: True yin is consumed by stubborn pathogenic heat or the pathogenic factor enters the *shaoyin* meridian and is transformed into yang heat that consumes true yin due to a prolonged deficiency of yin. Deficient kidney water fails to upwardly restrain heart fire that rises excessively with anxiety and insomnia, dry mouth and throat, red or dark-red tongue and minute, rapid pulse resulting.

Treatment: Replenish yin and check overactive fire with Coptis Root Decoction and Donkey-hide Gelation.[94]

10-4-6 *Jueyin* disease

Jueyin is the end of yin as well as the beginning of yang. It is the late stage to which a disease may develop. As the anti-pathogenic factor is exhausted and the yin and yang are unbalanced, there is intermingling of chills and fevers and extreme heat transforms into cold. If extremely-excessive yin cold transforms into the declining factor, and deficient yang *qi* changes into the flourishing factor, the disease will take a turn for the better; if yin cold is excessive, but yang *qi* is exhausted, the illness will become critical. If yang *qi* can still vie with excessive yin cold, the symptoms of intermingling chills and fever may appear.

Clinical picture: Persistent thirst, a stream of *qi* rushing upward affecting the heart, pain and heat in the heart, hunger with no desire for food, cold clammy extremities, diarrhea, vomiting or vomiting up roundworms.

Analysis of symptoms: The *jueyin* disease is due to the transference of the disease from one meridian to another, the attack of the pathogenic factor on the interior of the body or improper treatment and a trapped exogenous pathogenic factor and the development of disease into *jueyin*.[139] When a *jueyin* disease appears, the liver and pericardium are affected by the pathogenic factor and the liver's failure to perform its dispersing and discharging functions and *qi* movement is impeded, resulting in disordered *qi* and blood, disharmony between yin and yang and intermingling of chills and fever. Thirst and a stream of *qi* which rushes upward to affect the heart and pain and pernicious heat in the heart are caused by a combination of yang heat in the upper portion of the body. Hunger with no desire to eat, vomiting and diarrhea are due to the combination of yin and cold in the lower part of the body. A hot diaphragm and cold intestine lead to uneasiness and regurgitating roundworms or vomiting up the roundworms. As the *qi* mechanism is disordered and yin *qi* and yang *qi* cannot connect with each other smoothly, cold clammy extremities result.

Treatment: Regulate chills and fevers, moderate the stomach and expel roundworms with Black Plum Pills.[112]

10-5 Identification of syndromes according to the principle of *ying* (nutrition), *wei* (defence), *qi* (vital energy) and *xue* (blood) phases

Another way of identifying syndromes mainly used in acute febrile disease that are caused by exogenous pathogenic warm-heat, was advocated by Ye Tianshi in the Qing

Dynasty (1644-1911). It depends upon and supplements the identification of syndromes with the names of the six meridians of febrile diseases, in order to enrich the identification and treatment of exogenous diseases. *Ying, wei, qi* and *xue* are not only the four classifications of symptoms and signs of acute febrile disease, but also represent the four stages of different severities of acute febrile disease in the process of its development. Ye pointed out that the pathogenic factor entering from the *wei* phase to the *qi* phase, from the *qi* phase to the *ying* phase, and from the *ying* phase to the *xue* phase signifies that the pathogenic factor is invading the body deeper and deeper and the disease is becoming more severe. As far as the location of pathogenic change is concerned, the syndrome at the *wei* phase is superficial and lies in the lung, skin and hair; the syndrome at the *qi* phase, deep and lies in the chest, diaphragm, lung, stomach, intestines, and gallbladder. The syndrome at the *ying* phase indicates that pathogenic heat has entered the heart and lies in the heart and pericardium. The syndrome at the *xue* phase implies that pathogenic heat has entered the liver and kidney, exhausting and moving blood.

An acute febrile disease caused by the exogenous pathogenic factor occurs at the *wei* phase and then moves to the *qi, ying* and *xue* phases. Yet, this movement is not settled. Since the pathogenic factor varies, the classification and the severity of the disease and the patients' constitutions are different. There is also the case that begins from the *ying* or *qi* phase with characteristics of a relative excess of internal heat, but without symptoms at the *wei* phase. It may also be seen that the pathogenic factor at the *wei* phase has not been eliminated, although the disease has already entered the *qi* phase. If the heat spreads over not only the *qi* phase, but the *ying* and *xue* phases, serious heat at the *qi* and *ying* phases or *qi* and *xue* phases will form, or the disease at the *qi* phase will directly enter into the *ying* and *xue* phases by skipping the *qi* phase, i.e., the so-called "disorderly transference of exogenous diseases to the pericardium," etc. Hence, the disease condition can be grasped and a correct diagnosis made only when the practical condition is analysed accurately according to clinical signs.

Although both the acute disease caused by exogenous pathogenic warm-heat and the febrile disease caused by exogenous pathogenic cold belong to the category of exogenous disease, they are different in etiology, pathology, pulse, symptoms and treatment. The latter is caused by the affection of exogenous pathogenic cold and excess yin leads to a yang disease; the former is caused by the affection of exogenous pathogenic warm-heat and excess yang leads to a yin disease that easily produces pernicious dryness that consumes yin. It is advisable to treat a febrile disease at an early stage by diaphoresis with pungent drugs of a warm nature, so as to clear up exogenous pathogenic heat. For a febrile disease at the late stage, attention should be paid to restore the yang while for the acute febrile disease at the late stage, yin should be nourished.

Typical symptoms and signs at the *wei, qi, ying* and *xue* phases and their therapeutic principles are briefly introduced as follows.

10-5-1 The syndrome at the *wei* (defence) phase

The syndrome at the *wei* phase is manifest in symptoms of which exogenous pathogenic warm-heat invades the body surface, thus defensive *qi* becomes dysfunctional. It is commonly seen at the initial stage of an acute febrile disease. As the lung is concerned with skin and hair and defensive *qi* communicates with them, the syndrome at the *wei* phase is often accompanied by symptoms and signs of a pathological change of the Lung Meridian.

Clinical picture: Fever, slight aversion to cold, red tip and edge of the tongue, and superficial rapid pulse that are frequently associated with headache, dry mouth and mild thirst, cough, sore throat, etc.

Analysis of symptoms: An affection of pathogenic warm-heat or prolonged consumed body fluids complicated with the affection of exogenous pathogenic warm-heat results in abnormal defensive *qi* and a dysfunctional lung.

As a pathogenic factor invades the body surface and blocks defensive *qi*, fever and aversion to cold occur. Since exogenous pathogenic warmth is yang in nature, high fever and slight aversion to cold are seen. As exogenous pathogenic warm-heat lies in the exterior of the body, a red tongue with thin, white coating and superficial rapid pulse result. With yang heat upwardly disturbing the head, a headache appears. Since the lung is concerned with skin and hair and responsible for defensive *qi*, obstructed defensive *qi* would impede the spreading of lung *qi*, resulting in a cough. As the throat is the door of the lung, the lung affected by the warm-heat may cause a sore throat.

Treatment: Diaphoresis with pungent drugs of a cool nature and unobstruct defensive *qi* to promote sweating with Lonicra and Forsythia Powders[113] and Morus and Chrysanthemum Cold Decoction.[52]

10-5-2 The syndrome at the *qi* (vital energy) phase

The syndrome at the *qi* phase is the interior-heat syndrome in which exogenous pathogenic warm-heat enters the viscera and the anti-pathogenic factor vies with it violently and yang heat rises excessively. Since the viscera and location of the pathogenic factor invading the *qi* phase vary, symptoms vary too. The commonly-seen ones are characterized by heat accumulating in the lung, disturbance of the diaphragm by heat, excessive rise of stomach heat and obstruction of the intestinal tract by the heat, etc.

Clinical picture: Fever without aversion to cold, red tongue with yellow coating and rapid pulse that is often associated with anxiety, thirst, dark-red urine, etc. or asthmatic breath and cough, thoracalgia, yellow, mucoid expectoration, or anxiety and feeling of distress as well as a burning sensation in the chest and epigastrium, restlessness, or stomach fever, polydipsia and indulgence in cold drinks, hyperhidrosis, full large pulse, tidal fever and constipation, or thin watery diarrhea, full, firm and painful abdomen, yellow dry or dark thorny tongue coating and deep, substantive and forceful pulse.

Analysis of symptoms: The syndrome at the *wei* phase has not yet been relieved, but pathogenic heat has transferred inwardly and entered the *qi* phase.

As pathogenic heat enters the *qi* phase and the anti-pathogenic factor vies violently with it, when yang heat rises excessively, fever with aversion to heat, dark-red urine, yellow tongue coating and rapid pulse result. As the pathogenic factor has moved to the body surface, there is no aversion to cold. Owing to the consumption of fluids by excess heat, thirst appears. Disturbance of the heart (mind) by heat leads to restlessness. Since pernicious heat accumulates in the lung, the lung fails to perform its purifying function impeding the *qi* mechanism, and asthmatic breath, cough and thoracalgia result. As phlegm is formed by concentration of body fluids by the heat in the lung, yellow mucoid sputum occurs. As the heat disturbs the chest and diaphragm, but does not spread, anxiety and feelings of distress, as well as a burning sensation in the chest and epigastrium result. Since the burning heat affects the *yangming* meridian and excessively rising heat in the stomach spreads outwardly, persistent strong fever appears. Hyperhidrosis will follow if body fluids are forced to exude outward. Polydipsia and desire for drinking are caused by the consumption of body fluids by extreme heat. A full large pulse is due to excess heat obstructing the internal tract, and consumed body fluids causes pernicious dryness. Pathogenic dry-heat combines with the residue and *qi* in the yang viscera is blocked, so a full, firm and painful abdomen, and constipation with watery diarrhea result. As the yang viscera are hyperactive in a *yangming* disease, the dry-heat rises excessively internally and tidal fever in the afternoon, yellow dry or dark thorny coating of tongue, and deep substantive and forceful pulse occur.

Treatment: Mainly clear up pathogenic heat. For the heat accumulated in the lung, it is advisable to clear up pernicious heat and ventilate the troubled lung, with Decoction of Ephedra, Almond, Licorice and Gypsum.[53] For the disturbance of the chest and epigastrium by pernicious heat, it is advisable to clear up the stagnant heat with Capejasmine Fruit and Fermented Soybean Decoction.[114] For the *yangming* meridian affected by excessive pernicious heat in the stomach, it is advisable to clear up pernicious heat and produce body fluids with White Tiger Decoction.[109] For obstructed *qi* in the yang viscera, to excrete pernicious heat and promote bowel movements use Decoction for Increasing Body Fluids and Reinforcing *Qi*.[115]

10-5-3 The syndrome at the *ying* (nutrition) phase

The syndrome at the *ying* phase is a later or critical stage at which pathogenic warm-heat sinks inward. *Ying* (nutrients) is *qi* in blood and the "predecessor" of blood, communicated internally with the heart. Therefore, the syndrome at the *ying* phase is pathologically characterized by the impaired *ying* phase and disturbs the mind. The *ying* phase is between the *qi* and *xue* phases, indicating that the disease has taken a turn for the better if it moves from the *ying* phase to the *xue* phase or that it has worsened if it moves from the *ying* phase to the *qi* phase.

Clinical picture: Fever higher in the night, slight thirst, anxiety and insomnia, or even coma and delirium, faint skin rashes, dark-red tongue and minute rapid pulse.

Analysis of symptoms: The disease at the *qi* phase has not yet been relieved, but has moved inward into the *ying* phase, or the disease at the *wei* phase has moved into the *ying* phase. This is often caused by the patient's weak constitution and shortage of body fluids so that pathogenic heat is inwardly trapped in heart *ying*.[140] As pathological heat enters the *ying* phase and impairs *ying* (nutrition) so that true yin is deprived, fever higher at night, dry mouth with slight thirst and minute rapid pulse result. As pernicious heat at the *ying* phase must necessarily involve the *xue* phase, there is a dark-red tongue and faint skin rashes if the heat invades the blood vessel. Since nutritional *qi* communicates with the heart and the heart (mind) is disturbed by pernicious heat at the *ying* phase, anxiety and insomnia result. Coma and delirium may be seen if pathogenic heat enters the pericardium.

Treatment: Clear up pathogenic heat at the *ying* phase with *ying*-clearing Decoction[17] or clear up pathogenic heat from the heart or pericardium for resuscitation by taking *Bezoar* Resuscitation Pills[17] or Extremely Treasury Pills[78] and *Zixue* Pills[117] with Decoction for Clearing Heart Heat.[116]

10-5-4 The syndrome at the *xue* (blood) phase

The syndrome at the *xue* (blood) phase is the final stage of pathological change of the *wei*, *qi*, *ying* and *xue* phases as well as the most critical stage of acute febrile diseases. As the heart controls blood and the liver stores blood, pathogenic heat entering the *xue* phase must necessarily influence both the heart and liver on the one hand and on the other, if pathogenic heat stays for long, true yin will be consumed and water will be lost due to exhausted yin. The disease often affects the kidney, too. Hence, the syndrome at the *xue* phase is chiefly a pathological process of the heart, liver and kidney, clinically characterized by the consumption and aberration of blood, impairment of yin and movement of endogenous wind, as well as clinical manifestations of severe symptoms at the *ying* phase.

Clinical picture: In addition to symptoms at the *ying* phase, there is also high fever, restlessness and mania, skin rashes or hematemesis, epistaxis, blood stools, hematuria, irregular menstrual flow, and dark-purplish tongue. They may be accompanied by mental disturbance and restlessness, convulsions of the hands and feet, a stiff neck, opisthotonos, upward fixation of the eyes, lockjaw, or persisting low-grade fever, hot body in the evening, but cool in the morning, fever in the chest, palms and soles, dry mouth and throat, mental fatigue and deafness, dry tongue, or emaciation, atrophic lips and tongue, dry teeth, sunken eyes and blurred vision, lethargy, malar flush, convulsions of hands and feet when in peristalsis, vigorous heartbeat with empty sensation, and empty, rapid or minute hasty pulse.

Analysis of symptoms: The syndrome at the *ying* phase has not been relieved, but on the contrary, has moved to the *xue* phase or pathogenic heat has entered the *xue* phase.

The disease caused by pathogenic heat that has entered the *xue* phase is deeper and more severe than that one caused by pernicious heat that has entered the *ying* phase. As the heat in blood disturbs the heart (mind), mania even mental disturbance results. Since the heat in the blood goes wild, skin rashes are exposed or varieties of hemorrhages are seen. Owing to the burning heat in the blood, a dark-purplish tongue occurs. As the liver stores blood and the heat in the blood affects the Liver Meridian, the signs of the movement of endogenous pathogenic wind by liver heat, such as convulsions of hands and feet, stiff neck, opisthotonos, upward fixation of eyes, lock-jaw, etc. may be seen. If pathogenic heat is retained for long and affects liver and kidney yin, so that the yin is deficient and yang heat disturbs the interior of the body, a tidal fever and fever in the chest, palms and soles result. If yin *jing* (vital principle) fails to ascend, a dry mouth and lips and deafness may appear. If yin *jing* is consumed and *shen* (Spirit) is not nourished, mental fatigue and lethargy occur. If the true yin is consumed, the blood cannot nourish tendons and the tendons and vessels are rigid, and endogenous pathogenic wind due to deficiency will move internally and tremor of the hands and feet even clonic convulsion will result. If the true yin is severely consumed and not nourished by yin *jing* and blood, emaciation, atrophic lips and tongue, dry teeth, sunken eyes and blurred vision, vigorous heartbeat with an empty sensation may be seen. As the yin is too deficient to restrain the yang, and the yin and yang are in disharmony, an empty large and rapid or minute, small and hasty pulse results.

Treatment: Cool and dissipate blood with Rhinoceros Horn and Rehmannia Decoction[18] or cool the liver and subdue endogenous pathogenic wind with Decoction of Antelope's Horn and Uncaria Stem with Hooks[80] or replenish the yin and nourish blood, check the overactive liver and subdue exogenous wind with *Fumai* Decoction with Additives and Deductives[118] and Major Wind-eliminating Pearls.[119]

10-6 Identification of syndromes according to the triple energizer

Identification of syndromes according to the triple energizer is one of the ways of identifying acute febrile diseases. It was summed up by Wu Tang of the Qing Dynasty (1644-1911) according to the concept of the classification of the location of the triple energizer in *Internal Classic* on the basis of identification according to the principle of *wei, qi, ying* and *xue* phases in *Treatise on Acute Febrile Diseases* by Ye Tianshi in combination with the rule of transference and transformation of acute febrile diseases. In *More Discussions on Acute Febrile Diseases* Wu mainly explained pathological changes of the viscera pertaining to the triple energizer in the course of acute febrile diseases by applying the triple energizer as a guiding principle for identification of the diseases or syndromes of acute diseases and running through the *wei, qi, ying* and *xue* phases and characterizing various types of symptoms and signs in accordance with these changes. When differentiating the movement and transformation of acute febrile diseases with the triple energizer, the disease originates from the upper energizer, then moves to the middle energizer and finally reaches the lower energizer. The disease or syndrome of the upper energizer includes symptoms of the lung and pericardium; the syndrome of the middle energizer includes symptoms of the spleen and stomach; the syndrome of the lower energizer includes symptoms of the liver and kidney.

"The warm-heat" disease is a general term for an acute febrile disease caused by the affection of pathogenic warmth and heat that are different in the four seasons. As weather changes in four seasons, the pathogenic factor varies. An acute febrile disease has its own characteristics and various types can be seen.

But as far as pathological changes are concerned, there are two main types, namely the warm-heat type and the damp-heat type. Although the damp-heat and warm-heat diseases are common, they are different. It is advisable to identify a damp-heat disease according to the triple energizer. This is because pathogenic damp in the damp-heat disease is a major factor, which is yin in nature and easily injures yang *qi*. It is unlikely to injure the yin and form the heat at the *ying* and *xue* phases due to its persistent retention between the *wei* and *qi* phases. Damp often affects the body in the sequence of the upper, middle and lower energizers as it is heavy, turbid and downward moving. So far as an exogenous damp-heat disease is concerned, the identification of syndromes according to the triple energizer is determined in accordance with the characteristics of pathogenic damp and of the triple energizer, which can be a pathway of aqueous damp. According to the portions of the viscera that pathogenic damp-heat affects and the sequence of its affection, the triple energizer is divided into the upper, middle and lower sections, which are also the initial, advanced and late stages of a damp-heat disease.

The identification of a damp-heat disease according to the triple energizer is only briefly introduced since the contents of identification of acute febrile disease by the triple energizer are almost the same with that according to the principle of the *wei, qi, ying* and *xue* phases.

10-6-1 Damp-heat in the upper energizer

Damp-heat in the upper energizer is the initial stage at which pathogenic damp-heat affects the body, the symptoms of which pertain to the exterior syndrome and are located in the lung, skin and hair. As damp is internally related to the spleen, stomach, pathogenic damp-heat in the upper energizer is associated with damp symptoms of the spleen and stomach and muscles. At the initial stage, the hot signs are not so obvious, while the damp symptoms are more serious, but the hot symptoms will appear more markedly several days later.

Clinical picture: Severe aversion to cold, slight fever or no fever, or afternoon fever, sensation of a heavy head as if it were tightly bandaged, heavy limbs and trunk, chest distress and anhidrosis, mental dullness, mucoid mouth with no thirst, epigastric fullness and dyspepsia or borborygmi and loose stools, white glossy tongue coating and soft slow pulse.

Analysis of symptoms: Damp-heat is due to the affection of pathogenic damp, the damp stagnating in the body surface, and spleen *qi* obstructed by the damp. As pathogenic damp blocks the body surface and defensive yang *qi* is obstructed, severe aversion to cold without sweat results. Since pathogenic damp-heat is depressed in spreading, afternoon fever appears. The pathogenic damp obstructed in the upper portion of the body leads to a heavy feeling in the head, as if it were tightly bandaged. Owing to the damp stagnating in the body surface, immovable and heavy limbs and trunk occur. Because of the obstruction of chest yang by the damp and turbid matter, mental dullness results. As the damp is in excess, but body fluids have not yet been consumed, a mucoid mouth with no thirst appears. As the damp obstructs the spleen and stomach so that they fail to perform their functions, chest fullness and dyspepsia, borborygmi and loose stool result. When the disease is still at the initial stage, damp and the turbid matter have not yet completely changed into heat and the *qi* mechanism is blocked by the damp, a glossy tongue coating and soft slow pulse may be seen.

Treatment: Warmly dissipate the superficial pernicious damp with *qi* regulating Powders with Cablin Pachouli.[120] For the case with obvious hot signs, it is advisable to disperse and subdue pathogenic damp-heat with Decoction of Cablin Pachouli, Pinellia Tuber and Poria.[121]

10-6-2 Damp-heat in the middle energizer

The disease moving to the middle energizer is the middle stage of a damp-heat disease, chiefly manifested by the spleen and stomach injury by pathogenic damp. As the spleen dislikes dampness, but the latter is likely to obstruct the former, injury of the spleen and stomach would impede the spleen's transporting and digesting functions, as well as the stomach's receiving function. As the muscles and four extremities are controlled by the spleen, pathogenic damp-heat in the middle energizer is mainly manifested in pathological changes of the digestive tract, as well as sore and heavy limbs and muscles. Since the damp is mucoid, stagnant, and slow-moving, some of the symptoms of the upper energizer may be seen in pathogenic damp-heat in the middle energizer, although the pathological changes mainly occur in the middle energizer.

There may be three tendencies in the development of pathogenic damp-heat in the middle energizer. a. Pathogenic damp-heat in the middle energizer is influenced by yang, producing pernicious dryness or pathogenic heat consumes yin, forming pernicious heat in *ying* (nutrition) blood; b. Pathogenic damp-heat in the middle energizer is influenced by the yin, developing into a cold-damp syndrome; c. Pathogenic damp-heat in the middle energizer produces neither pernicious dryness nor cold, but moves to the lower energizer forming the damp-heat syndrome in the lower energizer.

Clinical picture: Obscure fever relieved by sweating that recurs or becomes higher in the afternoon, heavy limbs and trunk, full and distending chest and epigastrium, vomiting and nausea without hunger, thirst with no desire to drink, with red, yellow complexion, or light-coloured yellow face and eyes, mental retardation and little speech, even coma, dark-red scanty urine, loose stool possibly with white blisters, greyish-white-yellow tongue coating and soft, rapid pulse.

Analysis of symptoms: Pathogenic damp-heat in the upper energizer is caused by the spleen and stomach injured by pathogenic summer-heat and damp, or the damp-heat produced by improper food. As the heat is mixed with the damp, the damp-heat is depressed when spreading, and obscured fever aggravated in the afternoon results. Since the damp-heat is lingering and stubborn, recurrent fever relieved by sweating may appear. As the damp-heat is stagnant and obstructed *qi* ascends and descends abnormally, full and distending chest and epigastrium accompanied by vomiting without hunger result. As the heat consumes body fluids and the damp restrains the heat, thirst with no desire to drink or even no thirst occurs. Stagnation of the damp and spreading of the heat lead to a yellow face and eyes; obstructed sensitive organs lead to mental dullness and little speech or even coma. The damp-heat obstructed in the middle energizer, the spleen's failure to perform its transporting function and the failure of *qi* to flow smoothly result in dark-red scanty urine, loose stools with difficult defecation and white blisters exposed when the damp-heat spreads over the skin.

Treatment: Clear up damp-heat and regulate the *qi* mechanism with Detoxicating Pills for Universal Relief[63] or Three Seeds Decoction.[122]

10-6-3 Damp-heat in the lower energizer

Pathogenic damp-heat in the lower energizer moves from the middle energizer and its pathological change mainly occurs in the large intestine and urinary bladder. Its clinical symptoms are chiefly abnormal urination and defecation.

Clinical picture: Anuria, thirst with no desire for profuse drinking or constipation, firmness and fullness in the lower abdomen, distension of the head and dizziness, grey-white-yellow glossy tongue coating and soft, rapid pulse.

Analysis of symptoms: Pathogenic damp-heat that has moved to the lower energizer blocks the bladder and large intestine so that the bladder fails to perform its function and the large intestine *qi* is obstructed. As the bladder cannot perform its evaporating function due to stagnating damp-heat, anuria results. Since pathogenic damp accumulates in the lower portion of the body and body fluids cannot ascend, thirst with no desire for drinking occurs. As the large intestine fails to perform its transporting function and *qi* in the yang viscera is blocked due to obstruction of the large intestine by pathogenic damp, abnormal micturation and defecation and firmness and fullness in the lower abdomen appear. Since pathogenic damp and the turbid matter cannot be excreted outwardly but cloud sense organs due to stagnant damp-heat, distension of the head and dizziness, grey-white-yellow coating of tongue, and soft pulse result.

Treatment: Promote exudation and subdue pathogenic damp with Poria Skin Decoction[123] or remove the turbid matter and subdue the stagnant with Decoction for Spreading the Purified and Dispersing the Turbid.[124]

Notes

[1.] Ingredients: Ginseng, white atractylodes rhizome, poria and prepared licorice in equal amounts. Grind them into a rude powder. Take 2 *qian* after decocting them with water.

[2.] Ingredients: Astraglus root 5 *fen*, prepared licorice 5 *fen*, ginseng 5 *fen*, Chinese angelica root 2 *fen*, tangerine peel 2-3 *fen*, cimicifuga rhizome 2-3 *fen*, bupleurum root 2-3 *fen*, white atractylodes rhizome 3 *fen*.

[3.] Ingredients: Lindera root 3 *qian*, areca seeds 3 *qian*, eaglewood 1 *qian*, aucklandia root 2 *qian*, immature bitter orange 3 *qian*. Grind them into a thick juice with wine.

4. Ingredients: Sichuan Chinaberry 1 *liang*, cardialis tuber 1 *liang*. Take 3 *qian* once with wine.

5. Ingredients: Perilla seed 2 *liang* and 5 *qian*, pinellia tuber 2 *liang* and 5 *qian*, prepared licorice 2 *liang*, cinnamon bark 1 *liang* and 5 *qian*, peucedamum root 1 *liang*, magnolia bark 1 *liang*, tangerine peel 1 *liang* and 5 *qian*, Chinese angelica root 1 *liang* and 5 *qian*, fresh ginger 1 *liang* and 5 *qian*. Take 2 *qian* once.

6. Ingredients: Inula flower 3 *liang*, ginseng 2 *liang*, fresh ginger 5 *liang*, haematitum, 1 *liang*, prepared licorice 3 *liang*, pinellia tuber 0.5 *shen*, 12 dates.

7. Ingredients: Chinese angelica root, *Chuanxiong* rhizome, white peony root and prepared rehmannia root in equal amounts. Grind them into a rude powder and take 3 *qian* once.

8. Ingredients: Astraglus root 4 *liang*, Chinese angelica (tail) 2 *qian*, red peony root 1 *qian* and 5 *fen*, earthworm 1 *qian*, *Chuanxiong* rhizome 1 *qian*, peach kernel 1 *qian*, safflower 1 *qian*.

9. Ingredients: Chinese rehmannia root, Chinese angelica root, red peony root, *Chuanxiong* rhizome, peach kernel, and safflower.

10. Ingredients: Chinese angelica root 3 *liang*, cinnamon twig 3 *liang*, peony root 3 *liang*, asarum herb 3 *liang*, prepared licorice 2 *liang*, rice paper pith 2 *liang*, 15 dates. Take 1/3 once.

11. Ingredients: Evodia fruit 3 *liang*, Chinese angelica root 2 *liang*, *Chuanxiong* rhizome 2 *liang*, peony root 2 *liang*, ginseng 2 *liang*, cinnamon twig 2 *liang*, donkey-hide gelatin (melt) 2 *liang*, moutan bark 2 *liang*, fresh ginseng 2 *liang*, licorice 2 *liang*, pinellia tuber 0.5 *shen*, ophiopogon root 1 *shen*. Take 1/3 once.

12. Ingredients: Peach kernel 3 *qian*, Chinese angelica root 3 *qian*, peony root 3 *qian*, moutan bark 3 *qian*, rhubarb 5 *qian*, mirabilite 2 *qian*.

13. Ingredients: 30 pieces of leech, 20 gadflies, 25 peach kernels, rhubarb 3 *liang*. Take 1/3 once.

14. Ingredients: Rhubarb 4 *liang*, moutan bark 1 *liang*, 50 peach kernels, Benincasa seed 0.5 *shen*, mirabilite 3 *he* (pour boiling water on to it). Take it at one time.

15. Ingredients: Bupleurum root 9 *liang*, scutellaria root 3 *liang*, ginseng 3 *liang*, pinellia tuber 0.5 *shen*, prepared licorice 3 *liang*, fresh ginger 3 *liang*, 12 dates. Take 1/3 once.

16. Ingredients: Rhubarb 10 *fen*, scutellaria root 2 *liang*, licorice 3 *liang*, peach kernel 1 *shen*, bitter apricot seed 1 *shen*, white peony 4 *liang*, rehmannia root 10 *liang*, dried lacquer 1 *liang*, gadflies 0.5 *shen*, 100 leeches, grub 1 *shen*, cockroach 0.5 *shen*. Prepare them as pills with honey like a small bean, take 5 pills once with warm wine, three times per day.

17. Ingredients: Rhinoceros horn 3 *qian*, rehmannia root 5 *qian*, scrophularia root 3 *qian*, bamboo leaf (central part) 1 *qian*, ophiopogon root 3 *qian*, red sage root 2 *qian*, coptis root 1 *qian* and 5 *fen*, honeysuckle flower 3 *qian*, forsythia fruit 2 *qian*.

18. Ingredients: Rhinoceros horn 1 *liang*, rehmannia root 8 *liang*, peony root 3 *liang*, *moutan* bark 2 *liang*. Take 1/3 once.

19. Ingredients: Bupleurum root 1 *liang*, Chinese angelica root 1 *liang*, white peony root 1 *liang*, white atractylodes rhizome 1 *liang*, poria 1 *liang*, prepared licorice 1 *liang*. Grind them into a rude powder and take 2 *qian* once. Add a piece of ginger and a small amount of peppermint and decoct them with water.

20. Ingredients: Ginseng 1 *qian*, white atractylodes rhizome 1 *qian*, poria 1 *qian*, Chinese angelica root 1 *qian*, white peony root 1 *qian*, prepared rehmannia root 1 *qian*, *Chuanxiong* rhizome 1 *qian*, prepared licorice. Decoct them after adding ginger, dates and water.

21. Ingredients: Astraglus root 1 *liang*, Chinese angelica root 2 *qian*.

22. Ingredients: White atractylodes rhizome 1 *liang*, poria 1 *liang*, astraglus root 1 *liang*, longan aril 1 *liang*, stir-fried bitter apricot seed 1 *liang*, ginseng 5 *qian*, aucklandia root 5 *qian*, prepared licorice 2 *qian* and 5 *fen*. Grind them into rude powders. Take 4 *qian* once, add 5 pieces of fresh ginger and 1 date.

23. Ingredients: Ginseng 2 *liang*. Decoct it thoroughly and take it at one time.

24. Ingredients: Ginseng 1 *liang*, prepared aconite root 5 *liang*, add ginger and dates.

25. Ingredients: Scrophularia root 1 *liang*, ophiopogon root 8 *qian*, rehmannia root 8 *qian*.

26. Ingredients: Large-leaf gentian root 2 *liang*, gypsum 2 *liang*, licorice 1 *liang*, *Chuanxiong* rhizome 1 *liang*, scutellatia root 1 *liang*, white peony root 1 *liang*, Chinese angelica root 1 *liang*, prepared atractylodes rhizome 1 *liang*, rehmannia root 1 *liang*, prepared rehmannia root 1 *liang*, poria 1 *liang*, asarum herb 5 *qian*. Grind into a powder, take one *liang* once after decocting with water.

27. Ingredients: Trichosanthes fruit 1 *liang*, scutellaria root 1 *liang*, poria 1 *liang*, immature bitter orange 1 *liang*, bitter apricot seed 1 *liang*, tangerine peel 1 *liang*, prepared arisaema tuber 1 *liang* and 5 *qian*, prepared pinellia tuber 1 *liang* and 5 *qian*. Prepare them as pills with ginger juice. Take 2-3 *qian* once.

28. Ingredients: Mica schist 1 *liang*, scutellaria root 8 *liang*, rhubarb 8 *liang*, eaglewood 5 *qian*. Prepare them as pills with water. Take 1.5-2 *qian* once, 1-2 times per day.

29. Ingredients: Perulla seed, white mustard seed, radish seed (without definite amount). For obvious cough and asthmatic breath, the Perulla seed is mainly used; for profuse sputum, naustaid seed is mainly used; for food retention, radish seed is the main ingredient.

30. Ingredients: Pinellia tuber 5 *liang*, tangerine peel 5 *liang*, poria 3 *liang*, prepared licorice 1 *liang* and 5 *qian*. Grind them into powder. Take 4 *qian* once.

31. Ingredients: Mulberry leaf 3 *qian*, gypsum 2 *qian* and 5 *fen*, ginseng 7 *fen*, licorice 1 *qian*, stir-fried black sesamum 1 *qian*, donkey-hide gelatin (melt) 8 *fen*, ophiopogon root 1 *qian* and 2 *fen*, a piece of loquat leaf (stir-fried with honey), bitter apricot seed 7 *fen*. Take the decoction at one time.

32. Ingredients: Prepared rehmannia root 3 *qian*, rehmannia root 2 *qian*, the bulb of fritillary 1 *qian*, Chinese angelica root 1 *qian*, stir-fried peony root 1 *qian*, licorice 1 *qian*, scrophularia root 8 *fen*, platycodon root 8 *fen*, ophiopogon root 5 *fen*.

33. Ingredients: Poria 4 *liang*, cinnamon twig 3 *liang*, white atractylodes rhizome 2 *liang*, prepared licorice 2 *liang*. Take 1/3 once.

34. Ingredients: Genkwa flower, kansui root and reking spurge root in equal amount, 10 dates.

35. Ingredients: Kansui root, reking spurge root, white mustard seed in equal amount. Prepare them as pills like Chinese parasol seed. Take 5-9 pills once with ginger decoction.

36. Ingredients: Umbellate pore-fungus 18 *zhu*, alismatis rhizome 1 *liang* and 6 *zhu*, white atractylodes rhizome 18 *zhu*, poria 18 *zhu*, cinnamon twigs 5 *qian*. Grind them into powder. Take 1 *fangcunbi* once after pouring boiling water onto it or decoct it with water.

37. Ingredients: Mulberry bark, tangerine peel, fresh ginger skin, areca peel and poria in equal amount. Grind them into a powder. Take 3 *qian* once. Decoct it with water.

38. Ingredients: Ephedra 3 *liang*, white peony root 3 *liang*, asarum herb 3 *liang*, dried ginger 3 *liang* and cinnamon twigs 3 *liang*, schisandra fruit 0.5 *shen* and pinellia tuber 0.5 *shen*. Decoct them with water. Take 1/3 once.

39. Ingredients: Lepidium seed (thoroughly boil it to make it yellow, then prepare them as pills), 12 dates. First boil the dates, then add lepidium seed after taking the dates out, take the decoction at one time.

40. Ingredients: Prepared astraglus root, *Fushen* poria, poria, fermented pinellia tuber, Chinese angelica root, *Chuanxiong* rhizome 1 *qian* and 5 *fen* each; polygala root, stir-fried date kernel, cinnamon bark, arborvitae seed, schisandra fruit, ginseng 1 *qian* each, prepared licorice 5 *fen*, 5 pieces of fresh ginger and 2 dates.

41. Ingredients: Ginseng 2-3 *qian*, licorice 1 *qian*, cinnamon bark 5-7 *fen*, astraglus root 2-3 *qian*, and polished glutinous rice.

42. Ingredients: Rehmannia root 4 *liang*, schisandra fruit, Chinese angelica root, straglus root, ophiopogon root, arborvitae seed and date kernel 1 *liang* each, pilose asiobell root, scrophularia root, poria, polygala root, platycodon root 5 *qian* each. Prepare them as pills with honey, coated with cinnabaris. Take 3 *qian* once.

43. Ingredients: Rhubarb 2 *liang*, coptis root 1, *liang* and scutellaria root 1 *liang*.

44. Ingredients: Rehmannia root, licorice and rice-paper pith in equal amounts. Grind them into a rude powder and take 3 *qian* once after adding bamboo leaf and decocting it with water.

45. Ingredients: Prepared pinellia tuber 2 *qian*, tangerine peel 1 *qian* and poria 1 *qian*, licorice 5 *fen*, immature bitter orange 1 *qian*, prepared arisaema tuber 1 *qian*.

46. Ingredients: White atractylodes rhizome, aristolochia root, rhinoceros horn, cyperus tuber, cinnabar, chebula fruit, sandalwood, benzoin, eaglewood, musk, cloves and long pepper 2 *liang* each, borneol, storax (oil) and fumigated lysimachia foenum-graecum 1 *liang* each. Prepare them as pills like Chinese parasol seed with honey. Take four pills once.

47. Ingredients: Trichosanthes fruit, macrostem onion, cinnamon twigs, immature bitter orange, magnolia bark.

48. Ingredients: Red peony root 1 *qian*, *Chuanxiong* rhizome 1 *qian*, peach kernel 2 *qian*, safflower 2 *qian*, 3 scallions, 7 dates, fresh ginger 3 *qian*, and musk 5 *li*. Decoct them with wine and water.

49. Ingredients: Astraglus root 1 *qian*, ledebouriella root 1 *qian* and white atractylodes rhizome 2 *qian*. Grind them into powder, add 3 pieces of fresh ginger and decoct them with water.

50. Ingredients: Perilla leaf, pinellia tuber, poria, peucedanum root, platycodon root, bitter orange, licorice, fresh ginger, dates, pummelo peel and bitter apricot kernel.

51. Ingredients: Perilla seed, poria, mulberry bark, pummelo peel, bitter apricot kernel, ephedra 1 *liang* each, licorice 5 *qian*. Grind them into a rude powder. Take 2 *qian* once after being decocted with water.

52. Ingredients: Mulberry leaf 2 *qian* and 5 *fen*, chrysanthemum flower 1 *qian*, bitter apricot kernel 2 *qian*, forsythia fruit 1 *qian* and 5 *fen*, peppermint 8 *fen*, platycodon root 2 *qian*, licorice 8 *fen*, reed rhizome 2 *qian*.

53. Ingredients: Ephedra 5 *qian*, 50 stir-fried bitter apricot kernels, gypsum 0.5 *jin*, prepared licorice 2 *liang*. Grind them into a powder. Take 4 *qian* once, decoct them with water.

54. Ingredients: Reed rhizome 2 *shen*, coix seed 0.5 *shen*, benincasa seed 0.5 *shen*, 30 peach seeds. Take 1/3 once.

55. Ingredients: Mulberry leaf 1 *qian*, bitter apricot kernel 1 *qian* and 5 *fen*, radis adenophorae 2 *qian*, thunberg fritillary bulb, fermented soybean, capejasmine fruit, peach skin 1 *qian* each.

56. Ingredients: Puerarua root 0.5 *jin*, prepared licorice 2 *liang*, scutellaria root and coptis root 3 *liang* each. Take 1/3 once.

57. Ingredients: Pulsatilla root 2 *liang*, phellodendron bark, coptis root and ash bark 3 *liang* each. Take 1/2 once after decocting it.

58. Ingredients: Sesame 2 *shen*, peony root 0.5 *jin*, stir-baked immature bitter orange 0.5 *jin*, rhubarb 1 *jin*, stir-fried magnolia bark 1 *chi*, bitter apricot kernel 1 *shen*. Prepare them as pills with honey, shaped as Chinese parasol seeds. Take pills once, three times a day.

59. Ingredients: Tangerine peel 1 *qian*, pinellia tuber 1 *qian*, poria 2 *qian*, licorice 1 *qian*, ginseng 2 *qian* and white atractylodes rhizome 2 *qian*.

60. Ingredients: Ginseng, white atractylodes rhizome, prepared licorice and dry ginger 3 *liang* each. Prepare them as pills with honey. Take one pill once or decoct them with water and take 1/3 once.

61. Ingredients: White atractylodes rhizome, magnolia bark, areca seed tsaoko, aucklandia root, chaenomeles fruit, prepared aconite root, dried ginger and poria 1 *liang* each, prepared licorice 5 *qian*. Grind them into a powder, add 5 pieces of fresh ginger and one date. Decoct them with water.

62. Ingredients: Licorice, poria, atractylodes rhizome, tangerine peel, white atractylodes rhizome, cinnamon bark, alismatis rhizome, unbellate pore-fungus, and magnolia bark. Grind them into a powder. Take 5 *qian* once after adding ginger and dates and decocting.

63. Ingredients: Talcum, oriental wormwood, scutellaria root, grass-leaved sweetflag rhizome, rice-paper pith, tendrilled fritillary bulb, belamcanda rhizome, forsythia fruit, peppermint, round cardamom seed, agastache.

64. Ingredients: Magnolia bark 1 *liang*, dried ginger 7 *fen*, tangerine peel 1 *liang*, poria, kastsumadai seed, aucklandia root and prepared licorice 5 *qian* each. Grind them into powder and 5 *qianbi*, take them once after adding 3 pieces of fresh ginger and decocting them with water.

65. Ingredients: Gypsum 3-5 *qian*, prepared rehmannia root 3-5 *qian*, ophiopogon root 2 *qian*, anemarrhena rhizome and achyranthes root 1 *qian* and 5 *fen* each.

66. Ingredients: Hawthorn fruit 6 *liang*, medicated leaven 2 *liang*, pinellia tuber and poria 3 *liang* each, tangerine peel, forsythia fruit and radish seed 1 *liang* each.

67. Ingredients: Radis adenophorae 3 *qian*, ophiopogon root 5 *qian*, crystal sugar 1 *qian*, rehmannia root 5 *qian*, rhizome of Polygonatum odoratum 1 *qian* and 5 *fen*.

68. Ingredients: Tangerine peel and bupleurum root 2 *qian* each, peony root, and bitter orange 1 *qian* and 5 *fen*, stir-baked licorice 5 *fen*, *Chuanxiong* rhizome and cyperus tuber 1 *qian* and 5 *fen* each. Take it after decocting with water.

69. Ingredients: Prepared pinellia tuber 5 *liang*, poria 4 *liang*, magnolia bark 3 *liang*, perilla leaf 2 *liang*. Grind them into a powder. Take 4 *qian* once.

70. Ingredients: Sargassum, tendrilled fritillary bulb, tangerine peel, laminaria (or ecklonia),

green tangerine peel, *Chuanxiong* rhizome, Chinese angelica root, pinellia tuber, forsythia fruit, licorice and pubescent angelica root 1 *qian* each, kelp 5 *fen*.

71. Ingredients: Turtle shell 11 *fen*, belamcanda rhizome, scutellaria root, armadillidium vulgare, dried ginger, rhubarb, cinnamon twigs, pyrrosia leaf, magnolia bark, flos campsis and donkey-hide gelatin 3 *fen* each, bupleurum root and cockroach 5 *fen* each, dung beetle 6 *fen* each, Chinese pink and herbaceous peony, moutan bark and peach kernel 2 *fen* each, pinellia tuber, ginseng and lepidium seed 1 *fen* each, wasp's nest 4 *fen*, calcined cinnabar 12 *fen*. Take 7 pills once, three times per day.

72. Ingredients: Chinese angelica root 1 *liang*, Chinese gentian 5 *qian*, aloes, capejasmine fruit, coptis root, phellodendron bark, scutellaria root 1 *liang* each, rhubarb 5 *qian*, aucklandia root 2 *qian* and 5 *fen*, musk 5 *fen*. Prepare them with honey. Take 3 *qian* once.

73. Ingredients: Chinese gentian 3 *fen*, bupleurum root and alismatis rhizome 1 *qian* each, plantain seed and five leaf akebia 5 *fen* each, rehmannia root and Chinese angelica root 3 *fen* each.

74. Ingredients: Chinese angelica root, white peony root, *Chuanxiong* rhizome, prepared rehmannia root, date kernel, chaenomeles fruit, ophiopogon root, licorice.

75. Ingredients: Wolfberry fruit, chrysanthemum and moutan bark 30 g each, dogwood fruit and Chinese yam 60 g, alismatis rhizome and poria 45 g each, prepared rehmannia root 120 g. Prepare them as pills with honey. Take 9 g once, two times a day.

76. Ingredients: Gastrodia tuber, uncaria stem with hooks, prepared sea-ear shell, capejasmine fruit, scutellaria root, cyathul root, eucommia bark, motherwort, mulberry mistletoe, fleeceflower stem, *Fushen* (poria) mixed with cinnabaris.

77. Ingredients: Achyranthes root 30 g, hematite 30 g, dragon's bone, oyster shell, tortoise plastron, white peony root, scrophularia root and asparagus root 15 g each, Sichuan chinaberry, germinated barley and oriental wormwood 6 g each, licorice 4.5 g.

78. Ingredients: Rhinoceros horn, cinnabar, realgar, hawksbill shell and amber 1 *liang* each, musk and borneol 1 *fen* each, ox gallstone 5 *qian*, benzoin 1 *liang* and 5 *qian*. Prepare them as pills with honey like Chinese parasol seeds. Take 3-5 pills after they are decocted with ginseng.

79. Ingredients: Rehmannia root 3 *liang*, morinda root, dogwood fruit, cistanche, dendrobium, prepared aconite root, poria, grass-leaved sweetflag rhizome, polygala root, cinnamon bark and ophiopogon root 1 *liang* each, schisandra fruit 5 *qian*. Grind them into a powder. Take 3 *qian* once after adding fresh ginger, dates and peppermint.

80. Ingredients: Antelope's horn 1 *qian* and 6 *fen*, mulberry leaf 2 *qian*, tendrilled fritillary bulb 4 *qian*, rehmannia root 5 *qian*, uncaria stem with hooks, chrysanthemum, poria and white peony root 3 *qian* each, licorice 8 *fen*, fresh bamboo shavings 5 *qian*.

81. Ingredients: Ox gallstone, curcuma root, rhinoceros horn, coptis root, cinnabar, capejasmine fruit, realgar and scutellaria root 1 *liang* each, pearl 5 *qian*, borneol and musk 2 *qian* and 5 *fen* each.

82. Ingredients: Chinese angelica root, wolfberry fruit, fennel fruit, cinnamon bark, lindera root, agalloch eaglewood, poria and fresh ginger.

83. Ingredients: Oriental wormwood 6 *liang*, 12 capejasmine fruit, rhubarb 2 *liang*. Take 1/3 once.

84. Ingredients: Coptis root, pinellia tuber, tangerine peel, poria, licorice, fresh ginger, bamboo shavings and immature bitter orange.

85. Ingredients: Dried rehmannia root 8 *liang*, Chinese yam and dogwood fruit 4 *liang* each, alismatis rhizome, poria and moutan bark 3 *liang* each, cinnamon twigs (or cinnamon bark) and prepared aconite root 1 *liang* each. Prepare them as pills with honey. Take 6 *qian* once, two times a day with warm boiled water or slightly salty soup.

86. Ingredients: Prepared rehmannia root and Chinese yam 4 *liang* each, dogwood fruit 3 *liang*, wolfberry fruit, dodder seed, antler glue and eucommia bark 4 *liang* each, Chinese angelica root 3 *liang*, cinnamon bark 2-4 *liang*, prepared aconite root 2-6 *liang*. Prepare them as pills with honey. Take 2-3 pills at one time.

87. Ingredients: Dodder seed, Chinese chives (seeds), oyster shell, dragon's bone, schisandra fruit, mantis eggshell, white pottery clay and poria.

88. Ingredients: Poria, peony root and fresh ginger 3 *liang* each, white atractylodes rhizome 2 *liang*, 1 prepared aconite root.

^{89.} Ingredients: Rehmannia root 5 *qian*, Chinese yam, dogwood fruit, alismatis rhizome, poria and peony 1 *liang* each, cinnamon twigs 5 *qian*, plantain seed 1 *liang*. Prepare them as pills with honey. Take 3 *qian* once, 1-2 times a day.

^{90.} Ingredients: Prepared rehmannia root 8 *qian*, Chinese yam 4 *qian*, dogwood fruit 4 *qian*, poria 3 *qian*, alismatis rhizome 3 *qian*, peony bark 3 *qian*. Prepare them as pills with honey. Take 3 *qian* once, 2 times a day with boiled or slightly salty water.

^{91.} Ingredients: Prepared rehmannia root 8 *liang*, dogwood fruit and Chinese yam 4 *liang* each, peony bark, poria and alismatis rhizome 3 *liang* each, anemarrhena rhizome and phellodendron bark 2 *liang* each. Prepare them as pills with honey. Take 3 *qian* once, 2 times a day.

^{92.} Ingredients: Human placenta, ophiopogon root, asparagus root and achyrathes root 3 g each, phellodendron bark and eucommia bark 4.5 g each, prepared rehmannia root and tortoise shell 6 g each. Prepare them as pills with honey. Take 9 g once, 2 times a day.

^{93.} Ingredients: Chinese pink, common knotgrass, plantain root, talcum and capejasmine fruit, prepared licorice, Sichuan clematis stem and rhubarb (roasted with ashes) 1 *jin* each. Grind them into a powder, take 2 *qian* once after adding rush pith and decoct with water.

^{94.} Ingredients: Coptis root 4 *liang*, scutellaria root and peony root 2 *liang* each, 2 chicken egg-yolks, donkey-hide gelatin 3 *liang*. Decoct the first three ingredients with water, then add the melted donkey-hide gelatin and then stir in the yolks after the mixture cools. Take 1/3 once.

^{95.} Ingredients: Coptis root and cinnamon bark. Prepare them as pills with honey.

^{96.} Ingredients: Ginseng 1 *cun*, 3 pieces of peach. Decoct them after adding 5 pieces of fresh ginger into it.

^{97.} Ingredients: Eaglewood, prepared aconite root, fenugreek seed (stir-fried) psoralea fruit, nutmeg, Sichuan chinaberry and aucklandia root 1 *liang* each, cinnamon bark 5 *qian*, lead powder and sulphur 2 *liang* each. Prepare them as pastry pills like Chinese parasol seeds. Take 30-40 pills once.

^{98.} Ingredients: Prepared rehmannia root, dogwood fruit, Chinese yam, alismatis rhizome, peony bark, poria and schisandra fruit. Prepare as pills with honey. Take 3 *qian* once with slightly salty soup.

^{99.} Ingredients: Ginseng 5 *qian*, ophiopogon root and schisandra fruit 3 *qian* each.

^{100.} Ingredients: Prepared aconite root, ginseng, white atractylodes rhizome, dried ginger, prepared licorice 1 *liang* each. Prepare them as pills with honey. Take 3 *qian* once.

^{101.} Ingredients: Psoralea fruit 4 *liang*, nutmeg and schisandra fruit 2 *liang* each, evodia fruit 1 *liang*. Grind them into powder, add 8 *liang* of fresh ginger and 100 dates, stir the decoction and prepare it as pills like Chinese parasol seeds. Take 20 pills once.

^{102.} Ingredients: Stir-fried white atractylodes rhizome 3 *liang*, stir-fried white peony root 2 *liang*, lodebouriella root 1 *liang*, stir-fried tangerine peel 1 *liang* and 5 *qian*. Grind them into a powder, decoct them with water. Take 1/8 once or take it with water after grinding it into a powder or prepare it as pills.

^{103.} Ingredients: Tangerine orange peel 1 *qian* and 5 *fen* each, prepare licorice 5 *fen*, *Chuanxiong* rhizome and cyperus tuber 1 *liang*.

^{104.} Ingredients: Evodia fruit 1 *liang*, coptis root 6 *liang*. Prepare them as pills with water. Take 1 *qian* once.

^{105.} Ingredients: Calcined gecko 180 g and natural indigo 18 g. Grind them into a powder. Take 9-15 g once after decocting it with water and packing it with cloth.

^{106.} Ingredients: Mulberry bark and wolfberry bark 1 *liang* each, licorice 5 *qian*. Grind them into powders. Take 2-4 *qian* each. Decoct them with water after adding polished round-grained rice.

^{107.} Ingredients: Cinnamon twigs 3 *liang*, peony root 3 *liang*, prepared licorice 2 *liang*, fresh ginger 3 *liang*, and 12 dates. Take 1/3 once. Avoid wind after taking it. A few minutes later take thin porridge to strengthen the action of the drugs and promote slight sweating.

^{108.} Ingredients: Ephedra 3 *liang*, cinnamon twigs 2 *liang*, 70 bitter apricot kernels, prepared licorice 1 *liang*. Take 1/3 of the decoction once.

^{109.} Ingredients: Anemarrhea rhizome 6 *liang*, gypsum 1 *jin*, prepared licorice 2 *liang*, polished round-grained rice 6 *he*. Take 1/3 once.

^{110.} Ingredients: Rhubarb 4 *liang* (decocted later), magnolia bark 8 *liang*, immature bitter orange (5 fruits), mirabilite 3 *he* (melt).

111. Ingredients: Prepared licorice 2 *liang*, dried ginger 1 *liang* and 5 *qian*, one fresh aconite.

112. Ingredients: 300 black plum seeds, asarum herb 6 *liang*, dried ginger 10 *liang*, coptis root 6 *liang*, prickly-ash peel 4 *liang*, cinnamon twigs 6 *liang*, ginseng 6 *liang*, phellodendron bark 6 *liang*. Prepare them as pills with honey like Chinese parasol seeds. Take 10 pills once, three times per day.

113. Ingredients: Honeysuckle flower and forsythia fruit 1 *liang* each, platycodon root, peppermint and arctium fruit 1 *liang* each, bamboo leaf and ashizone peta (ear) 4 *qian* each, fermented soybean and licorice 5 *qian* each. Grind them into powder. Take 6 *qian* once after adding fresh reed rhizome and decocting with water. Take the decoction when the fragrant vapour spreads.

114. Ingredients: 14 capejasmine fruits, fermented soybean 4 *he*. Take 1/2 of the decoction once.

115. Ingredients: Scrophularia root 1 *liang*, ophiopogon root and rehmannia rhizome 8 *qian* each, rhubarb 3 *qian* and minabilite 1 *qian* and 5 *fen* (melt). Take 1/3 once.

116. Ingredients: Scrophularia (the central part), forsythia fruit (central part) and tip of rhinoceros horn 2 *qian* each (ground into juice and taken after pouring boiling water onto it), forsythia fruit (central part) ophiopogon root 3 *qian* each. Decoct them with water.

117. Ingredients: Gypsum, mirabilite (crystal) magnetite, talcum, 3 *jin* each, rhinoceros horn, antelope's horn, radix aristolochiae and eaglewood 5 *liang* each, scrophularia root and cimicifuga rhizome 1 *jin* each, licorice 8 *liang*, cloves 1 *liang* and 2 *qian* and 5 *fen*, nitre 4 *shen*, musk 1 *liang*, prepared mirabilite, cinnabar 3 *liang*. Take 1/2 *qian* (powder) once.

118. Ingredients: Prepared licorice, rehmannia rhizome and white peony root 6 *qian* each, ophiopogon root 5 *qian*, donkey-hide gelatin 3 *qian*, hempseed 3 *qian*.

119. Ingredients: White peony root, rehmannia rhizome and ophiophon root 6 *qian* each, donkey-hide gelatin 3 *qian*, fresh tortoise plaston, fresh oyster shell, fresh turtle shell and prepared licorice 4 *qian* each, hempseed and schisandra *fruit* 2 *qian* each. Decoct them and remove their residues, add a chicken yolk, stir it evenly. Take 1/3 once.

120. Ingredients: Areca peel, dahuria angelica root, perilla and poria 1 *liang* each, fermented pinellia tuber, white atractylodes rhizome, pummelo peel, magnolia bark and platycodon root 2 *liang* each, agastache 3 *liang*, licorice 2 *liang*, and 5 *qian*. Grind them into a powder. Take 2 *qian* once after adding 3 pieces of fresh ginger and 1 date and decocting with water.

121. Ingredients: Agastache 2 *qian*, magnolia bark 1 *qian*, pinellia tuber 1 *qian* and 5 *fen*, poria 3 *qian*, bitter apricot kernel 3 *qian*, coix seed 4 *qian*, round cardamom seed 6 *fen*, umbellate pore-fungus 1 *qian* and 5 *fen*, fermented soybean 3 *qian*, alismatis rhizome 1 *qian* and 5 *fen*.

122. Ingredients: Bitter apricot kernel 5 *qian*, talcum 6 *qian*, rice paper, round cardamom seed, bamboo leaf and magnolia bark 2 *qian* each, coix seed 6 *qian*, pinellia tuber 5 *qian*.

123. Ingredients: Poria bark and round cardamom seed 5 *qian*, umbellate pore-fungus 3 *qian*, areca peel and rice paper 3 *qian* each, bamboo leaf 2 *qian*.

124. Ingredients: Umbellate pore-fungus 5 *qian*, poria 5 *qian*, mirabilite (crystal) 6 *qian*, silkworm excrement 4 *qian*, Chinese honey lotus (seed) 3 *qian*.

125. A collective term for the parts of the body connected with respiration (e.g., lung, trachea, larynx, nose, etc.)

126. A type of *bi* (blockage) syndrome caused by an excess of pathogenic damp and characterized by a heavy feeling and numbness of the limbs and body with localized swelling and pain.

127. Autumn dry (the disease due to exposure to pathogenic dryness in autumn). There are two types: Cool Dry and Heat Dry with the main symptoms of headache, fever, chills, no swelling, dryness of the nasal cavity and lips, etc.

128. It is autumn dry of a hot nature with the main symptoms of headache, fever, dry cough, dry throat, nasal cavity and lips, anxiety, and thirst, etc.

129. A collective term for sweat, mucus, tears, *yan* (a kind of saliva closely related to the spleen) and *tuo* (another kind of saliva closely related to the kidney).

130. The large blood vessels directly connected with the heart, i.e., the heart connections.

131. Fever due to deficient yin, as if the heat is spreading from the inside of the bone to the outside of the skin. It is usually accompanied by night sweating, and frequently seen in pulmonary tuberculosis.

132. Gangrene of the fingers or toes with excruciating pain at first, and after rather a long time necrosis and sloughing off the skin, subcutaneous tissues, muscles and bones, resembling throm-

boangitis obliteration.

[133.] A *bi* (blockage) syndrome mainly characterized by symptoms of pain in the bones, a heavy feeling and limp body and limbs.

[134.] Suppuration of the lung with purulent and bloody expectoration, i.e., lung abscess and gangrene of the lung.

[135.] A hysteria condition where the patient feels a foreign body, like the stone of a plum obstructing the throat and has difficulty swallowing. There is neither redness nor swelling of the throat.

[136.] The reservoir of the blood (referring to the liver or Strategic Vessel Meridian).

[137.] A collective term for the five signs representing the delayed development of an infant, namely, delayed standing, walking, hair growth, growth of the teeth and speech.

[138.] A collective term for the five symptom complexes in infancy, namely, softness of the head, softness of the neck, softness of the arms and legs, softness of the muscles and softness of the mouth.

[139.] A collective term for a group of meridians, which means that yin *qi* is at the final stage of its development.

[140.] Yin fluid of the heart.

[141.] An unpleasant sensation that mimics pain and hunger. It is often seen in peptic ulcer, gastritis, etc.

[142.] Ravenous appetite and excessive hunger.

Notes:

1 *jin* = 500 g	1 *fen* = 0.3123 g
1 *shen* = 193.7 cc	1 *chi* = 32 cm
1 *liang* = 31.25 g	1 *li* = 0.031 g
1 *he* = 19.37 cc	1 *qianbi* = 2 g
1 *qian* = 3.123 g	1 *cun* = 3.2 cm
1 *zhu* = 1/6 *fen*	1 *fangcunbi* = 0.27 mm

11. GENERAL RULES OF PREVENTION AND TREATMENT

11-1 Prevention

In TCM disease prevention is emphasized. As early as in *Internal Classic*, disease prevention and measures to prevent a disease from taking a turn for the worse were discussed.

11-1-1 Prevention against disease

The occurrence of disease involves two aspects. The pathogenic factor is an important cause of disease, while the body's weak anti-pathogenic factor is the internal cause of disease. The two factors must be considered in disease prevention.

11-1-1-1 Building up health and strengthening body resistance against the pathogenic factor

Whether the anti-pathogenic factor is strong or not depends upon the constitution. In general, if one has a strong constitution, the anti-pathogenic factor will be strong; if not, it will be weak. Hence, maintaining the health and strengthening the constitution are very important to enhance the anti-pathogenic factor. In keeping up one's health, attention should be paid to the following:

a. Regulating or harmonizing Spirit: The TCM system maintains that mental and emotional activities are closely related to physiopathological changes. Rapid or repeated and persistent mental stimuli can impede the *qi* mechanism and cause disharmony of *qi*, blood, yin and yang, resulting in disease. Emotional stimuli can weaken the anti-pathogenic factor and cause the invasion of the exogenous pathogenic factor. In the course of disease, negative or excess emotion can aggravate a disease, whereas balanced emotions and a good mood will promote recovery. A strong anti-pathogenic factor within the body prevents disease from occurring and developing. So, regulating and harmonizing the emotions can strengthen the ability of the anti-pathogenic factor against the pathogenic factor and prevent disease.

b. Physical exercise: The constitution can be strengthened by regular physical exercise. According to the principle of "Running water never stales and a door hinge never gets worm-eaten," Hua Tuo, a medical expert of the Han Dynasty (206 B.C.-A.D. 220), created the "five animal games"[1] to promote blood circulation, making joints more flexible and regulating the *qi* mechanism in order to maintain health and treat disease. In addition, varieties of exercises derived from the "five animal games" in later generations, such as *Taijiquan*,[2] *Baduanjin*,[3] etc. not only maintain health and prevent disease, but also can be used to treat a number of chronic diseases.

c. Leading a regular life: In order to keep healthy and vigorous and live long, one should understand natural changes, adapt himself to changes of the geographical environment and arrange work, rest and daily habits to maximum benefit. One should not drink too much alcohol, overwork and carry on sexual activity after drinking alcohol lest *jing* (vital principle) should be exhausted and primordial *qi* severely consumed.

d. Prevention with drugs and artificial immunology: As early as in *Internal Classic*, it was recorded that a "pestilential disease can be prevented after taking 10 pills of Minor Golden Pillets," which explains that prevention against smallpox with the variola vaccination method[4] invented by Chinese medical experts in the 16th century was the vanguard to immunology for later generations. In addition, Chinese atractylodes, realgar, etc. are used for preventing disease. In recent years, favourable effects have been obtained by applying Chinese herbal medicines to prevent disease. For example, the rhizome of cyrtomium and dyers woad root or dyers woad leaf are used to prevent flu, and capillary artemisia and the capejasmine fruit, etc. are used to prevent hepatitis, and purslane (herb) is used to prevent bacterial dysentery.

11-1-1-2 Prevention against the invasion of the pathogenic factor

Since a pathogenic factor causes disease, maintaining health and enhancing the level of body resistance is emphasized in TCM, for instance, paying attention to personal hygiene, the environment, avoiding the "six excesses," pestilential factor, "seven emotions," improper diet, fatigue and lack of physical exercise, etc. External injuries and animal bites should also be closely observed to prevent infection.

11-1-2 Prevention against disease from developing and changing

When illness does occur, early diagnosis and treatment is best so as to prevent the disease from worsening.

11-1-2-1 Early diagnosis and treatment

If the exogenous pathogenic factor that has invaded the body is not diagnosed and treated early, it may move from the exterior to the interior of the body, so that the internal organs are invaded and the disease becomes more complex, severe and difficult to treat. Hence, in treating a disease, the development of the disease and its changes must be grasped, in order to diagnose it early and treat it effectively.

11-1-2-2 Reinforcement of the unaffected part according to the rule of movement and transformation of disease

"The 77 Difficult Problems," a chapter in *Classic on Difficult Medical Problems* states, "A superior medical worker treats the person before he or she is sick and an average one, the person who has been ill." In disease treatment the interconnection of the organs is considered, for example, if the liver is affected, the trouble will affect the spleen. As the liver corresponds to wood and the spleen, earth, the liver can overact upon the spleen so the therapy of reinforcing the spleen and harmonizing the stomach is frequently used in coordination in clinical treatment of liver trouble. This is a practical application of the principle of preventing the disease from spreading. Take another example. Ye Tianshi, a medical expert from the Qing Dynasty (1644-1911), advocated certain salty, cold drugs to replenish the kidney and emphasized the principle of prevention and treatment, "the viscus that has not yet been affected must be reinforced." This is an example of the principle of preventing the disease from spreading.

11-2 General rules of treatment

General rules of treatment are formulated under the guidance of a holistic concept and *bianzheng* and *lunzhi* (planning treatment according to diagnosis) are significant for therapies and the application of drugs. The reinforcement of the anti-pathogenic factor and elimination of the pathogenic factor are general therapeutical principles. Reinforcing *qi*, nourishing blood, replenishing yin and reinforcing yang, etc. are guided by these general rules. Diaphoresis, emesis and purgation, etc. are therapies to eliminate the pathogenic factor.

Since symptoms of a disease vary, the pathological process is complex and varies with severity, time and environment. The doctor must grasp the essence of the pathological changes of a disease and treat it by tracing its primary cause. The anti-pathogenic factor should be reinforced and the pathogenic one eliminated according to the (deficiency and excess) changes occurring in the struggle between the anti-pathogenic and pathogenic factors. Yin and yang should be regulated according to the disharmony between them. Visceral function and the relation between *qi* and blood should be regulated and harmonized. The disease should be treated according to the season, environment and individual.

11-2-1 Treating a disease by treating its primary cause

Treating a disease by treating its primary cause is a basic principle of *bianzheng* and *lunzhi* (planning treatment according to diagnosis). *Ben* is the primary cause and *biao* is the secondary cause. An old and primary disease is *ben*, but a newly-encountered and secondary disease is *biao*.

Only by completely collecting and understanding various aspects of the disease, tracing its primary cause and analysing the symptoms under the guidance of the basic theories of TCM can the cause of the disease be found and proper therapies determined. For example, a headache can be caused by an exogenous pathogenic factor and internal injury. A headache caused by exogenous pathogenic wind-cold should be treated by diaphoresis with pungent drugs of a warm nature; a headache caused by exogenous pathogenic wind-warmth should be treated by diaphoresis with pungent drugs of a cool nature. Headache from internal injury is ascribed to deficient blood, congealed blood, pathogenic phlegm-damp, overactive liver yang and liver fire, etc. Hence, it is treated by applying therapies, such as nourishing blood, promoting blood circulation and subduing congealed blood, removing pathogenic damp and eliminating phlegm, checking an overactive liver and restraining the yang, etc.

11-2-1-1 Regular (or routine) and contrary treatments

a. Regular (or routine) treatment is a common therapeutic principle where a disease is treated by applying the medications which have features contrary to those of the disease, i.e., different therapies, such as "heating the cold," "cooling the heat," "tonifying the deficiency," "purging the excess," etc. suit the disease whose symptoms accord with its essence. Since most symptoms of a disease accord with its characteristics, e.g., cold signs seen in a cold disease, hot signs seen in a heat disease, deficiency signs seen in a deficiency disease, excess signs seen in an excess disease, etc. This is a common therapy in clinic.

b. Contrary treatment is a therapy in which a disease is treated by applying drugs which accord with false symptoms of a disease. It is a therapy using the guidance of the principle of treating the disease by tracing its primary cause. For example, contrary treatment treats heat with heat, cold with cold, obstruction by tonification, diarrhea by purgation, etc.

"Treating heat with heat" is to treat a disease or syndrome with false hot symptoms with drugs of a hot nature. In true-cold and false-heat syndromes yin cold is so excessive internally that yang is excluded with hot signs seen. For instance, a *shaoyin* disease manifested by aqueous diarrhea, coldness in the interior and hotness in the exterior of the body, cold clammy extremities, faint pulse, no aversion to cold and flushed face is treated with *Shini* Decoction of Unobstructing Meridian. Since deficient yang and excess *yin* are the essence of disease, false heat may spontaneously disappear by treating true cold with drugs of a warm and hot nature.

"Cooling the cold" is to treat the disease or syndrome of false cold symptoms with drugs of a cold nature. It suits true-heat and false-cold syndromes where internal heat is so extremely excessive that yin is excluded by excess yang, with cold signs seen. For instance, in "heat-*jue*" syndrome cold clammy extremities and deep pulse appear resembling a cold syndrome, but "strong fever" and anxiety, thirst and preference for cold drinks, dark-red scanty urine, etc. exist because yang is internally excessive but yin is excluded. As excess heat is the essence of the disease, drugs of a cold-cool nature must be used to treat true heat, so that false signs can disappear.

"Treating obstruction by tonification" is to treat the disease with obstruction symptoms with tonics. It suits the true-deficiency and false-excess disease of obstruction due to deficiency, e.g., for the patient with a weak spleen, abdominal distension and fullness at intervals that are not relieved by pressure, dyspepsia, light-coloured tongue, empty and forceless pulse, and no sign of aqueous damp and food retention, etc. often appear and are treated by reinforcing the spleen and nourishing *qi*. Abdominal distension will spontaneously disappear if spleen *qi* performs its transporting function normally. In addition, dysuria due to deficient *jing* (vital principle), and blood and severely impaired amenorrhea due to exhausted blood and severely impaired Strategic Vessel Meridian and Conception Vessel Meridian, etc. are treated with tonics.

"Treating diarrhea with purgation" is to treat diarrhea[5] with purgatives. This treatment suits abdominal pain due to food retention, irregular bowel movements, fecal impaction with watery diarrhea, metrorrhagia caused by congealed blood, frequent micturition, urgent urination and urethralgia caused by the bladder affected by pathogenic heat, promoting blood circulation and eliminating congealed blood and clearing up pathogenic damp-heat in the bladder, etc. may be applied respectively.

11-2-1-2 Treatment of *biao* (secondary) and *ben* (primary) diseases

In complex and changeable diseases or syndromes, some are primary but others are secondary. They should therefore be distinguished in treatment. The treatment of *biao* and *ben* diseases is generally the treatment of disease by tracing its primary cause. Under certain cases, a *biao* disease is acute. If it is not solved in time, the patient will die or treatment will be influenced. Thus, the principles of treating the *biao* aspect for emergency and the *ben* aspect for chronicity should be adopted. If the secondary and primary diseases are equally severe, both of them may be treated simultaneously.

a. Treating the *biao* (secondary) aspect for emergency: "*Biaoben* and *Huanji*," a chapter in *Plain Questions* states, "For the patient first suffering from fever and then abdominal fullness and distension, treat the *biao* (secondary) aspect for emergency. For the one who is first sick and suffers from abdominal fullness and distension, treat the *biao* (secondary) aspect for emergency. For difficulty in defecation and micturation, treat the *biao* (secondary) aspect for emergency." Abdominal fullness and distension and difficulty in defecation and micturation are all acute symptoms and should be first treated. For example, for the ascites patient, when ascites increase, the abdomen is distending and full, the respiration is asthmatic and defecation and micturation are difficult, and ascites of the *biao* (secondary) disease should be first treated. Difficulty in defecation and micturation may be treated by diuresis and the *ben* (primary) one, by regulating the liver and spleen after ascites are relieved and the disease improved.

b. Treating the *ben* (primary) aspect for chronicity is significant for chronic diseases or the rehabilitation period of acute disease, e.g., a cough due to pulmonary tuberculosis. Since its *ben* (primary) aspect is usually yin deficiency of the lung and kidney, it should not be treated by a cough-relieving therapy to treat the *biao* (secondary) aspect for emergency, but by replenishing lung yin and kidney yin to treat the primary aspect for chronicity. Take another example. Yin consumption at the advanced and late stages of an acute febrile disease should be treated by nourishing the stomach and replenishing the kidney, etc.

c. Simultaneous treatment of *biao* and *ben* aspects: If the secondary and primary diseases are equally severe, they should be treated simultaneously. For example, the case with fever, firmness, fullness and pain in the abdomen, constipation, dry and thirsty mouth, dry tongue with yellowish coating, etc. is ascribed to internally-stagnant pathogenic heat (the secondary aspect) and consumed yin fluid (the primary aspect) and both of them are treated simultaneously with Fluid-increasing and *Qi*-replenishing Decoction. If purgation and yin-replenishing therapies are used simultaneously, the yin can be preserved by purging heat and purgation promoted by replenishing the yin and removing pathogenic dryness. Take another example. The asthmatic person who frequently suffers from colds is treated by reinforcing *qi* and moving the pathogenic factor in the superficial part of the body. Reinforcing *qi* is to treat the *ben* aspect for chronicity and diaphoresis and the *biao* aspect for emergency.

11-2-2 Reinforcing the anti-pathogenic factor and eliminating the pathogenic factor

Disease is the struggle between the anti-pathogenic and pathogenic factors. The reinforcement of the anti-pathogenic factor and elimination of the pathogenic factor are the important principles guiding clinical treatment.

11-2-2-1 Reinforcing the anti-pathogenic factor and eliminating the pathogenic factor

Reinforcing the anti-pathogenic factor means to assist the anti-pathogenic factor, strengthen the constitution, and enhance the immune system. In reinforcement of the anti-pathogenic factor, tonification for a weak body is frequently used, including acupuncture and moxibustion, *qigong* and exercise. Regulating emotions and supplementing dietary nutrition are important for the reinforcement of the anti-pathogenic factor.

The therapy of purging the excess is usually used for eliminating the pathogenic factor, but it varies according to different pathogenic factors in different locations.

11-2-2-2 The principle of reinforcing the anti-pathogenic factor and eliminating the pathogenic factor

When applying the principle of reinforcing the anti-pathogenic factor and eliminating the pathogenic factor, the flourishing and decline of the anti-pathogenic and pathogenic factors should be observed and analysed and whether the reinforcement of the anti-pathogenic factor or elimination of the pathogenic factor is primary is determined according to the struggle between them. In general, there are the following conditions:

Reinforcement of the anti-pathogenic factor suits the deficiency disease (syndrome) where the anti-pathogenic factor is weak, but the pathogenic factor is not so predominant.

For example, the patient with deficient *qi* and yang should be treated by tonifying the *qi* and yang; the patient with deficient yin and blood, by replenishing the yin and tonifying the blood.

Elimination of the pathogenic factor suits the excess disease (or syndrome) where the pathogenic factor is mainly substantive, but the anti-pathogenic factor has not yet declined. For example, the patient affected by a violent pathogenic factor in the superficial part of the body should be treated by diaphoresis. The patient affected by the pathogenic factor in the chest and epigastrium, such as profuse obstructed phlegm and saliva, food retention, or food poisoning, etc. should be treated with emesis. The patient affected by the pathogenic factor in the intestine and stomach, such as pathogenic heat combining with intestinal residues should be treated by purgation; the patient affected by substantive heat and fire, by clearing up the heat and fire; the cold syndrome, by warming the middle energizer to eliminate pathogenic cold; the damp syndrome, by subduing pathogenic damp and diuresis; food retention and abdominal distension and fullness, by promoting digestion and relieving the stagnant; phlegm affection, by eliminating phlegm; congealed blood, by promoting blood circulation and subduing congealed blood, etc.

Reinforcement of the anti-pathogenic factor and elimination of the pathogenic one in coordination suits the disease (or syndrome) where the anti-pathogenic factor is weak, but the pathogenic one, substantive. For the case where the anti-pathogenic factor is comparatively urgent and weak, it is reinforced in association with elimination of the pathogenic factor. For the case where the pathogenic factor is urgent and more substantive, elimination is used in association with reinforcement of the anti-pathogenic factor.

Prior-elimination of the pathogenic factor and post-reinforcement of the anti-pathogenic factor suits the disease (or syndrome) where the weak anti-pathogenic factor can still resist the violent pathogenic factor or the pathogenic factor would be resisted when the anti-pathogenic factor is reinforced, e.g., in metrorrhagia caused by congealed blood, if congealed blood is not eliminated, metrorrhagia will not stop. So, promoting blood circulation and eliminating congealed blood should first be used and then blood tonified.

Prior-reinforcement of the anti-pathogenic factor and post-elimination of the pathogenic factor suit the patient whose anti-pathogenic factor is weak, but the pathogenic factor is strong. As the anti-pathogenic factor is extremely weak and will be further injured if it is reinforced in association with the elimination of the pathogenic factor, it should be first reinforced and then the pathogenic factor eliminated. For example, for patients with parasites, their spleens should first be reinforced to regain the anti-pathogenic factor to a certain extent and then parasites will be eliminated.

11-2-3 Regulating yin and yang

A disease will result from a loss of the equilibrium between yin and yang (excess of one and deficiency of the other). Hence it is one of the primary principles in treatment that the yin and yang should be regulated and their equilibrium regained in order to promote "yin flourishing smoothly and yang vivified steadily."

11-2-3-1 Reducing a relative excess

This chiefly implies that an excess of yin or yang can be treated by reducing the excess, e.g., the excess-heat syndrome due to external excess of yang heat should be treated by cooling the heat, so as to clear it up; the cold excess syndrome due to internal excess of yin cold, by heating the cold so as to warmly dissipate it.

In the pathological change due to a relative excess of yin or yang, an excess of one may lead to a deficiency of the other. Excess yang heat easily consumes yin fluids and excess yin cold easily injures yang *qi*. So, when regulating an excess of yin or yang, any corresponding decline of yin or yang should be noted. If an excess of one causes a deficiency of the other, it should also be treated in association with reinforcing the yang or replenishing the yin.

11-2-3-2 Reinforcing a relative decline

For declining yin or yang, the therapy of reinforcing the deficiency is adopted. If deficient yin fails to restrain yang, which is often manifested as the deficiency heat syndrome due to deficient yin and excess yang, the yin should be replenished to restrain yang; if it leads to impaired kidney yin, it should be treated by "strengthening the master of water to counteract the brilliance of yang."[6] If it is ascribed to deficient yin and yang, both the yin and yang should be reinforced. It should be pointed out that since the yin and yang are interdependent, excess yin and yang may also impair each other. Therefore, yang-tonifying drugs are used in treating the yin and yin-tonifying ones are used in treating the yang when treating a disease (or syndrome) caused by excess yin or yang.

11-2-4 Regulating the function of the viscera

The viscera are interdependent. When a yin or yang viscus is affected, it influences the other. Hence, during the treatment of pathological changes of the viscera, one cannot only consider the affected viscus, but should pay attention to regulating the relation of the viscera. For instance, pathological changes of the lung can be caused not only by the pathogenic factor, but also by pathological changes of the heart, liver, spleen, kidney and large intestine. If asthmatic breath and cough due to the failure of lung *qi* to descend are caused by deficient heart *qi* and a blocked Heart Meridian, then they should be treated by chiefly warming heart yang. If hematemesis is caused by hyperactive liver fire and adversely ascending *qi* fire, it should be treated by reducing liver fire. If a cough with profuse phlegm due to the lung's failure to perform its dispersing and clearing functions is caused by accumulated damp and production of phlegm due to a weak spleen and phlegm-damp stagnating in the lung, it should be treated by warmly reinforcing the spleen and removing the pathogenic damp. A dry cough and dry mouth and throat caused by deficient kidney yin and a shortage of lung fluid should be treated by replenishing the kidney and moisture to absorb *qi* and regurgitation of lung *qi* should be treated by mainly warming the kidney and making it absorb *qi*. Asthmatic breath due to pathogenic heat stagnating in the large intestine and the failure of lung *qi* to descend should be treated by unobstructing the yang viscera to purge substantive heat in the large intestine. Take another example. The pathological change of the spleen can also be caused by pathological change of the liver, heart, kidney and stomach besides spleen trouble. The spleen's failure to perform its functions should be treated by mainly soothing the liver. It is advisable to reinforce the spleen (earth) and inhibit the liver (wood) for the case when the weak spleen is overacted upon by the liver; the case that the spleen (earth) is not promoted by the liver (fire) due to declining *mingmen* (vital portal) fire should be treated by reinforcing fire (liver) to promote earth (spleen). The case where the stomach fails to propel downward and the spleen fails to carry on its transporting function should be treated by mainly harmonizing the stomach in order to promote the harmony between the ascending and descending functions of the spleen and stomach.

11-2-5 Regulating the relation between *qi* and blood

Qi can generate blood, promote blood circulation and control blood. Blood supplies a material basis for *qi* activities and carries *qi*. When they fail to supplement and promote each other, a variety of diseases or disharmony between *qi* and blood may appear. The principle of regulating the relation between *qi* and blood is reducing excess and reinforcing deficiency.

Qi can generate blood. When *qi* is enriched, blood is generated; when it is weak, blood is insufficiently generated, leading to blood deficiency or *qi* is insufficiently generated, leading to blood deficiency or *qi* and blood are deficient which is treated by mainly reinforcing *qi* in association with tonifying and nourishing blood, but not only tonifying blood.

Qi promotes blood circulation. Deficient or stagnant *qi* may lead to a lowering of blood circulation and congealed and obstructed blood called blood congealment due to *qi* deficiency or stasis. It is advisable to treat it by reinforcing *qi* and promoting blood circulation or regurgitating *qi*, promoting blood circulation and subduing congealed blood. Disorders of the *qi* mechanism would lead to blood disorders. Blood ascends adversely together with liver *qi*, often resulting in fainting or hemoptysis that may be treated by checking adversely-ascending *qi* and normalizing blood circulation.

Qi can control blood. If deficient, it will fail to control blood, leading to hemorrhage due to extravasation of blood which is treated by reinforcing *qi* to control blood.

Deficient blood will lead to deficient *qi*. In the case of exhausted blood, *qi* is often exhausted together with blood. It is advisable to treat it by reinforcing *qi* to arrest the exhausted blood according to the principle of first nourishing *qi* to treat exhausted blood.

11-2-6 Treatment of a disease according to season, environment and individual constitution

The treatment of disease according to the season, environment and individual constitution refers to the therapy established according to the above factors. The occurrence and change of disease are influenced by these various factors, particularly the constitution of an individual. Therefore these factors must be taken into consideration in treatment.

11-2-6-1 Treatment of a disease according to the season

Seasonal changes influence physiological functions and pathological changes. The principle of treatment and practical application of drugs are considered according to different seasons and weather. In general, in spring and summer when it gets warmer, yang *qi* elevates and flourishes. The junction between the skin and muscle becomes loose and open. In such a case, for the patient affected by exogenous pathogenic wind-cold, pungent and warm drugs with a dissipating action are not used lest the junction should open excessively and yin *qi* should be consumed. Yin flourishes but yang declines, the junction gets closer and yang *qi* withdraws into the body. In such a case, unless severe febrile disease occurs cold-cool drugs are not prescribed lest the yang should be injured. Since the affection of pathogenic summer-heat is obviously seasonal and it is usually accompanied by pathogenic damp, attention should be paid to relieving pathogenic summer-heat and removing pathogenic damp in the treatment of disease in summer. It is advisable to treat the external affection of autumn pathogenic dryness by moistening the body with pungent-cool drugs in dry autumn, which is not entirely the same as the application of drugs in the treatment of wind-warm affection in spring and wind-cold affection in autumn. It is advisable to treat the wind-warmth affection by diaphoresis with pungent-cool drugs and wind-cold affection by diaphoresis with pungent-warm drugs.

11-2-6-2 Treatment of a disease according to the geographical environment

Treatment is considered according to the geographical characteristics of different areas. As the climate and way of life vary in different areas, physiological processes and pathological changes are not entirely the same. The treatment and application of drugs should accord with the local geographical environment and way of life. For example, on the northwest plateau of China, it is cold and dry with little rainfall, so, the exogenous pathogenic factor can hardly invade the body and internal injuries occur frequently. Southeast China is near the sea, flat, with marshlands and its terrain is low. The climate is warm and hot and rainy. People there prefer fish and salty food, the junctions between the skin and muscles are loose, and they are likely to have carbuncles and sores, or be easily affected by an exogenous pathogenic factor. It is cold in northwest China and the affections of external cold and internal heat usually occur. They should be treated by dissipating exogenous pathogenic cold and cooling endogenous pathogenic heat; since it is warm and hot in southwest China, and yang *qi* discharges outward, exogenous pathogenic cold occurs easily. So, it should be treated by arresting outward-discharging yang *qi* and warming the body to remove the cold. It is because of different weather conditions that the physician cures the same patient with different therapies. For example, a disorder due to exogenous wind-cold affection is treated in cold northwest China with a large amount of pungent diaphoretics of a warm nature, such as Ephedra-sinica equisetina and cinnamon (barks), and in warm and hot southeast China it is treated with a small amount of pungent diaphoretics of a hot nature, such as Nepeta japonica and radix sileris.

11-2-6-3 Treatment of a disease according to the individual

Treatment and application of drugs are considered according to the age, sex, constitution and way of life of the individual.

a. Age: People of different ages have different physiological states of *qi* and blood. The treatment and application of drugs differ accordingly. Senile people are short of vitality and their *qi* and blood are deficient. They are likely to have a deficiency or deficiency-excess syndrome; it is advisable to treat it by tonification, and the substantive pathogenic factor should be eliminated cautiously with smaller quantities of drugs that are milder than those used for the young and middle-aged. Young children are full of vigour, but their *qi* and blood have not yet been enriched. Their viscera are delicate and likely to be affected by pathogenic cold and heat and their disease condition changes rapidly. So, drugs of drastic action are prohibited, tonics used less and a small amount of drugs should be used in treatment.

b. Sex: In treatment and prescription, menstrual-flow, leukorrhea, pregnancy and delirium, etc. of women should be considered. For example, the drastic congealed-blood-removing, lubricating and fetus-injuring drugs must be prohibited or used with caution during pregnancy and postpartum *qi* and blood deficiencies and lochia, etc. should be considered.

c. Constitution: People's constitutions are strong or weak, cold or hot. For patients with excess yang or deficient yin, warm-hot drugs are used carefully; for those with deficient yang or excess yin, the cold-cool ones which injure yang are used cautiously. In addition, attention should be paid to certain chronic or occupational diseases, emotional factors and lifestyle, etc. in diagnosis and treatment.

To sum up, individual treatment means that a disease (or syndrome) cannot be treated in isolation, but the individual constitution must be taken into consideration. In treatment of disease according to season and geographical environment, the influence of the natural environment upon the body is stressed. The therapeutic principle of treatment according to season, environment and the individual shows that the holistic concept and *bianzheng* and *lunzhi* are flexible. Only by viewing a disease from all perspectives and analysing it according to the season, environment and individual can an ideal therapeutic effect be obtained.

11-2-7 Application of the general rules of treatment

11-2-7-1 Application of the eight principal therapies

Diaphoresis, emesis, purgation, harmonization, warming nourishment, purification, tonification and elimination are the eight principal therapies applied in treatment. All of them are most commonly used in clinic except emesis.

a. Diaphoresis: This is a therapy which opens up the pores and expels the pathogenic factor from the body. Its chief action is to eliminate the exogenous pathogenic factor that has invaded the body surface.

Range of its application: Early stages of all the diseases due to external affection, those of edema and sores and the stage at which measles begins to occur.

Applications: Chiefly suitable for all diseases (or syndromes) where the pathogenic factor is in the superficial part of the body. As an exterior syndrome of external-cold and external-heat types, its application may be classified into: Diaphoresis with pungent drugs of warm nature which suits the exterior-cold syndrome; diaphoresis with pungent drugs of a cool nature, which suits the exterior-heat syndrome. The above-mentioned methods are primary. As patients have different constitutions or suffer from chronic diseases so that the internal and external causes combine and the disease becomes complicated, these methods cannot be used mechanically but according to the following conditions: Diaphoresis by nourishing yin suits the patient who is usually weak in yin and is affected by the superficial pathogenic factor; diaphoresis by reinforcing yang suits the patient who is usually weak in yang and is affected by superficial pathogenic factor. Eliminating *yin* (excess exudates) and subduing phlegm suit the patient who usually suffers from *tan-yin* (phlegm and excess exudates) and is affected by the superficial pathogenic factor.

In addition, there are also *qi*-regulating and food-digesting therapies used in coordination with diaphoresis, which may also be called a "simultaneous treatment of exterior and interior," etc.

b. Emesis: A therapy used to get the pathogenic factor or poisonous substance out of the body by vomiting. It is for first aid which works by chiefly making the substantive pathogenic factor stagnate in the upper energizer and it is then vomited to eliminate it.

Range of its applications: It suits disorders such as excessive phlegm and saliva, food retention in the stomach that tends to ascend, or stagnant poisonous food mistaken in the stomach, etc.

Applications: It is used for the excess syndrome when something stagnating in the body must be rapidly vomited in emergency cases. Since the pathogenic factor is of the cold and hot types and varies when the anti-pathogenic factor has (or not yet) been injured, its application may be generally divided into cold emesis which suits the disorder where pathogenic heat stagnates in the upper part of the body; hot emesis which suits pathogenic cold stagnating in the upper part of the body; drastic emesis suiting the excessive pathogenic factor in the upper part of body that makes the disorder acute; mild emesis suits the case where the pathogenic factor is violent but the anti-pathogenic factor is weak and the disorder located in the upper energizer must be treated with emesis.

The above-mentioned methods are general principles for the application of emesis. But, the drugs that may be used for emesis can also be divided into pungent, sweet, sour, bitter and salty and those of a cold, hot, warm and cool nature, which can induce vomiting. At the same time, there exists a difference between extremely poisonous and mild poisonous drugs in emetics. Therefore, the above-mentioned therapies cannot be used mechanically, but according to the condition in treatment.

c. Purgation: A therapy to expel the stagnant material from the body and promote bowel movements, and regulate the *qi* mechanism.

Ranges of its application: It suits the case of pathogenic heat stagnating in the stomach and intestine, pathogenic heat stagnating inside the body, and cases such as stagnant water, congealed blood, stagnant phlegm, retention of parasites, etc.

Applications: It chiefly suits the interior-excess syndrome, which varies with cold, heat, water, blood, phlegm, parasites, and can be new or prolonged, mild or acute. It is therefore divided into: cold purgation for disorders such as the interior, excess and heat syndromes characterized by constipation and dysentery due to fecal impaction with watery diarrhea, stagnation in the intestine, etc., pathogenic cold accumulated in the spleen and stomach, excess cold, pathogenic cold accumulated in the spleen and stomach, excess cold knotting in the chest and constipation, etc.; excessive water suits the excess syndrome of yang water; the subduing purgation suits constipation due to insufficient body fluids and constipation due to impaired yin and deficient blood. Subduing the congealed blood suits the internal stagnation syndrome of congealed blood. Eliminating phlegm suits the phlegm-stagnating syndrome; destroying parasites suits parasite retention.

d. Harmonization: A therapy to eliminate the pathogenic factor and reinforce the anti-pathogenic factor by harmonization.

Ranges of its application: It is widely used, for instance, in a *shaoyang* disease, in disharmony between the liver and stomach, irregular menstruation due to stagnant liver *qi*, abdominal pain and diarrhea due to the overactive liver and weak spleen, etc.

Applications: It suits the case where the pathogenic factor lies between the superficial and deep parts of the body or where both parts are simultaneously ill, and cases in which therapies, such as diaphoresis, emesis and purgation, etc. are not suitable.

e. Warming nourishment: A therapy to eliminate pathogenic cold and tonify yang *qi*, of which the chief action is to revive the yang for resuscitation, warm the middle energizer and dissipate pathogenic cold so as to eliminate persistent cold and tonify yang *qi*.

Range of its applications: It suits the case in which pathogenic cold attacks the three yin meridians or when a heat syndrome has changed into a cold one.

Applications: It is used for an interior-cold syndrome, but there is usually deficient yang in the patient affected by endogenous pathogenic cold. So, methods of eliminating pathogenic cold and of tonifying the yang are used jointly.

Its applications are generally divided into: reviving yang from deficient real yang, attack of pathogenic cold on the three yin meridians or excessive use of cold drugs with a clearing action so that the pathogenic factor enters the three yin meridians.

Eliminating pathogenic cold by warming the middle energizer suits the mild case in which the patient's yang is weak so that exogenous pathogenic cold invades the middle energizer.

f. Purification: A therapy for treating febrile disease, having the action of clearing up pathogenic heat, removing fire, promoting body fluids and relieving polydipsia.

Ranges of its application: It can be used for treating all the febrile diseases where pathogenic heat is at the *qi* (vital energy), or *ying* (nutrition) or *xue* (blood) phase, and where the superficial pathogenic factor has been eliminated, but the internal heat is still in excess, with nothing substantial. It may also be used for treating the case where both the superficial and deep parts of the body are affected by pathogenic heat according to the condition.

Applications: As a heat syndrome is located in different *qi*, *ying* and *xue* phases, it may be generally classified into: clearing up pathogenic heat and producing body fluids, which is suitable for the disease where burning heat is at the *qi* phase and body fluids are impaired by it; clearing up the pathogenic heat and purging fire, which is suitable for the excess-heat syndrome with pathogenic heat at the *qi* phase; clearing up pathogenic heat at the *ying* phase, which is suitable for the disorder where pathogenic heat has entered the *xue* phase; nourishing the yin and clearing up pathogenic heat, which is suitable for the disorder where pathogenic heat consumes yin so that body fluids are impaired and fire flares up and is suitable for the disorder of persistent high fever and mental disturbance.

There are also the therapies, such as clearing up heat fire, clearing up liver fire, clearing up lung fire, clearing up stomach fire, etc. besides the above-mentioned therapies. Since purification has a wide range, it should not be used mechanically.

g. Tonification: A therapy for tonifying deficient yin, yang, *qi* and blood or weak and impaired viscera. Tonifying supplements deficient *qi* and blood, harmonizes yin and yang so as to balance them. In addition, under certain circumstances where the body constitution is too weak to clear up a stubborn pathogenic factor, the application of tonification not only helps body resistance, but can also clear up the pathogenic factor indirectly.

Ranges of its application: It suits the patient with a weak constitution and lacking physical exercise, e.g., those with deficient *qi*, deficient blood, deficient yin, deficient yang and weak body resistance who fail to eliminate the pathogenic factor.

Applications: It is used by applying tonics of nourishing *qi*, reinforcing yang, tonifying *jing* (vital principle) and replenishing blood. In general, it may be chiefly classified into the four following types.

Qi-tonification: Used for the disorder, such as the deficiencies of spleen *qi* and lung *qi* manifested by lassitude, feeble and short breath, spontaneous sweating, empty and large pulse, etc. For example, for trapped *qi* in the middle energizer, prolapse of rectum, hernia, prolapse of uterus, collapse due to apoplexy, etc. may be treated with this therapy. The patient suffering from a great loss of blood should be treated by first tonifying blood because blood is produced by tonifying *qi*, i.e., the principle of "yang flourishing smoothly and yin vivified steadily."

Blood-tonification: Used for the syndrome caused by deficient and impaired blood, e.g., withered yellowish complexion, pale mouth, lips and nails, dizziness, tinnitus, blurred vision, even amenorrhea, etc. When tonifying blood, the hot or cold blood must be differentiated. In the hot blood syndrome, pathogenic heat is cleared up by replenishing the yin and cooling blood; in the cold blood syndrome, pathogenic cold is alternated by warming the meridian and nourishing blood.

Yin-tonification: Used for the disorder caused by deficient yin *jing* (vital principle) or body fluids, blurred vision, palpitation, restlessness and insomnia due to deficiency, night sweats, nocturnal emission, hematemesis, hemoptysis, "wasting and thirst" disease, etc. It may be generally divided into: tonifying *jing* (vital principle) used for the disorder of body fluids injured by extreme heat.

Yang-tonification: Used for the disorder caused by deficient yang of the spleen and stomach, e.g., cold sensation below the loin, pain in the loin and knees, weak lower limbs, occasional pain in the lower abdomen, diarrhea, frequent urination, impotence, prospermia, etc.

Attention should be paid to which viscus is deficient when applying a tonifying therapy, and it should also be tonified besides the above-mentioned therapies.

h. Elimination: A therapy to eliminate various substantial pathogenic factors that stagnate in the body. It seems to be the same as, but is actually different from the purgation and pain, which cannot be purged, but can be gradually subdued.

Ranges of its application: It suits chronic abdominal tumours causing distension and pain, etc., which are formed by *qi*, blood, diet, phlegm and *yin* (excess exudates).

Applications: It should be applied according to etiology, pathology and disorders. In general, it is classified into the following:

Eliminating the solid and subduing the stagnant suits abdominal tumours causing abdominal distension and pain; promoting digestion and subduing the stagnant suits excessive food intake and a hypoactive spleen and retention of food in the stomach. Promoting *qi* circulation and subduing congealed blood suits the disorder of stagnant *qi* and blood. Subduing *tan-yin* (phlegm and excess exudates) suits the disorder of accumulating *tan-yin*. Subduing edema that suits the disorder due to the failure of *qi* to subdue *yin* (excess exudates) and overflowing aqueous *qi*.

In addition, disorders, such as accumulated parasites, subcutaneous fruit or stone-shaped masses[7] recurrent metastatic abscesses[8] in the deep part of the body, etc. may be treated with it.

11-2-7-2 Application of the eight principal therapies in coordination

The eight principal therapies should be applied according to the disorder, but not used in isolation because alone they cannot relieve various disease conditions. The coordinated application of the therapies may be divided into the following:

Coordinated diaphoresis and purgation: For the exterior syndrome accompanied by an interior syndrome, such as the acute case with an excess and accumulation both inside and outside of the body, one must not mechanically adhere to the routine that the former is first treated and then the latter, but rather adopt diaphoretic and purgative therapies simultaneously.

Coordinated warming nourishment and purification: If diseases or syndromes with pathogenic heat mixed with pathogenic cold are treated with the warming nourishment or purification solely, an unfavourable change will result. Hence, only when they are adopted in cooperation can pathogenic cold mixed with pathogenic heat be solved. While using this therapy, the mild or severe condition of pathogenic cold and heat and the deep or superficial, upper or lower location of the disorder must be analysed and then dealt with appropriately.

Coordinated purgation and tonification: If all the disorders due to a weak anti-pathogenic factor and a violent pathogenic factor are treated only by tonification, the pathogenic factor will stagnate further; if only purgation is used, again the pathogenic factor will stagnate further; if only purgation is used, the anti-pathogenic factor will probably be impaired, resulting in collapse. Under such circumstances, neither prior-purgation and post-tonification nor prior-tonification and post-purgation can be used, but the purgation and tonification should be adopted simultaneously. If it is used inappro-priately, the anti-pathogenic factor will be impaired. So, the degree of deficiency and excess must be examined carefully and purgation and tonification applied in coordination in order to eliminate the pathogenic factor and strengthen the anti-pathogenic factor.

Coordinated purgation and elimination: They can be adopted for all cases where asthenic patients suffer from stagnation of some sort which needs to be treated by gradually eliminating the pathogenic factor. At the initial stage, it cannot be adopted for the case due to a prolonged illness and abdominal masses that have been subdued.

Notes

[1] Physical fitness exercises for promoting health which imitate the movements of the tiger, deer, bear, monkey and bird as devised by the famous physician Hua Tuo in the Three Kingdoms (220-260).

[2] A popular Chinese folk exercise. With soft, slow movements, which can be used not only for defence against an attack, but also to maintain health and prevent disease.

[3] Chinese folk fitness exercises which consist of eight kinds of movements. The first movement is holding the hand straight towards the sky for regulating the function of the triple energizer; the second is extending the left hand to the right of the body and the right one to the left; the third is holding up one arm for regulating the function of the spleen and stomach; the fourth is turning the head backward for treating strains; the fifth is moving the head and arms to get rid of heart fire; the sixth is holding the feet with the hands by bending the waist for strengthening the kidney and loin; the seventh is making a fist and opening the eyes wide to increase qi; the eighth is jumping with both hands on the waist which helps eliminate a number of illnesses.

[4] The method discovered by the Chinese medical experts to prevent smallpox during the Long Qing Reign (1556) in the Ming Dynasty (1368-1644) which is a vaccination using the thick fluid of smallpox to immunize a healthy person. Nowadays, it has been replaced by vaccination using a vaccinal virus.

[5] The disease or syndrome manifested by diarrhea of an excess type.

[6] The method of treating the syndrome of excess yang caused by yin deficiency, by tonifying and nourishing the kidney.

[7] A collective term for subcutaneous fruit-stone shaped masses.

[8] Recurrent metastatic abscesses in the deep layer of muscle.